MODERN ESSENTIALS USAGE GUIDE

A Quick Guide to the Therapeutic Use of Essential Oils

PEPPERMINT
Mentha piperita

Essential Oil
LAVENDER
Lavandula angustifolia

Essential Oil
LEMON
Citrus limon

Sixth Edition

Published and Distributed by:

AromaTools
  1351 W. 800 N.
  Orem, UT 84057

Phone: 1-866-728-0070 • 801-798-7921

Internet: www.AromaTools.com

E-mail: Webmaster@AromaTools.com

Copyright:

© **2014 AromaTools.** 6th Edition, 1st Printing, September 2014. All rights reserved. No part of this book may be reproduced or transmitted in any form or by any means, electronic or mechanical, including photocopying, recording, or by any other information storage or retrieval system, without written permission from AromaTools.

ISBN Number:

978-1-937702-22-9

Disclaimer:

This book has been designed to provide information to help educate the reader in regard to the subject matter covered. It is sold with the understanding that the publisher and the authors are not liable for the misconception and misuse of the information provided. It is not provided in order to diagnose, proscribe, or treat any disease, illness, or injured condition of the body. The authors and publisher shall have neither liability nor responsibility to any person or entity with respect to any loss, damage, or injury caused, or alleged to be caused, directly or indirectly by the information contained in this book. The information presented herein is in no way intended as a substitute for medical counseling. Anyone suffering from any disease, illness, or injury should consult a qualified health care professional.

Printed and Bound in the U.S.A.

Table of Contents

Personal Guide

Science & App.

Single Oils

Appendix

Index

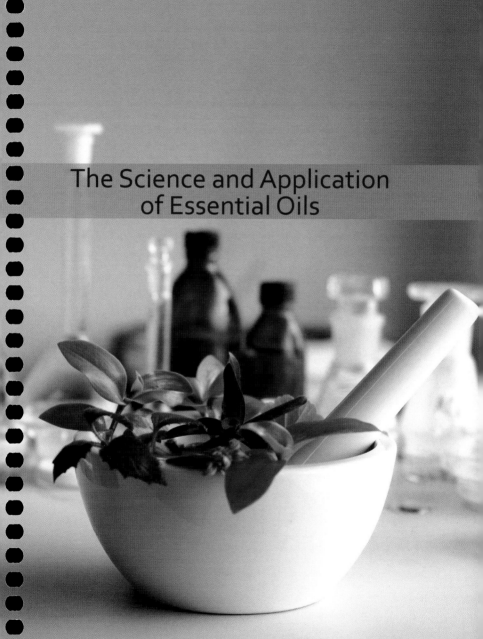

The Science and Application
of Essential Oils

An Introduction to Essential Oils

What are essential oils?

Essential oils are the volatile liquids that are distilled from plants (including their respective parts such as seeds, bark, leaves, stems, roots, flowers, fruit, etc.). One of the factors that determines the purity and therapeutic value of an oil is its chemical constituents. These constituents can be affected by a vast number of variables: the part(s) of the plant from which the oil was produced, soil condition, fertilizer (organic or chemical), geographic region, climate, altitude, harvest season and method, and distillation process (Andradea et al., 2011; Sell, 2006; Pengelly, 2004). For example, common thyme, or thyme vulgaris, produces several different chemotypes (biochemical specifics or simple species) depending on the conditions of its growth, climate, and altitude (Thompson et al., 2003). High levels of thymol depend on the time of year in which the oil is distilled. If distilled during mid-summer or late fall, there can be higher levels of carvacrol, which can cause the oil to be more caustic or irritating to the skin (Hudaib et al., 2002).

As we begin to understand the power of essential oils in the realm of personal holistic health care, we comprehend the absolute necessity of obtaining pure, therapeutic-grade essential oils. No matter how costly pure, therapeutic-grade essential oils may be, there can be no substitute. Chemists can replicate some of the known individual constituents (Sell, 2006), but it would be difficult, if not impossible, to successfully recreate complete essential oils in the laboratory.

The information in this book is based on the use of pure, therapeutic-grade essential oils. Those who are beginning their journey into the realm of aromatherapy and essential oils must actively seek for the purest quality and highest therapeutic-grade oils available. Anything less than pure, therapeutic-grade essential oil may not produce the desired results and can, in some cases, be extremely toxic.

Why is it so difficult to find pure, therapeutic-grade essential oils?

Producing the purest of oils can be very costly because it may require several hundred pounds, or even several thousand pounds, of plant material to extract one pound of pure essential oil. For example, one pound of pure melissa oil sells for thousands of dollars. Although this sounds quite expensive, one must realize that three tons of plant material are required to produce that single pound of oil. Because the vast majority of all the oils produced in the world today are used by the perfume industry, the oils are being purchased for their aromatic qualities only. Unnecessary high pressure and high temperature, rapid processing, and the use of chemical solvents are often employed during the distillation process so that a greater quantity of oil can be produced at a faster rate. These oils may smell just as good and cost much less, but they will lack most, if not all, of the chemical constituents necessary to produce the expected therapeutic results.

What benefits do pure, therapeutic-grade essential oils provide?

Essential oils embody the regenerating, protective, and immune-strengthening properties of plants.

Essential oil constituents are both small in molecular size and are also lipid soluble, allowing many of them to easily and quickly penetrate the skin (Onocha et al., 2011; Kohlert et al., 2000). The lipid solubility of essential oil constituents also allows the constituents to penetrate cell membranes, even if these membranes have hardened because of an oxygen deficiency (Onocha et al., 2011). In fact, essential oil constituents have the potential to affect every cell of the body within twenty minutes and then be metabolized like other nutrients (Jager et al., 1992; Jager et al., 1996).

Simple Diffusion Across the Cell Membrane

When water and oil are mixed together in a cup, they eventually separate, forming two layers. A similar phenomenon results in the formation of the cell membrane. The hydrocarbon tails of the lipid membrane form an oily barrier separating extracellular fluid from the intracellular fluid of the cell. Essential oils are able to penetrate the oily barrier because the barrier and the essential oil have similar lipophilic properties. Hydrophilic molecules, like ions, are reluctant to enter the lipophilic interior created by the hydrocarbon tails (Alberts et al., 2013). The smaller the molecule and the more lipophilic, or nonpolar, it is, the more rapidly it will diffuse across the membrane (Alberts et al., 2013).

Essential oils are very powerful antioxidants. Antioxidants neutralize or quench free radicals (Lobo et al., 2010). Free radicals are atoms with at least one unpaired electron and are created naturally by the body during metabolism. The body uses free radicals to perform important roles in gene transcription, cell signaling, and other regulatory functions (Fang et al., 2002). Free radicals can also be created by environmental factors such as pollution, radiation, and cigarette smoke. In these situations, free radicals outnumber the body's natural antioxidants and may cause cell injury and death (Fang et al., 2002). This imbalance between free radicals and antioxidants is called oxidative stress and occurs when antioxidants are unable to neutralize free radicals (Urso et al., 2003). If a free radical is not properly managed, it can cause "domino-like" damage by creating new free radicals out of normal atoms. Consequences of oxidative stress may include damage to proteins, DNA, and tissue, as well as the triggering of a number of human diseases (Fang et al., 2002; Lobo et al., 2010). Essential oils, omega-3 fatty acids found in fish oil, and certain vitamins have been shown to act as inhibitors of free radical generation (Fang et al., 2002) and can help diminish oxidative stress and harmful free radical production, helping the body fight disease and damage.

Many essential oil constituents have antibacterial, antifungal (Aguiar et al., 2014), anti-infectious, antimicrobial, antitumor, antiparasitic, antiviral, and antiseptic properties. Essential oils have been shown to destroy many harmful bacteria and viruses while simultaneously providing immune system support (Serafino et al., 2008).

Some essential oils can support the liver in detoxifying the blood. For example, rosemary essential oil constituents have been shown to induce enzyme activity in the liver, suggesting a possibility of increased ability to remove toxins (Debersac et al., 2001).

Essential oils are volatile, aromatic, and possess powerful antimicrobial activity (Tyagi et al., 2010). When vaporized, some essential oils, including peppermint, produce stronger antimicrobial properties than when used in the liquid phase (Tyagi et al., 2010). This increased antimicrobial action occurs because vaporized essential oils combine with negative ions in the air for synergistic air purification and disinfection (Tyagi et al., 2010). Furthermore, essential oils fill the air with a fresh aromatic scent while destroying odors.

Essential oils help promote emotional, physical, and spiritual healing.

How long have essential oils been around?

From the beginning of early civilization, aromatic plants have been used for their therapeutic properties. Egyptian papyri and Chinese manuscripts describe the medicinal use of aromatics employed thousands of years ago. The Egyptians placed a great value on aromatic oils and even included thirty-five alabaster jars for the oils in King Tutankhamen's tomb. Similarly, the Greeks attributed the invention of perfumes to the gods and believed all aromatic plants to be of divine origin. Additionally, there are many references to aromatics, ointments, and incenses (such as frankincense, myrrh, rosemary, etc.) in the Bible and Torah. For more on the history of essential oils, please refer to the history section on page 11.

How do essential oils affect the brain?

The blood-brain barrier is the filtering mechanism between the circulating blood and the brain that prevents certain damaging substances from reaching brain tissue and cerebrospinal fluid. A common misconception is that all small molecules cross the blood-brain barrier. However, an astounding 98% of small molecule drugs cannot cross the blood-brain barrier (Pardridge, 2009). Dr. William M. Pardridge, an expert in blood-brain barrier research, determined that "The development of new drugs for the brain has not kept pace with progress in the molecular neurosciences, because the majority of new drugs discovered do not cross the blood-brain barrier" (2003). The ability to cross the blood-brain barrier is essential for the treatment of brain diseases and disorders. Chemical constituents known as sesquiterpenes—commonly found in essential oils such as frankincense and sandalwood—are known to be able to go beyond the blood-brain barrier (Wang et al., 2012; Zhang et al., 2009). Therefore, sesquiterpenes can directly interact with brain cells, unlike most pharmaceutical drugs, and can impact the brain therapeutically. In fact, sesquiterpenes are known to interact with neurotransmitter receptors, specifically glycine, dopamine, and serotonin receptors (Wang et al., 2012; Okugawa et al., 2000).

The Limbic System

The limbic system is composed of many brain structures, including the olfactory bulb and the amygdala.

Even if the chemical constituents of an essential oil cannot cross the blood-brain barrier, the essential oil can still affect the brain through activation of the olfactory bulb. Odors and emotions are processed in similar brain structures located in the limbic system (Pause et al., 2003). The limbic system is a group of related structures in the brain that are responsible for processing emotion, memory, and smell. The sense of smell is unique in the fact that "No other sensory system makes this kind of direct and intense contact with the neural substrates of emotion and memory, which may explain why odor-evoked memories are unusually emotionally potent" (Herz et al., 1996)..

Also present in the limbic system of the brain is a gland called the amygdala. In the 1980s, it was discovered that the amygdala plays a major role in the storing and releasing of emotional trauma (LeDoux, 2003; LeDoux et al., 1988; Iwata et al., 1986; LeDoux et al., 1989). One way to stimulate this gland is with fragrance or the sense of smell (Kadohisa, 2013). Therefore, essential oils can be a powerful key to help unlock and release emotional trauma.

What enables essential oils to provide such incredible benefits?

The benefits of an essential oil depend greatly on the oil's diversity of chemical constituents—and not only on the existence of specific constituents but also on their amounts in proportion to other constituents present in the same oil. Some individual oils may have hundreds of different chemical constituents (Miguel, 2010; Sell, 2006). Many of these constituents have yet to be identified. Although not everything is known about all the different constituents, most of them can be grouped into a few distinct families, each with some dominant characteristics. The essential oil constituent section beginning on page 30 provides greater insights into these constituent families.

How are essential oils extracted?

There are two ways in which pure, therapeutic-grade essential oils are extracted:

—Steam Distillation

In order to understand why and how steam distillation works, it is important to be aware of two central characteristics of essential oils: First, essential oils are volatile. This means that they evaporate easily when exposed to the air. And second, essential oils are hydrophobic, which means that they do not mix with water.

Steam distillation is the method most commonly used to extract essential oils; in fact, 93% of essential oils are extracted by steam distillation (Masango, 2005). In this method, plant material is placed in an extraction chamber and then steam (produced by boiling water in another chamber) is released into the bottom of the extraction chamber where the plant material is. As the steam passes through the plant material, both the steam and the essential oil rise to the top (this is because essential oils are volatile). The steam and essential oil are directed to another chamber where they are allowed to cool. Since essential oils are hydrophobic, as the oil/steam mixture cools, the essential oil rises to the top of the chamber while the water stays at the bottom. The essential oil can then be easily separated from the water.

Schematic of the steam distillation of plant material to produce essential oil.

—Expression

Cold expression, or cold pressing, is the method most commonly used for extracting essential oils from citrus fruits. Mechanical pressure is used to "press" the oils out of the plant material—most often from the peel or rind.

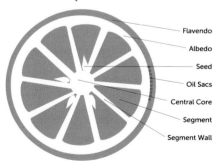

Orange essential oil is contained in oil sacs found in the peel. The peel consists of a thin colored outer layer called the flavedo and a thicker fibrous inner layer called the albedo. The oil sacs are located in the flavedo of the peel. Expression requires the breaking of these oil sacs in order to release the essential oil they contain.

A Brief History of Essential Oils

Aromatic plants have long played an important role in human civilizations. They have been a part of religion, marriage ceremonies, dating and courtship, cosmetics, funerary services, medicine, and many other aspects of human life. Although the use of essential oils has evolved over the years, the basic principles remain the same. From the beginning of time, oils extracted from aromatic plants have been recognized as the most effective medicine known to mankind.

Egypt

The Egyptians are most often credited with being the first to use essential oils. Although there is still some debate, most historians believe that the oils used anciently were not identical to the steam distilled essential oils used today. Rather, the oils used by the

ancient Egyptians appear to be animal fats and vegetable oils into which the aromatic essential oils from the plants had been extracted—typically by steeping the plant material in the hot oils or fats[1]. Although not as concentrated as the steam distilled oils used at present, they were, nonetheless, used for their aromatic and therapeutic properties and are considered the precursors to pure essential oils.

—Portion of the Ebers Papyrus

For the Egyptians, the distinction between medicines and perfumes was not always clear. Often a single scented oil served both purposes. Common aromatics of the time included frankincense, myrrh, cedarwood, spikenard, juniper, coriander, bitter almond, henna, calamus, and origanum[2].

One of the oldest and best–preserved documents that we know of, the Ebers Papyrus, documents the Egyptians' use of frankincense and other aromatics in treating a variety of different ailments. This papyrus is thought to have been composed somewhere between 1553 and 1550 BC[3].

In 1922, archeologist Howard Carter and his team discovered the tomb of the ancient Egyptian king Tutankhamen. Despite evidence of some robbery and the tomb having been resealed, the majority of the original treasures remained in the tomb[4].

---

1   Tisserand. 22.
2   Tiserand. 22.
3   Hill. 44.
4   Carter. 33–44.

As Howard Carter surveyed the contents of the tomb, he discovered thirty-five alabaster jars that had been used to hold scented oils and unguents, but every single one of them had been emptied. It soon became evident to Carter that two separate robberies had taken place in the tomb—the first robbery was for precious metals, and the second robbery was for the oils and unguents[1]. Carter marveled that in the presence of so many other precious objects the thieves would have chosen to steal the oils. The only thing Carter could conclude was that "The greases, or oils, that they contained had, no doubt, a far greater value in those days than possibly we imagine." [2]

China

The ancient Chinese are also believed to have been masters of the use of aromatic plants for healing. Some speculate that the Chinese may have begun studying aromatics at the same time as the Egyptians did—or even before. An ancient Chinese text "Pen T'Sao," which is believed to have been written by Emperor Shen Nung around 2500 BC, identifies medicinal uses for over 300 different plants[3]. Chinese aromatherapists believed that extracting a plant's fragrance represented freeing the plant's soul[4].

The Chinese upper classes used fragrances lavishly during the T'ang dynasties, scenting their homes, clothing, temples, ink, paper, and cosmetics with aromatics. Huge statues of Buddha were even carved from fragrant camphor wood[8].

Greece

The Greeks learned a lot about perfumery from the Egyptians. When Herodotus and Democrates visited Egypt in the fourth century BC, they declared that the people were "masters of the art of perfumery."[5]

The Greeks believed all aromatic plants to be of divine origin, and they attributed the invention of perfumes to the gods[6].

The Greek physician Marestheus recognized that aromatic plants had either stimulating or sedative properties. He identified rose and hyacinth as refreshing and invigorating. Another Greek, Theophrastus, wrote that he wasn't surprised that perfumes should have medicinal properties when taking into consideration the other virtues of perfumes[7].

Without fully understanding the composition or chemical processes of essential oils, the Greeks were still able to profit from the antiseptic properties of the oils. Hippocrates used aromatic essences to fumigate the city of Athens to fight off the plague epidemic. Hip-

---

1 Carter. 248-50.
2 Carter. 249.
3 Petrovska. 1–5.
4 Keville, 2012
5 Tisserand. 25.
6 Tisserand. 25.
7 Tisserand. 27.

pocrates also suggested that the key to good health is found in taking a daily aromatic bath and receiving a daily scented massage[1].

Rome

The Romans also used aromatics—even more lavishly than the Greeks did. They used aromatics to scent everything—their hair, their clothes, their beds, their bodies, their military flags, the walls of their houses, and everything else they could think of. They also used the oils and unguents in massage and baths[2].

The Romans, who were famous for their preoccupation with public health and for their public baths, were said to have embraced aromatherapy. Roman soldiers were also known to carry pouches filled with the seeds of aromatic plants on their military campaigns[3].

Israel

The value of aromatics to the ancient people of Israel is clearly evident throughout many historical texts.

The writings of the Old Testament/Torah contain numerous references to aromatics, ointments, and incenses that were used by the ancient Israelites.

The New Testament also includes additional references to the use of aromatics and aromatic ointments by the Israelites, including the gifts of frankincense and myrrh given by the wise men who came to worship the Christ child[4] and the use of spikenard for anointing[5].

Arabia

Between 1000 BC and 400 BC, Arabia was the center of a lucrative spice trade route. During this time, frankincense was by far the biggest trade commodity and brought great wealth to Arabia. The trade route extended from the Dhofar region of Omar to Petra in Jordan—approximately 2400 miles—and was commonly referred to as the Frankincense Trail. This trail was used so many times that modern day satellite images still show faint marks on the ground where the camel caravans passed over[6].

The Arabs are also credited with being the first to discover steam distillation as a method

—Satellite images of the Frankincense Trail

1   Gawronski. 142.
2   Tisserand. 28.
3   Gawronski. 142.
4   St. Matthew 2:11.
5   St. John 12:3–5.
6   Hill. 44–46

of extracting essential oils from plants around 1000 AD. The Arabian physician 'Abu 'Ali al-Husian Ibn 'Abd Allah Ibn Sina, more commonly known as Avicenna, is said to be the inventor of this method of distillation. Avicenna distilled both essences and aromatic waters[1].

Europe

With the invention of distillation, the use of aromatic essential oils in perfumes quickly migrated to Europe, and by the end of the end of the twelfth century, the Europeans were distilling their own essential oils and manufacturing their own perfumes[2].

When the Great Plague became widespread in Europe, fumigations with aromatics were often employed to try and drive the sickness from the cities. It was found that those who were most in contact with aromatics, especially the perfumers, were virtually immune to the plague while so many died around them[3]. In London, houses and workplaces were fumigated on a daily basis to try and keep away the plague. Frankincense was among the aromatics used[4].

By the 1500s physicians such as Hieronymus Brunschwig (who wrote one of the earliest printed books on essential oil distillation and use, *Liber de Arte Distillandi*) were distilling and using essential oils for their medicinal benefits.

The Reintroduction of Essential Oils

Essential oils regained popularity in the mid 19th century largely because of their desirable fragrances. As the cosmetic, soap, and food industries grew, so did the demand for essential oils to be used to scent and flavor these products[5]. These essential oils weren't necessarily of a therapeutic grade, but they did call back the attention to essential oils.

—*Title Page of* Liber de Arte Distillande, *by Brunschwig (c. 1512)*

With the help of research and several key individuals, essential oils became recognized once again for their therapeutic and medicinal properties, and aromatherapy and pure, therapeutic-grade essential oils were reintroduced to the general public.

---

1 Tisserand. 30.
2 Tisserand. 30.
3 Tisserand. 38–39.
4 Porter. 42.
5 Başer et al. 184.

—René-Maurice Gattefossé

René-Maurice Gattefossé was a French chemist born in 1881. He is known as the "father of aromatherapy" because of his extensive research of essential oils and is credited with coining the term "aromatherapy." [1]

Gattefossé is most famous for his work and personal experience with lavender essential oil. While working in his laboratory one day, there was an explosion that covered Gattefossé with "burning substances," which he extinguished by rolling on the grass outside. Gattefossé says of the experience, "Both my hands were covered with a rapidly developing gas gangrene. Just one rinse with lavender essence stopped 'the gastification of the tissue.' This treatment was followed by profuse sweating and healing began the next day."[2] Gattefossé was only partly surprised by the healing power of the lavender essential oil because Gattefossé had been researching essential oils long enough to know of their powerful antiseptic and healing properties[3].

Although René-Maurice Gattefossé was not the first to use essential oils, nor was he the first to write about their therapeutic use, his vision was unlike that of any of his contemporaries. Gattefossé saw aromatherapy as a discipline of its own and recognized the great value of essential oils in healthcare. There were others researching essential oils at the same time as Gattefossé, but none of them equaled Gattefossé in their enthusiasm and dedication to the subject[4]. Gattefossé was instrumental in helping essential oils to be seen for their therapeutic properties and not just for their pleasant smell.

—Jean Valnet

Jean Valnet, MD, was a French army physician and surgeon. During World War II in Tokin, China, Valnet used his limited supply of essential oils in the treatment of injured soldiers and was very satisfied with the consistency of the results he achieved[5].

Valnet recognized the drawbacks of modern medications and antibiotics with their harmful side effects and the need to continually increase their dosages as the body's tolerance increases[6], and for this reason he turned to essential oils as a natural alternative.

Valnet very strongly believed that there was always something more that could be done for a patient before condemning him or her to death[7], and essential oil use was that "something more" that Valnet turned to.

---

1 Gattefossé. 134.
2 Gattefossé. 87.
3 Tisserand. 41–42.
4 Gattefossé. v.
5 Valnet. 66.
6 Valnet. 49–50.
7 Valnet. 227.

—Robert B. Tisserand

Robert Tisserand searched for 20 years to obtain a copy of *Gattefossé's Aromatherapy*. After searching for so long, Tisserand began to doubt that the book even existed[1]. Once he found the book, he edited it and added his own introduction to the 1993 printing. He calls *Gattefossé's Aromatherapy* the "missing link for 20th century aromatherapy."[2]

Tisserand's own research delves into the history, use, properties, and therapeutic benefits of essential oils. Tisserand was also very instrumental in making information about the therapeutic use of essential oils available to the general public.

Essential Oils Today

Today, scientists, physicians, researchers, and many individuals concerned with managing their own personal health are just beginning to explore and discover some of the amazing benefits pure, therapeutic grade essential oils have to offer.

Science & App.

---

1   Gattefossé. v.
2   Gattefossé. vi.

Essential Oil Constituents

In general, pure essential oil constituents can be subdivided into two distinct groups: the hydrocarbons, which are made up almost exclusively of terpenes (monoterpenes, sesquiterpenes, and diterpenes), and the oxygenated compounds, which are mainly esters, aldehydes, ketones, alcohols, phenols, and oxides.

Terpenes

Terpenes are the largest family of natural products and are found throughout nature. High concentrations of terpenes are found directly after flowering[1]. The basic molecular structure of a terpene is an isoprene unit (which has a C_5H_8 molecular formula).

Classes of terpenes are named according to how many isoprene units are present.

- Monoterpenes (C10) = two isoprene units
- Sesquiterpenes (C15) = three isoprene units
- Triterpenes (C30) = six isoprene units
- Tetraterpenes (C40) = eight isoprene units

Terpenes may also have oxygen-containing functional groups. Terpenes with these oxygen-containing functional groups are referred to as terpenoids[2].

Isoprene Unit
(C_5H_8)

Isoprene Unit
(C_5H_8)

Figures such as the one shown at left represent the bonds between carbon (C) atoms in a molecule. Single lines represent a single bond, while double lines represent a double bond. Each intersecting point and the end of each line represents a carbon molecule along with any hydrogen molecules it is bonded to. Since each carbon molecule can have up to four bonds with other atoms, the number of hydrogen atoms can be determined by subtracting the number of bonds (lines) coming to each carbon atom from four. Thus the shorthand figure at top represents the same molecule shown below it.

◯ = carbon
● = hydrogen

—Monoterpenes

Monoterpenes occur in practically all essential oils and have many different activities. Most tend to inhibit the accumulation of toxins and help discharge existing toxins from the liver and kidneys. Some are antiseptic, antibacterial, stimulating, analgesic (weak), and expectorant; while other specific terpenes have antifungal, antiviral, antihistaminic, antirheumatic, antitumor (antiblastic, anticarcinogenic), hypotensive, insecticidal, purgative, and pheromonal properties. Monoterpenes, in general, have a stimulating effect and can be very soothing to irritated tissues as well. Most citrus oils (not bergamot) and conifer oils contain a high proportion of terpenes.

Found as a Significant Constituent in ALL Essential Oils Except: Basil, birch, cassia, cinnamon, clary sage, clove, geranium, sandalwood, vetiver, wintergreen, and ylang ylang.

Examples of Monoterpenes:

---

1 Paduch et al., 2007.
2 McGarvey et al., 1995.

– Pinenes (α- & β-)

α- and β- pinene are isomers (meaning they have the same chemical formula but differing structures). They get their name because they are major constituents in pine resin or pine oil. They give off a resiny, piney smell. Pinenes have strong antiseptic, antibacterial, antifungal, and expectorant properties.

α- Pinene

β- Pinene

Bone Resorption Inhibition: α- and β-pinene (found in pine oil) were found in animal studies to inhibit bone resorption. Bone resorption is the process by which osteoclasts—macrophage cells that reside in the bones—break down bone and release the minerals, which can lead to the loss of bone, such as in osteoporosis. Further studies have indicated that while α- and β-pinene may not directly influence osteoclast activity and bone resorption rates, a metabolite (a product created by the body from the original molecule when taken internally) of the pinenes, cis-verbenol, did directly inhibit bone resorption and the formation of osteoclasts[1,2].

Mosquito Larvicide: α-pinenes found in *Alpinia speciosa* and *Rosmarinus officinalis* (ginger and rosemary) demonstrated effective larvicidal activity against the mosquito *Aedes aegypti L.* The *A. aegypti* is a carrier of the dengue virus that causes dengue fever in tropical areas of the world[3].

Antibacterial: It has been observed that the larvae of the Douglas fir tussock moth have digestive systems that are relatively clear of bacterial flora. These larvae feed on terpenes found in the bark of Douglas fir trees, of which α-pinene is a major constituent. α-pinene inhibits the growth of *Bacillus* species (gram-positive bacteria). The concentration needed for maximum inhibition is well below the concentrations of α-pinene found in Douglas fir pine trees. Bacterial inhibition occurs because α-pinene disrupts the cytoplasmic membranes of the bacterial species. α-pinene seems to perform more effectively against gram-positive bacteria than gram-negative bacteria due to the extra outer membrane found in the cell walls of gram-negative bacteria[4,5].

Anti-inflammatory: NF_KB is an important transcription factor in the body that regulates proinflammatory responses (signals proteins, specifically cytokines, to cause inflammation). When NF_KB is activated, it goes to the nucleus of the cells, binds to DNA, and activates transcription needed to produce cytokines, chemokines, and cell adhesion molecules. These molecules all help in producing inflammation in the body.

α-pinene has been shown to inhibit/block NF_KB from going to the nucleus. LPS (lipopolysaccharide, an endotoxin produced by gram-negative bacteria

1   Eriksson et al., 1996.
2   Muhlbauer et al., 2003.
3   Freitas et al., 2010.
4   Andrews et al., 1980.
5   Uribe et al., 1985.

that causes inflammation in the body) was introduced to the cell culture of THP-1 cells to induce the activation of $NF_\kappa B$. However, when α-pinene was present, activation was markedly reduced.

α-pinene inhibits $NF_\kappa B$ by blocking the degradation of $I_\kappa B\alpha$. $I_\kappa B\alpha$ is a protein that binds to $NF_\kappa B$ to prevent it from constantly transcribing proinflammatory genes. If LPS, a virus, or some stimulant of the immune system is recognized, $I_\kappa B\alpha$ will degrade and release/activate $NF_\kappa B$. $NF_\kappa B$ will then transcribe genes to make proteins that cause inflammation at the site of "invasion," such as a cut, scrape, or burn.

Even in the presence of an immune system stimulant (LPS), α-pinene blocks $I_\kappa B\alpha$. During experimentation, it was also noted that the THP-1 cells received no cytotoxicity from the addition of α-pinene[1,2].

– Camphene

Camphene is found in many oils, such as cypress, citronella, neroli, ginger, and others. It is an insect repellent. According to the *Phytochemical Dictionary*, it is "used to reduce cholesterol saturation index in the treatment of gallstones."

Camphene

– β-Myrcene

β-Myrcene is found in oils such as lemongrass, verbena, and bay. It has cancer–preventative properties.

Antioxidant: Studies have elucidated that β-myrcene can reverse and prevent the damaging effects of TCDD (2,3,7,8-Tetrachloro-p-dibenzodioxin) to the liver of rats by increasing GSH (glutathione), SOD (superoxide dismutase), and catalase activation[3,4].

β-Myrcene

– d-Limonene

d-Limonene is found in 90% of the citrus peel oils and in caraway seeds and dill. It is anticancer, antibacterial, antifungal, antiseptic (5x phenol), and highly antiviral.

Cancer Cell Inhibition: d-limonene has been found to be cancer-preventive in vitro and in human mammary cells. It acts as a selective isoprenylation inhibitor. d-Limonene specifically inhibits small g-proteins known as Ras p21 (or p21ras). p21ras is a critical protein for oncogenesis (formation of cancer cells) in the body. In order for

Broken lines such as this represent a bond that bends 90° inward (towards the book).

d-Limonene

1   Zhou et al., 2004.
2   Weaver, 2008.
3   Ciftci et al., 2011.
4   Gaetani et al., 1996.

oncogenesis to commence, the p21ras protein must be transferred within the cell to the plasma membrane. Once p21ras is able to interact with the plasma membrane of the cell, it causes abnormal cell growth, intracellular localization, and transformations.

d-limonene inhibits the transferral of p21ras within the cell, blocking its access to the plasma membrane.

Researchers also found that d-limonene is selectively inhibitive. It targets only the transferral of Ras proteins and leaves all other ordinary cell functions alone. This makes d-Limonene a potentially effective chemopreventive agent because it targets areas of high oncogenic susceptibility and has no harmful side effects against critical cell components (low toxicity)[1,2,3].

Researchers have also observed that a continuous dose of limonene in the diets of rats with chemical-induced cancer helps inhibit the formation of secondary tumors and reduces the size of primary tumors. However, when limonene was removed from the rat's daily diet, tumors were more likely to return. This gives evidence that limonene works as a cytostatic agent (an agent that stops the tumor cells from creating new tumor cells) rather than a cytotoxic agent (an agent that kills the tumor cells). These researchers also observed that little toxicity occurred to the rats from the high doses of d-limonene[4].

Cholesterol Suppression: Researchers have discovered that when d-limonene is included in the daily diet of rats treated with a chemical (7,12-dimetylbenzantracene) that induced high cholesterol, there was a 45% decrease in hepatic HMG-CoA reductase activity. HMG-CoA reductase is an enzyme that converts HMG-CoA (93-hydroxy-3-methylglutaryl coenzyme A) to mevalonic acid, which acts as a precursor to the production of cholesterol. Inhibiting HMG-CoA reductase halts this process and, in effect, lowers cholesterol rates[5,6].

—Sesquiterpenes

Sesquiterpenes are found in great abundance in essential oils. They are antibacterial, strongly anti-inflammatory, slightly antiseptic and hypotensive, and sedative. Some have analgesic properties, while others are highly antispasmodic. They are soothing to irritated skin and tissue and are calming. They also work as liver and gland stimulants. Research from the universities of Berlin and Vienna shows that sesquiterpenes increase oxygenation around the pineal and pituitary glands. Further research has shown that sesquiterpenes have the ability to surpass the blood-brain barrier and enter the brain tissue. They are larger molecules than monoterpenes and have a strong aroma.

Found as a Major Constituent In: Ginger, myrrh, sandalwood, vetiver, and ylang ylang.

1   Kato et al., 1992.
2   Crowell et al., 1991.
3   Morse et al., 1993.
4   Haag et al., 1992.
5   Sorentino et al., 2005.
6   Qureshi et al., 1988.

Found as a Minor Constituent In: Bergamot, cinnamon, clary sage, clove, cypress, white fir, frankincense, geranium, helichrysum, lavender, lemongrass, melaleuca, and peppermint.

Examples of Sesquiterpenes:

–β-Caryophyllene

β-caryophyllene is found in clove and cinnamon essential oils and is found in high proportions in plants from the Labiatae family. It is antiedema, anti-inflammatory, antispasmodic, and an insect and termite repellent.

β-Caryophyllene

Anesthetic: β-caryophyllene has been shown to act as a local anesthetic in vitro and in vivo. In an in vitro experiment, β-caryophyllene reduced the number of contractions electrically invoked in rat phrenic nerve-hemidiaphragms. Phrenic nerves are found in the spine, specifically at the 3rd, 4th, and 5th cervical vertebrae. These nerves provide sole motor control to the diaphragm. In this experiment, electrical impulses through the phrenic nerves induced diaphragm contractions, but the addition of β-caryophyllene reduced the number of contractions[1].

In an in vivo (real life) experiment, researchers performed a conjunctival reflex test on rabbits in which the conjunctival sac, found in the eye, was stimulated with a cat whisker to promote palpebral closure (or blinking). β-caryophyllene acted as a local anesthetic: when it was applied to the eye, more stimulation with the cat whisker was required in order to promote blinking in the rabbit[2].

–Chamazulene

Chamazulene is found in chamomile oil and is very high in anti-inflammatory and antibacterial activity.

Chamazulene

–Farnesene

Farnesene refers to several isomers with the chemical formula $C_{15}H_{24}$. Farnesene is found in ylang ylang, valerian, and German chamomile oil and is antiviral in action.

α-Farnesene   β-Farnesene

Alcohols

Alcohols are any organic molecule with a carbon atom bound to a hydroxyl group. A hydroxyl group is an oxygen and hydrogen molecule (-OH).

---

1 Bulbring, 1946.
2 Ghelardini et al., 2001.

Alcohols are commonly recognized for their antibacterial, anti-infectious, and antiviral activities. They are somewhat stimulating and help to increase blood circulation. Because of their high resistance to oxidation and their low toxicity levels, they have been shown in animal studies to revert cells to normal function and activity. They create an uplifting quality and are regarded as safe and effective for young and old alike.

Methanol (CH$_3$OH)

—OH

Methanol (CH$_3$OH)

Shorthand model of methanol, the simplest alcohol, and the molecular model it represents, below.

= carbon
= hydrogen
= oxygen

Found as a Significant Constituent in ALL Essential Oils Except: Birch, cassia, clove, white fir, grapefruit, myrrh, oregano, and wintergreen.

—Monoterpene Alcohols (or Monoterpenols)

Like monoterpenes, monoterpene alcohols are comprised of two isoprene units but have a hydroxyl group bound to one of the carbons instead of a hydrogen. Monoterpene alcohols are known for their ability to stimulate the immune system and to work as a diuretic and a general tonic. They are antibacterial and mildly antiseptic as well.

Examples of Monoterpene Alcohols:

–Linalool

Linalool is found in rosewood, bergamot, coriander, rose, jasmine, and lavender essential oils. It has a flowery aroma and is used to scent soaps, shampoos, and perfumes. Linalool can help relieve discomfort. It has antibacterial, antifungal, antiseptic (5x phenol), antispasmodic, antiviral, and sedative properties.

OH

Linalool

Anti-inflammatory: Linalool has been used to reduce paw swelling induced by carrageenan in mice. The effects of linalool work against swelling in a dose-dependent manner[1,2]. Linalool also mediates pain caused by inflammation. In a particular study, acetic acid was administered to mice via intraperitoneal (gut) injections. Mice that received a dose of linalool following administration of acetic acid exhibited less writhing (due to pain) than mice that acted as controls[3].

Antifungal: *Candida albicans* is the primary fungus responsible for yeast infections. Yeast infections are commonly exhibited as vulvovaginal candidiasis and thrush (oropharyngeal candidiasis, in the mouth). Thrush is commonly expressed in newborns and AIDS patients.

Candida albicans is also becoming a concern due to its emergence as a nosoco-

1   Peana et al., 2002.
2   Skold et al., 2002.
3   Peana et al., 2003.

mial infection (an infection contracted in a hospital) and its increasing resistance to fluconazole—an antifungal drug. *C. albicans* can form biofilms (aggregated colonies) on medical devices such as catheters and dentures[1,2].

Topical application of linalool to colonies of the polymorphic fungus *Candida albicans* results in growth inhibition and fungal death. Linalool affects growth by blocking passage beyond the G1 (cell growth) phase of the cell cycle[3].

Sedative: Linalool is a common sedative used in Brazilian folk medicine. According to studies using mice, inhaled linalool induces sleep or sedation[4,5].

Antiepileptic/Anticonvulsant: Epilepsy is characterized by seemingly spontaneous spasms of electrical activity in the brain. These spasms can cause seizures and convulsions. One hypothesis for the cause of epilepsy is excessive glutamate levels in neurons (nerve cells)[6,7,8,9]. Glutamates are a common form of neurotransmitter that are stored in special vesicles (storage containers) near nerve synapses (locations where nerve cells come close to each other in order to pass along electrical impulses and signals). Impulses along the nerve cause one nerve cell to release glutamate across the synapse where it is received by receptors on the second nerve cell, opening channels in that cell to allow it to pass ions through the cell membrane, changing the electrical potential of that cell[10].

Studies have shown that the release of large concentrations of glutamate will lead to too many open channels, which will cause high, intense depolarization sequences of the action potential. Disproportionate depolarizations are the basis for seizures and convulsions in epilepsy[11,12,13].

Using mouse models, researchers have found that applications of linalool on cortical synaptosomes (isolated nerve terminals, or synapses) significantly inhibited glutamate uptake. Inhibition of glutamate is a method to reduce occurrences of epileptic seizures. These observations provide significant evidence for linalool acting as a possible antiepileptic agent[14,15].

1   Mukherjee et al., 2003.
2   Microbiology. 9th ed, 2007.
3   Zore et al., 2011.
4   Linck et al., 2009.
5   de Almeida et al., 2009.
6   Chapman et al., 2000.
7   Meldrum et al., 1999.
8   Meldrum, 1994.
9   Chapman, 1998.
10 Medical Physiology. 10th ed, 2000.
11 Chapman et al., 2000.
12 Meldrum et al., 1994.
13 Paolette et al., 2007.
14 Silva Brum et al., 2001a.
15 Silva Brum et al., 2001b.

Nerve Cells

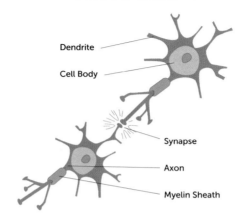

Dendrite

Cell Body

Synapse

Axon

Myelin Sheath

Synapse

Axon Terminal of
Presynaptic Cell

Glutamate Vesicle

Glutamate

Synaptic Cleft

Glutamate Receptors

Dendrite Terminal of
Postsynaptic Cell

−Citronellol

Citronellol is found in citronella, rose, melissa, and eucalyptus essential oils. It has antibacterial, antifungal, antiseptic (3.8x phenol), and sedative properties.

Anticonvulsant Activity: Administered doses of citronellol given via the intraperitoneal cavity (gut) to rodents have been observed to reduce the convulsive effects in induced epileptic attacks. Epilepsy is studied in animal models by inducing convulsions with compounds such as pentylenetetrazol (PTZ) and picrotoxin. Citronellol, over time, reduces the amplitude of the compound action potential (CAP) in neurons. This decreases the effect and intensity of convulsions[1].

OH

Citronellol

Blood Pressure: Injections of citronellol into the blood were found by researchers to reduce blood pressure in animal models. Citronellol is theorized to decrease the flux of Ca^{2+} ions into smooth vascular muscle cells by deactivating VOCCs (voltage-operated calcium channels).Calcium is the principle regulator of tension in vascular smooth muscle (blood vessels). When the transport of Ca^{2+} into the cell is blocked, smooth muscle relaxation occurs. This leads to increased vasodilation (an increase in the diameter of the blood vessels, allowing a higher volume of blood flow) and, thus, lowered blood pressure[2,3,4].

−Geraniol

Geraniol is found in rose, citronella, and lemon essential oils. It has antifungal, antiseptic (7x phenol), cancer preventative, and sedative properties.

Geraniol

OH

−Other Monoterpene Alcohols:

Borneol, menthol, nerol, terpineol (which Dr. Gattefossé considered to be a decongestant), vetiverol, and cedrol.

—Sesquiterpene Alcohols (Sesquiterpenols)

Like sesquiterpenes, sesquiterpene alcohols are comprised of three isoprene units but have a hydroxyl group bound to one of the carbons instead of a hydrogen. Sesquiterpene alcohols are known to be antiallergic, antibacterial, anti-inflammatory, ulcer-protective (preventative), and liver and glandular stimulant.

Examples of Monoterpene Alcohols:

---

1   de Sousa et al., 2006.
2   Bastos et al., 2009.
3   Gurney, 1994.
4   Munzel et al., 2003.

−Farnesol

Farnesol is found in rose, neroli, ylang ylang, and Roman chamomile essential oils. It is known to be good for the mucous membranes and to help prevent bacterial growth from perspiration.

Farnesol

−Bisabolol

Bisabolol is found in German chamomile essential oil. It is one of the strongest sesquiterpene alcohols.

−Other Sesquiterpene Alcohols:

Others include nerolidol and zingiberol.

Bisabolol

Esters

Esters are the compounds resulting from the reaction of an alcohol with an acid (known as esterification). Esters consist of a carboxyl group (a carbon atom double bonded to an oxygen atom) bound to a hydrocarbon group on one side and bound to an oxygen and a hydrocarbon group on the opposite side. Esters are very common and are found in the mildest essential oils. Mostly free of toxicity and irritants, they tend to be the most calming, relaxing, and balancing of all the

Methyl Acetate
(CH₃OOCH₃)

Methyl Acetate
(CH₃OOCH₃)

Methyl acetate (shown here) is a simple organic ester molecule.

○ = carbon
● = hydrogen
= oxygen

essential oil constituents. They are also antifungal and antispasmodic. They have a balancing or regulatory effect, especially on the nervous system. Some examples are linalyl acetate, geranyl acetate (with strong antifungal properties), and bornyl acetate (effective on bronchial candida). Other esters include eugenyl acetate, lavendulyl acetate, and methyl salicylate.

Found as a Major Constituent In: Birch, bergamot, clary sage, geranium, helichrysum, lavender, wintergreen, and ylang ylang.

Found as a Minor Constituent In: Cassia, clove, cypress, white fir, lemon, lemongrass, marjoram, and orange.

Aldehydes

Aldehydes are often responsible for the fragrance of an oil. They exert powerful aromas and are often calming to the emotions. They are highly reactive and are characterized by a carboxyl group (a carbon atom double bonded to an oxygen atom) with a hydrogen atom on one side and a hydrocarbon group on the opposite side.

In general, they are anti-infectious, anti-inflammatory, calming to the central nervous system, fever-reducing,

Acetaldehyde
(CH₃CHO)

Acetaldehyde
(CH₃CHO)

Acetaldehyde (shown here) is a simple organic aldehyde molecule.

⚪ = carbon
⚫ = hydrogen
🔘 = oxygen

hypotensive, and tonic. Some are antiseptic, antimicrobial, and antifungal, while others act as vasodilators. They can be quite irritating when applied topically (citrals being an example). However, it has been shown that adding an essential oil with an equal amount of d-Limonene can negate the irritant properties of a high citral oil.

Found as a Major Constituent In: Cassia, cinnamon, and lemongrass.

Found as a Minor Constituent In: *Eucalyptus radiata*, grapefruit, lemon, myrrh, and orange.

Examples of Aldehydes:

—Citrals

Citrals (like neral, geranial, and citronellal) are very common and have a distinct antiseptic action. They also show antiviral properties (as is the case with melissa oil) when applied topically on herpes simplex.

Geranial

—Other Aldehydes

Benzaldehyde, cinnamic aldehyde, cuminic aldehyde, and perillaldehyde.

Ketones

Ketones are organic compounds characterized by a carboxyl group (a carbon atom double bonded to an oxygen atom) with a hydrocarbon on both sides.

Ketones are sometimes mucolytic and neurotoxic when isolated from other constituents. However, all recorded toxic effects come from laboratory testing on guinea pigs and rats. No documented cases exist where oils with a high concen-

Acetone
(CH₃COCH₃)

Acetone
(CH₃COCH₃)

Acetone (shown here) is a simple ketone molecule.

⚪ = carbon
⚫ = hydrogen
🔘 = oxygen

tration of ketones (such as mugwort, tansy, sage, and wormwood) have ever caused a toxic effect on a human being. Also, large amounts of these oils would have to be consumed for them to result in a toxic neurological effect. Ketones stimulate cell regeneration, promote the formation of tissue, and liquefy mucous. They are helpful with conditions such as dry asthma, colds, flu, and dry cough and are largely found in oils used for the upper respiratory system, such as hyssop, rosemary, and sage.

Found as a Major Constituent In: rosemary
(CT verbenon).

Found as a Minor (but significant) Constituent In: Fennel, geranium, helichrysum, lemongrass, myrrh, peppermint, and vetiver.

Examples of Ketones:

—Thujone

Thujone is one of the most toxic members of the ketone family. It can be an irritant and upsetting to the central nervous system and may be neurotoxic when taken internally, such as in the banned drink absinthe. Although oils containing thujone may be inhaled to relieve respiratory distress and may stimulate the immune system, they should usually be used in dilution (1–2%) and/or for only short periods of time.

α-Thujone

—Jasmone

Jasmone is found in jasmine essential oil and is nontoxic.

Jasmone

—Fenchone

Fenchone is found in fennel essential oil and is nontoxic.

—Other Ketones:

Camphor, carvone, menthone, methyl nonyl ketone, and pinocamphone.

Fenchone

Phenols

Phenols are a diverse group of compounds derived from a phenol group, which is comprised of a benzene ring (six carbon atoms bound in a circle) and a hydroxyl group (oxygen and hydrogen).

Phenols comprise some of the most powerful antibacterial, anti-infectious, and antiseptic constituents in the plant world.

Phenol (C_6H_6OH)
OH

Phenol (C_6H_6OH)

Phenol (shown here) is a simple phenol molecule.

○ = carbon
● = hydrogen
◯ = oxygen

They are also very stimulating to both the nervous and immune systems. They contain high levels of oxygenating molecules and have antioxidant properties. However, they can be quite caustic to the skin, and they present some concerns regarding liver toxicity. Essential oils that contain a high proportion of phenols should be diluted and/or used only for short periods of time.

Found as a Major Constituent In: Basil, birch, cinnamon, clove, fennel, melaleuca, oregano, peppermint, thyme, and wintergreen.

Found as a Minor Constituent In: Cassia, marjoram, and ylang ylang.

Examples of Phenols:

—Eugenol

Eugenol is found in clove, nutmeg, cinnamon, bay, and basil essential oils. It has analgesic, anesthetic (in dentistry), anticonvulsant, antifungal, anti-inflammatory, antioxidant, antiseptic, cancer-preventative, and sedative properties.

Eugenol

Vasodilator: Eugenol was found to increase vasodilation (increase the diameter of the opening through the blood vessels) in animal models. When blood vessels expand, the result is larger amounts of blood flow and, thus, a decrease in heart rate. In these particular studies, it was observed that heart rate decreased in conjunction with increased vasodilation, as compared to controls[1,2].

Eugenol is thought to increase vasodilation by inhibiting the action of calcium (Ca^{2+}) in voltage-operated calcium channels (VOCCs). Ca^{2+} is the main regulator of vascular smooth muscle (blood vessel) tension. When Ca^{2+} is blocked, blood vessels relax and widen, allowing for an increase in blood flow[3,4].

—Thymol

Thymol is found in thyme and oregano essential oils. It may not be as caustic as other phenols. It has antibacterial, antifungal, anti-inflammatory, antioxidant, antiplaque, antirheumatic, antiseptic (20x phenol), antispasmodic, deodorizing, and expectorant properties.

Antibacterial: Thymol has been shown to inhibit the growth of microorganisms such as *Escherichia coli*, *Campylobacter jejuni*, *Porphyromonas gingivalis*, *Staphylococcus aureus*, and *Pseudomonas aeruginosa*. Thymol is thought to disrupt (or impair) the cytoplasmic membranes of microbes, causing cell leakage. Without the

Thymol

---

1   Lahlou et al., 2004.
2   Damiani et al., 2003.
3   Gurney, 1994.
4   Munzel et al., 2003.

protective barrier of the cytoplasmic membrane, viability of these microorganisms significantly decreases[1,2,3,4].

—Carvacrol

Carvacrol is a product of auto-oxidation of d-Limonene. It is antibacterial, antifungal, anti-inflammatory, antiseptic (1.5x phenol), antispasmodic, and expectorant. Researchers believe it may possibly have some anticancer properties as well.

—Other Phenols

Carvacrol

Methyl eugenol, methyl chavicol, anethole, and safrole.

Oxides

An organic oxide typically refers to an organic molecule (one that contains carbon and hydrogen) that has been oxidized, meaning an oxygen atom has become bound between two carbon atoms. According to the *American Heritage® Dictionary of the English Language*, an oxide is "a binary compound of an element or a radical with oxygen." Oxides act as expectorants and are mildly stimulating.

Found as a Major Constituent In: *Eucalyptus radiata* and rosemary.

Found as a Minor Constituent In: Basil, lemongrass, melaleuca, thyme, and ylang ylang.

Examples of Oxides:

—1,8-Cineol (Eucalyptol)

1,8-cineol is, by far, the most prevalent member of the oxide family and virtually exists in a class of its own. It is anesthetic, antiseptic, and works as a strong mucolytic as it thins mucus in respiratory tract infections.

1,8-Cineol
(Eucalyptol)

Anti-Inflammatory: Researchers found in an animal experiment that rats that were given oral doses of 1,8-cineole before injection with lambda carrageenan (a sweetener that causes inflammation) had markedly decreased swelling when compared to rats that were given the injection without a dosage of 1,8-cineole.

It has been suggested by scientists that 1,8-cineole inhibits cytokine production. Inhibiting cytokine production would decrease inflammation despite having a stimulant present (such a carrageenan)[5,6].

Asthma: Asthma is a chronic inflammatory disease that restricts air flow to the lungs (specifically in the bronchial tubes). A double-blind, placebo-controlled study was

1   Shapiro et al., 1995.
2   Xu et al., 2008.
3   Lambert et al., 2001.
4   Evans et al., 2000.
5   Santos et al., 2000.
6   Juergens et al., 2003.

performed to test the ability of 1,8-cineole to alleviate asthmatic symptoms. All subjects in the study suffered from bronchial asthma and required daily administration of oral glucocorticosteroids in order to maintain stable conditions.

At the conclusion of the study, which lasted over a course of 12 weeks, patients who received daily doses of 1,8-cineole were able to maintain stable conditions despite significantly reduced oral doses of glucocorticosteroids, as compared to the placebo group. Proper lung function was also maintained four times longer in the test group than in the placebo group[1,2].

Pain: In one study, mice were injected in the hind paw with a dose of 1% formalin (a common substance used to model pain in experimental studies)/99% saline solution. A portion of mice were given 1,8-cineole. It was observed that mice given the 1,8-cineole licked their paw substantially less (meaning they did not feel as much pain) than mice that did not receive 1,8-cineole treatment. In this study, researchers found that 1,8-cineole treatment produced antinociceptive (pain-blocking) effects comparable to those observed for morphine[3,4].

—Other oxides

Linalool oxide, ascaridol, bisabolol oxide, 1,4-cineol, and bisabolone oxide.

---

1   Juergens et al., 2003.
2   Goodwin et al., 1986.
3   Santos et al., 2000.
4   Shibata et al., 1989.

Essential Oil Application Methods: Topical

Topical application is the process of placing an essential oil on the skin, hair, mouth, teeth, nails, or mucus membranes of the body. Applying essential oils directly on the body without any kind of dilution is commonly referred to as applying the oil "neat." Since essential oils are so potent, and because some essential oils may irritate the skin or other areas of the body, they are often diluted with a pure vegetable oil (usually called a "carrier oil") such as fractionated coconut oil, almond oil, olive oil, jojoba oil, etc. Several topical application methods are outlined below.

Direct Application:

Direct application is applying the oils directly on the area of concern. Because essential oils are so potent, more is not necessarily better. To achieve the desired results, 1–3 drops of oil are usually adequate. A few guidelines for direct application of the oils are as follow:

– The feet are the second fastest area of the body to absorb oils because of the large pores. Other quick-absorbing areas include behind the ears and on the wrists.

– To produce a feeling of peace, relaxation, or energy, 3–6 drops per foot are adequate.

– When massaging a large area of the body, always dilute the oils by 15% to 30% with fractionated coconut oil.

– When applying oils to infants and small children, dilute with fractionated coconut oil. Use 1–3 drops of an essential oil to 1 tablespoon (Tbs) of fractionated coconut oil for infants and 1–3 drops of an essential oil to 1 teaspoon (tsp) fractionated coconut oil for children ages 2–5.

– Use caution when creating blends for topical therapeutic use. Commercially-available blends have been specially formulated by someone who understands the chemical constituents of each oil and which oils blend well. The chemical properties of the oils can be altered when mixed improperly, resulting in some undesirable reactions.

– Layering individual oils is preferred over mixing your own blends for topical use. Layering refers to the process of applying one oil, rubbing it in, and then applying another oil. There is no need to wait more than a couple of seconds between each oil, as absorption occurs quite rapidly. If dilution is necessary, fractionated coconut oil may be applied on top. The layering technique is not only useful in physical healing but also in emotional clearing.

Massage:

Massage is the stimulation of muscle, skin, and connective tissues using various techniques to help promote healing, balance, and connection. Massages can be invigorating, relaxing, stimulating, or soothing, and essential oils applied using massage can help enhance these benefits. There are many different massage techniques currently in use, and to explore all of the various techniques would be beyond the scope of this book.

Unless you are a certified massage therapist and have a thorough understanding of anatomy, it is best to use only light to medium massage strokes for applying oils and to avoid the spine and other sensitive areas of the body. Extreme caution must also be used when massaging pregnant women and others with certain health conditions.

To create a simple massage oil that includes the benefits of essential oils, combine 3–10 drops of your desired essential oil or blend with 1 tablespoon (15 ml) of fractionated coconut oil or another carrier oil. Apply a small amount of this mixture on location, and massage it into the skin using light to medium-light strokes of the hand or fingers.

Reflexology/Reflex Therapy:

Reflex therapy is a simple method of applying oils to contact points (or nerve endings) in the feet or hands. A series of hand rotation movements at those control points create a vibrational healing energy that carries the oils along the neuroelectrical pathways. The oils either help remove any blockage along the pathways or travel the length of the pathway to benefit the particular organ. Refer to the reflex hand and foot charts on the following pages for more details.

Auricular Therapy

Auricular therapy is a method of applying the oils to various points on the rim of the ears to effect changes on internal body parts. Small amounts of the oil are applied to the point, and then the point is stimulated with the fingers or with a glass probe. See the Auricular Body Points chart on the following page for more details.

Compresses

1. Basin. Fill a wash basin with 2 quarts of hot or cold water, and add the desired essential oils. Stir the water vigorously; then lay a towel on top of the water. Since the oils will float to the top, the towel will absorb the oils with the water. After the towel is completely saturated, wring out the excess water (leaving much of the oils in the towel), and place the towel over the area needing the compress. For a hot compress, cover with a dry towel and a hot water bottle. For a cold compress, cover with a piece of plastic or plastic wrap. Finally, put another towel on top, and leave for as long as possible (1–2 hours is best).

2. Massage. Apply a hot, wet towel and then a dry towel on top of an already massaged area. The moist heat will force the oils deeper into the tissues of the body.

Baths

1. Bathwater. Begin by adding 3–6 drops of oil to the bathwater while the tub is filling. Because the individual oils will separate as the water calms down, the skin will quickly draw the oils from the top of the water. Some people have commented that they were unable to endure more than 6 drops of oil. Such individuals may benefit from adding the oils to a bath and shower gel base first. Soak for 15 minutes.

2. Bath and Shower Gel. Begin by adding 3–6 drops of oil to ½ oz of a bath and shower gel base; add to the water while the tub is filling. Adding the oils to a bath and shower gel base first allows one to obtain the greatest benefit from the oils as they are more evenly dispersed throughout the water and not allowed to immediately separate.

3. Bath Salts. Combine 3–10 drops essential oil with ¼–½ cup of bath salts or Epsom salts. Dissolve the salt mixture in warm bathwater before bathing.

4. Washcloth. When showering, add 3–6 drops of oil to a bath and shower gel base before applying to a washcloth and using to wash the body.

5. Body Sprays. Fill a small spray bottle with distilled water, and add 10–15 drops of your favorite oil blend or single oils. Shake well, and spray onto the entire body just after taking a bath or shower.

Auricular Internal Body Points

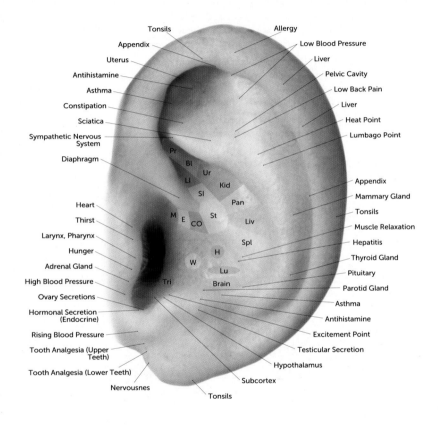

Bl: Bladder	Liv: Liver	Spl: Spleen
CO: Cardiac Orifice	Lu: Lungs	ST: Stomach
E: Esophogus	M: Mouth	Tri: Triple Warmer
H: Heart	Pan: Pancreas	Ur: Ureter
Kid: Kidney	Pr: Prostate	W: Windpipe/Trachea
LI: Large Intestine	SI Small Intestine	

Reflexology Hand Chart

Reflex points on this hand chart correspond to those on the feet. Occasionally the feet can be too sensitive for typical reflex therapy. Working with the hands will not only affect the specific body points but may also help to provide some pain relief to the corresponding points on the feet.

Reflexology Feet Charts

Sinus
Brain
Pineal
Pituitary
Parathyroid
Thyroid
Trachea
Bronchial
Lung
Thymus
Spine
Esophogus
Stomach
Transverse Colon
Adrenal
Kidney
Small Intestine
Rectum
Coccyx
Sciatica

Sinus
Ears
Eyes
Shoulder
Heart
Spleen
Pancreas
Descending Colon

Ears
Eyes
Shoulder
Liver
Gallbladder
Ascending Colon
Appendix

Right Foot

Left Foot

Uterus
Ovaries
Shoulder

Colon (Secondary Point—Inside of Shin from Knee to Ankle)
Testes
Prostate
Shoulder

Bronchial Tubes

Autonomic Nervous System

Sympathetic Nervous System

- Dilates Pupils
- Inhibits Salivation
- Accelerates Heart Rate
- Dilates Bronchi
- Dilates Skeletal Muscle Blood Vessels to Increase Blood Flow to Muscles
- Constricts Other Blood Vessels to Increase Overall Blood Pressure
- Inhibits Gastric Juice Production
- Stimulates Secretion of Epinephrine and Norepinephrine
- Inhibits Digestive Process
- Contracts Rectum
- Relaxes Bladder Muscles

Parasympathetic Nervous System

- Constricts Pupils
- Stimulates Salivation
- Slows Heart Rate
- Constricts Bronchi
- Constricts Skeletal Muscle Blood Vessels to Decrease Blood Flow to Muscles
- Dilates Other Blood Vessels to Decrease Overall Blood Pressure
- Stimulates Gastric Juice Production
- Stimulates Digestive Process
- Relaxes Rectum
- Contracts Bladder Muscles

Essential Oil Application Methods: Aromatic

Aromatic application involves inhaling either a fine mist of the oil, or a vapor of volatile aromatic components that have evaporated from the oil. Inhalation of the oil, or the aroma from the oil, can be a powerful way to affect memory, hormones, and emotions through the olfactory system (see the following page for further discussion on this topic). Inhalation of oils can also be a quick and effective way to affect the sinuses, larynx, brochial tubes, and lungs.

Diffusion:

The easiest and simplest way of putting a fine mist of the whole oil into the air for inhalation is to use a nebulizing diffuser. A cool-air nebulizing diffuser uses room-temperature air to break the oils into a micro-fine mist that is then dispersed into the air, covering hundreds of square feet in seconds. An ultrasonic nebulizer uses ultrasonic vibrations to convert oil mixed with water into a fine water vapor. When diffused in this manner, the oils, with their oxygenating molecules, will then remain suspended for several hours to freshen and improve the quality of the air. The antiviral, antibacterial, and antiseptic properties of the oils kill bacteria and help to reduce fungus and mold.

Other diffusers may use cool-air blowing through a pad containing the oil, or a low level of heat to quickly evaporate the volatile oil molecules into the air. This type of diffusion is beneficial, but may not be as effective for some therapeutic uses as nebulizing the whole oil can be.

Diffusers that use an intense heat source (such as a light bulb ring or candle) may alter the chemical makeup of the oil and its therapeutic qualities, and are typically not recommended.

Essential oils, when diffused, have been found to reduce the amount of airborne chemicals and to help to create greater physical and emotional harmony. The greatest therapeutic benefit is received by diffusing oils for only 15 minutes out of an hour so that the olfactory system has time to recover before receiving more oils. The easiest way to do this is by using a timer that can be set to turn the diffuser on in 15-minute increments over a 24-hour period.

Direct Inhalation:

Direct inhilation is the simplest way to inhale the aroma of an essential oil in order to affect moods and emotions. Simply hold an opened essential oil vial close to the face, and inhale. You may also apply 1-2 drops of oil onto your hands, cup your hands over your mouth and nose, and inhale.

Cloth or Tissue:

Put one to three drops of an essential oil on a paper towel, tissue, cotton ball, handkerchief, towel, or pillow case; hold it close to your face, and inhale.

Hot Water Vapor:

Put one to three drops of an essential oil into hot water, and inhale. Again, heat may reduce some of the benefits.

Vaporizer or Humidifier:

Put oil in a vaporizer or a humidifier. The cool mist types are best, since heat reduces some of the benefits. There are some commercially available diffusers that utilize ultrasonic vibration to vaporize water into a cool mist. These work well with essential oils since they produce a very fine mist that helps suspend the oil particles in the air for extended periods of time.

Fan or Vent:

Put oil on a cotton ball, and attach to ceiling fans or air vents. This can also work well in a vehicle since the area is so small.

Perfume or Cologne.

Wearing the oils as a perfume or cologne can provide some wonderful emotional support and physical support as well—not just a beautiful fragrance. Apply 1-2 drops of oil to the wrists or neck, or create a simple perfume or cologne by dissolving 10-15 drops essential oil in 20 drops alcohol (such as vodka, or a perfumer's alcohol) and combining this mixture with 1 tsp. distilled water. Apply or mist on wrists or neck.

Nose and Olfactory System

Olfactory System

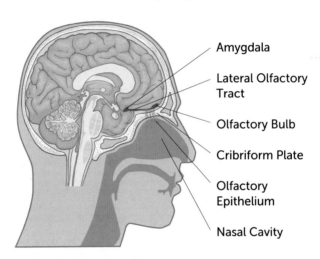

- Amygdala
- Lateral Olfactory Tract
- Olfactory Bulb
- Cribriform Plate
- Olfactory Epithelium
- Nasal Cavity

When an odor molecule is inhaled into the nasal cavity, it is first sensed by the olfactory cells that are part of the olfactory epithelium. The olfactory epithelium is comprised of two small patches of olfactory nerves (each about 1 cm square) that lie on the roof of the nasal cavity. The olfactory cells within the olfactory epithelium are specialized nerve cells that extend cilia (small hair-like structures) from their dendrites into the nasal cavity. Each of these cilia have receptors that bind to a specific type of odor molecule. When an odor molecule binds to a receptor on the cilia of an olfactory cell, the olfactory cell passes the signal through the cribriform plate (the bone at the roof of the nasal cavity) to the olfactory bulb. The olfactory bulb, in turn, sends those impulses along the lateral olfactory tract to five different structures in the brain, including the amygdala (which is responsible for storing and releasing emotional trauma), the anterior olfactory nucleus (which helps process smells), the olfactory tubercle, the piriform cortex (which passes the signal on to other structures that create a conscious perception of the odor), and the entorhinal cortex (which processes stimuli before sending them on to the hippocampus, the long-term memory center of the brain). Anatomically, the olfactory system is closely connected to the limbic system of the brain. The limbic system includes structures such as the hippocampus (long-term memory), the amygdala (emotions), the hypothalamus (autonomic nervous system and hormones), and the cingulate gyrus (regulates blood pressure, heart rate, and attention). It is due to the fact that the olfactory system is so closely connected to the limbic system that essential oils have such profound physiological and psychological effects.

The Art of Blending

Blending essential oils is an art and usually requires a little bit of training and experimentation. If you choose to create your own blends, it is important to understand that the order in which the oils are blended is key to maintaining the desired therapeutic properties in a synergistic blend. An alteration in the sequence of adding selected oils to a blend may change the chemical properties, the fragrance, and thus the desired results. The "Blend Classification" and "Blends With" listings under each oil in the Single Oils section of the book, *Modern Essentials*, should assist one in the blending process. In general, oils that are from the same botanical family usually blend well together. In addition, oils with similar constituents also mix well.

Another method utilizes four blending classifications. The following information explains the characteristics of each classification, the order in which they should be added to the blend (i.e. Personifiers first, Enhancers second, Equalizers third, and Modifiers fourth), and the amount of each type of oil as a percentage of the blend.

1st—The Personifier (1-5% of blend) oils have very sharp, strong, and long-lasting fragrances. They also have dominant properties with strong therapeutic action.

Oils in this classification may include birch, cinnamon, clary sage, clove, coriander, ginger, helichrysum, orange, peppermint, rose, wintergreen, and ylang ylang.

2nd—The Enhancer (50-80% of blend) oil should be the predominant oil as it serves to enhance the properties of the other oils in the blend. Its fragrance is not as sharp as the personifiers and is usually of a shorter duration.

Oils in this classification may include basil, bergamot, birch, eucalyptus, frankincense, geranium, grapefruit, lavender, lemon, lemongrass, marjoram, melaleuca, orange, oregano, rose, rosemary, thyme, and wintergreen.

3rd—The Equalizer (10-15% of blend) oils create balance and synergy among the oils contained in the blend. Their fragrance is also not as sharp as the personifier and is of a shorter duration.

Oils in this classification may include basil, bergamot, cypress, fennel, white fir, frankincense, geranium, ginger, lavender, lemongrass, marjoram, melaleuca, myrrh, oregano, rose, sandalwood, and thyme.

4th—The Modifier (5-8% of blend) oils have a mild and short fragrance. These oils add harmony to the blend.

Oils in this classification may include bergamot, coriander, eucalyptus, fennel, grapefruit, lavender, lemon, myrrh, rose, sandalwood, and ylang ylang.

Depending upon the topical application of your blend, you will want to add some carrier/base oil. When creating a therapeutic essential oil blend, you may want to use about 28 drops of essential oil to ½ oz. of fractionated coconut oil. When creating a body massage blend, you will want to use a total of about 50 drops of essential oils to 4 oz. of fractionated coconut oil. Remember to store your fragrant creation in dark-colored glass bottles.

As essential oils can vary in thickness, the following are approximate measurements:

25-30 drops	= 1/4 tsp.	= 1-2 ml	= 5/8 dram
45-50 drops	= 1/2 tsp.	= 2-3 ml	= 1 dram
75-80 drops	= 3/4 tsp.	= 3-4 ml	= 1/8 oz.
100-120 drops	= 1 tsp.	= 5 ml	= 1/6 oz.
160 drops	= 1½ tsp.	= 6-8 ml	= 1/4 oz.
320-400 drops	= 3 tsp.	= 13-15 ml	= 1/2 oz.
600-650 drops	= 6 tsp.	= 25-30 ml	= 1 oz.

Learn to trust your nose as it can help you decide which classification an oil should be in. More detailed information about these methods of blending is beyond the scope of this revision of the book. For additional information on using these classifications in your blending, we highly recommend Marcel Lavabre's *Aromatherapy Workbook*. Another very simple book about blending, with recipes and easy-to-follow guidelines, is Mindy Green's *Natural Perfumes*, which uses perfume notes (top, middle, base), odor, and odor intensity to help guide you in making your own fragrant blend creations.

Essential Oil Application Methods: Internal

Internal use is the process of consuming or otherwise internalizing an essential oil into the body. Only pure, therapeutic-grade essential oils should be used for internal consumption, as other essential oils on the market may be diluted or processed using harmful chemicals.

The U.S. Food and Drug Administration (FDA) has approved some essential oils generically for internal use and given them the following designations: GRAS (Generally Recognized As Safe for human consumption), FA (Food Additive), or FL (Flavoring Agent). These designations are listed for each oil that is safe for human consumption in the Single Essential Oils section of this book under Oral Use As Dietary Supplement. Oils without this designation should never be used internally without first consulting a certified health care professional.

—Understanding GRAS, FA, and FL Status

In 1938, the United States Congress passed The Federal Food, Drug, and Cosmetic Act (FFDCA), giving authority to the FDA to regulate the food, drug, and cosmetic industries. To increase the FDA's regulatory authority, the Food Additives Amendment to the FFDCA was added in 1958. This amendment requires all food additives to be approved by the FDA. To eliminate unneeded and duplicate testing, the FDA also released a list of substances considered Generally Recognized As Safe (GRAS) for human consumption. The designation of a substance as GRAS means that the substance, when intentionally added to food under the conditions of its intended use, is recognized by competent experts as being safe. Substances obtain GRAS status through scientific procedures or through experience based on common use in food before 1958.

Substances designated as GRAS are listed in the US Code of Federal Regulations (CFR). Most essential oils that are considered GRAS can be found under 21 CFR § 182.20. This section of the CFR was completed shortly after the passing of the 1958 Food Additives Amendment. Additionally, some GRAS substances are listed under section 184, including clove oil (found under 21 CFR § 184.1257) and dill oil (found under 21 CFR § 184.1282). Section 184 was added in the 1970s as part of the FDA's comprehensive review of GRAS substances.

Not all essential oils are GRAS substances. Some essential oils, like birch oil and cedarwood oil, are not recommended for internal use. Other essential oils, including frankincense oil and melaleuca oil, have been granted Food Additive (FA) or Flavoring Agent (FL) status. Food additives are used to maintain food safety, freshness, and nutritional value. Ingredients added to foods to improve the aroma or quality of taste are considered flavoring agents. A list of substances, including essential oils, that maintain Food Additive and Flavoring Agent status can be found under 21 CFR § 172.510.

Essential oils with GRAS, FA, or FL status are considered by the FDA as safe to consume and can be used internally via several routes of administration.

Common Essential Oils Designated at GRAS:	Angelica, Anise, Basil, Bay, Bergamot, Black Pepper, Chamomile, Cardamom, Cassia, Celery, Cinnamon, Citronella, Citrus (all), Clary Sage, Coriander, Cumin, Fennel, Geranium, Ginger, Grapefruit, Helichrysum, Jasmine, Juniper Berry, Lavender, Lemon, Lemongrass, Lime, Mandarin, Marjoram, Melissa, Neroli, Orange, Oregano, Palmarosa, Peppermint, Rose, Rosemary, Sage, Spearmint, Tangerine, Thyme, Vanilla, Ylang Ylang
Common Essential Oils Designated at FA/FL:	Dill, Frankincense, Melaleuca, Myrrh, Patchouli, Sandalwood, Vetiver, White Fir

Sublingual

One of the most effective ways to take essential oils internally is sublingually, or by placing a drop or two of an essential oil under the tongue. Because the blood capillaries are so close to the surface of the tissue under the tongue, many essential oil constituents are able to pass directly into the bloodstream, from which they can then quickly travel to the different areas of the body where they are needed. This method provides a faster therapeutic effect than oral administration (Turley, 2009). The sublingual method enables rapid absorption and bypasses the first-pass drug metabolism in the liver, meaning that a higher dosage of chemical constituents is delivered to the body than by most other internal routes (Brenner et al., 2009). Low dosages should be given to avoid irritation to the tissue and to ensure that the essential oil is not washed away by saliva or swallowed before absorption (Brenner et al., 2009).

Capsules

One common way to take essential oils internally is by placing 1–10 drops of essential oil inside an empty capsule, closing the capsule, and then swallowing it. It is also common to dilute the pure essential oil by filling the remainder of the capsule with olive oil before closing and swallowing. This can be an effective way to take oils internally that have a less desirable taste.

Beverage

An easy way to take essential oils internally is by adding them to a beverage. This is done by placing 1 drop of essential oil in 1–4 cups of rice milk, almond milk, or water, before drinking.

Cooking

Essential oils can easily be incorporated into your cooking, as long as you remember that they are very concentrated. Usually only 1 drop is necessary, and sometimes even less. Use a toothpick to help control the addition of smaller amounts of oil by dipping the toothpick into the oil (more oil on the toothpick = stronger flavor, etc.) and then stirring it into the food. For more information on cooking with essential oils, see the Essential Lifestyle section on page 54.

Vaginal Insertion

There are three main ways to insert essential oils vaginally. First, the oils can be diluted in 2–3 tsp of a carrier oil, inserted using a vaginal syringe, and then held in place using a tampon. Alternately, the oils can be diluted in 1–2 tsp of carrier oil, and then a tampon can be used to soak up the mixture. This is then inserted and retained, typically all day or overnight. The third method is to add a few drops of oil to warm water and then to use a vaginal syringe to irrigate and rinse internally using the oil and water mixture. In each case it is important to ensure that the oil is evenly dispersed to avoid irritation (Tisserand et al., 2014).

Rectal Insertion

Rectal oil insertion is often recommended to aid various respiratory problems and other internal conditions. Two ways are often recommended for implanting the oils rectally. First, a rectal syringe can be used to deposit the oils into the rectum. Second, the oils can be placed in capsules and the capsules be inserted into the rectum. The oils are typically retained inside the rectum for several hours or overnight. Assure that the oil is evenly dispersed to avoid irritation. Rectal insertion is an important method that can produce systemic effects at a slow rate of absorption (Schellack, 2011). Rectal insertion should be used when a higher systemic concentration is needed. This higher concentration is possible because rectal insertion avoids the first-pass metabolism in the liver (Brenner et al., 2009).

Daily Tips for An Essential Lifestyle

Essential oils can be used in many different ways throughout the day. Pure, therapeutic-grade essential oils are a safe, natural alternative to many of the artificial chemicals that are often used in the typical daily routine. While by no means comprehensive, this section outlines a few tips on how to use essential oils as part of everyday living. See the Personal Usage Guide chapter for supporting research and for more ways essential oils and blends can be used. See the Supplements and the Essential Living chapters for additional essential oil–inspired supplements and natural personal care items that can be used every day as well.

Essential oils are great for adding flavor or spice to your favorite meal. Essential oils can impart the natural, fresh taste of fresh herbs and spices but are more concentrated and can easily be used year-round when fresh herbs are not available. Essential oils are also a great substitute for dried or powdered spices, since dried spices have lost many of the liquid essential oils that impart much of the flavor and aroma found in the natural plant. Additionally, while many commercially available flavoring extracts use artificial flavors or are diluted in alcohol or propelyne glycol, essential oils provide a concentrated, pure flavor that is extracted naturally from the plant.

Essential Oil Cooking Tips:

Many great essential oil cookbooks are available that can help you get started using essential oils in cooking. But it is fairly easy (and a lot of fun) to substitute essential oils into your own favorite recipes in place of spices, flavoring extracts, and fresh or dried herbs. There are a few tips to keep in mind when substituting essential oils in recipes:

Amount to Use: Essential oils are extremely concentrated, so you won't use as much oil as you would dried spices or extracts. Start with a drop or two instead of a teaspoon; then adjust the amount according to taste.

When to Add: The preferred time to add essential oils is at the end of cooking or when the the food has cooled a bit. This is so the volatile oils don't evaporate out and also so the heat of cooking doesn't affect the oil's natural constituents. If you need to add the oils sooner in the recipe, you may need to add a bit more oil to account for any oil that will evaporate during cooking.

Recipes

Below are a few sample recipes to get you started using essential oils in your everyday cooking!

Lemon Tarragon Dressing

1 Tbs. fresh tarragon diced, or 1 tsp. dried tarragon
1 Tbs. fresh or 1 tsp. dried basil leaves
1 c. organic, cold-pressed olive oil
Dash of black pepper
Dash of red pepper
6 drops lemon essential oil

Mix well, and drizzle on salad or fish or anything! Keep unused portion in the fridge.

Luscious Lemon Bars

2 c. flour	1 tsp. baking powder
½ c. sugar	Dash of salt
1 c. butter	½ c. water
¼ tsp. salt	½ c. lemon juice
4 eggs	3 drops lemon ess. oil
6 Tbs. flour	1 Tbs. powdered sugar
1½ c. sugar	Lemon zest (optional)

Preheat oven to 350° F. Mix together flour, sugar, and salt. Cut in the butter until the dough reaches a fine crumb consistency. Press the dough into the bottom of a 9" x 13" pan. Bake for 20 minutes till golden. While crust is baking, beat eggs in a large mixing bowl. In a separate dish, stir together flour, sugar, baking powder, and salt. Add flour mixture to eggs, and stir till smooth. Gradually stir in lemon juice, water, and lemon oil. Pour mixture over baked crust, and return to the oven. Bake 30 minutes or until set. Allow to cool completely, and sift powdered sugar over the top. Garnish with zest if desired.
*Substitute orange oil and orange juice to make orange bars.

Strawberry Citrus Breakfast Ice Cream*

¼ ripe avocado	1 Tbs. honey or agave
1 c. frozen strawberries	1 drop ea. orange and lime essential oils
2 Tbs. plain yogurt	

Place all ingredients minus oils into a food processor, and puree on high. Remove from food processor, and stir in oils. Serve immediately. *Prepare the night before and freeze in ice-pop molds for a quick, on-the-go breakfast.

Creamy, Creamless, Raw, Tomato Soup*

6 ripe tomatoes, seeded and chopped
½ c. water
1 tsp. minced garlic (1 clove)
½ tsp. onion powder

1 tsp. sea salt
1 ripe avocado, chopped
2 Tbs. extra-virgin olive oil
2 drops basil essential oil

Place tomatoes, water, garlic, onion powder, and salt in blender, and blend until smooth. Add the avocado and olive oil, and blend again until smooth. Pour soup into a ceramic or wooden bowl, and add basil oil, stirring to combine. Serve immediately. For a chilled soup, refrigerate for 2 hours. For warm soup, heat over stove.

Rosemary Roasted Red Potatoes*

16–24 red potatoes, washed and dried
½–3/4 c. all-natural ranch dressing
1 drop ea. rosemary and oregano ess. oils

2 Tbs. garlic powder
1–2 tsp. smoked paprika
Sea salt and black pepper to taste

Preheat oven to 450° F. Dice potatoes into 1" pieces and place in 9" x 13" pan. Blend essential oils with ranch dressing and toss with potatoes to coat. Sprinkle potato mixture with garlic, paprika, salt, and pepper. Cover with aluminum foil, and bake for 25–40 minutes. Remove foil, stir potatoes, and bake uncovered for 15–20 minutes, stirring once more, until golden.

Peppermint Healthy Fudge*

1½ c. coconut oil
1¼ c. agave
1 c. organic cocoa powder
½ tsp. sea salt
1/8 scraped out vanilla bean (or 1 tsp. vanilla extract)
1–2 drops peppermint essential oil

Warm coconut oil until liquid. Combine all ingredients in blender, and blend until smooth. Pour into baking dish and spread evenly. Place in fridge to set up; then cut and enjoy.

*These recipes were adapted from *The Slimmed and Sassed Cookbook* by Natalie Albaugh & Kristyan Williams, ©2011. Used with permission.

Sleeping/Relaxing and Waking Up/Energizing

Essential oils are perfect for helping soothe and calm the mind and body at the end of a stressful day. Unlike synthetic sleep aids that can have unwanted side effects, pure essential oils are a natural way to help the mind and body relax.

Soothing Essential Oils:

Soothing Oils: lavender, Serenity, ylang ylang, Roman chamomile, clary sage, orange, Citrus Bliss, vetiver, geranium, melissa, sandalwood, bergamot, rose.

Sleeping/Relaxation Tips:

Diffusion: Diffuse soothing essential oils or blends to help you feel calm and relaxed before going to sleep.

Pillow: Place a drop or two of a soothing essential oil or blend on a pillow or stuffed animal before you sleep to help calm your mind and body.

Linen Spray: Make a soothing linen spray by mixing 5–6 drops of a soothing essential oil or blend with 1 oz. water in a small misting spray bottle. Shake, and spray lightly onto pillows, sheets, blankets, curtains, or into the air. (Note: Since some essential oils can clog spray bottles, it may help to dissolve the essential oil in 1 tsp. of grain alcohol before adding water to the spray bottle.)

Relaxing Bath: Mix 1–3 drops of a soothing essential oil with bath salts or directly in warm bathwater for a relaxing bath.

Essential oils can also help invigorate and energize the body in the morning or whenever you feel tired and lethargic—without the addictive rise/crash cycle and other side effects that come with many energy drinks and other caffeinated beverages.

Invigorating Essential Oils:

Invigorating Oils: peppermint, eucalyptus, white fir, lemon, basil, wintergreen, thyme.

Energizing/Invigorating Tips:

Difusion: Diffuse an invigorating oil in the morning. Some individuals like to use a diffuser or appliance timer to start their diffuser a few minutes before their alarm clock goes off to help the body begin to wake up naturally.

Morning Beverage: Add a few drops of peppermint, lemon, or orange to water, a fresh fruit/vegetable smoothie, or another healthy beverage.

Invigorating Shower: Place a few drops of an energizing essential oil or blend on the floor of a shower or in a bath and shower gel for an invigorating morning shower.

Bath and Shower Tips

Using essential oils in the bath or shower instead of products with artificial perfumes and fragrances allows one to simultaneously enjoy the topical and aromatic benefits of an essential oil or blend.

Bath and Shower Tips

Bathwater: Add 3–6 drops of oil to the bathwater while the tub is filling. Because the individual oils will separate as the water calms down, the skin will quickly draw the oils from the top of the water. Some people have commented that they were unable to endure more than 6 drops of oil. Such individuals may benefit from adding the oils to a bath and shower gel base first. Soak in the tub for 15 minutes.

Bath Oil: Add 1–5 drops of essential oil to 1 oz. (2 Tablespoons) of fractionated coconut oil (or another carrier/vegetable oil). Add a small amount of this bath oil to bathwater, and stir before bathing.

Bath and Shower Gel: Add 3–6 drops of oil to ½ oz. of a natural bath and shower gel base; add to the water while the tub is filling. Adding the oils to a bath and shower gel base first allows one to obtain the greatest benefit from the oils, as they are more evenly dispersed throughout the water and not allowed to immediately separate.

Bath Salts: Combine 3–10 drops essential oil with ¼–½ cup of bath salts or Epsom salts. Dissolve the salt mixture in warm bathwater before bathing.

Washcloth: When showering, add 3–6 drops of oil to a bath and shower gel base before applying to a washcloth and using to wash the body.

Body Sprays: Fill a small spray bottle with distilled water, and add 10–15 drops of your favorite essential oil or blend. Shake well, and spray onto the entire body just after taking a bath or shower.

Foot Bath: Add enough hot water to a basin to cover the ankles. Add 1–3 drops of your desired essential oil. Soak feet for 5–10 minutes, inhaling the aroma of the oils.

Hand Bath: Pour enough hot water in a basin to cover hands up to the wrists. Add 1–3 drops of your desired essential oil. Soak hands for 5–10 minutes while bending, pulling, and massaging the fingers and hands to stimulate. Try combining essential oils with 1 Tbs. honey in a hand bath or regular bath to help moisturize the skin.

Shower: With the water turned on, drop peppermint, rosemary, or Breathe on the shower floor as you enter to help invigorate and open the nasal passages. Use soothing oils at night to help promote a feeling of calmness and relaxation. Alternately, fill a tub/shower combo with about an inch or two of water; then place oils in the water before turning on the shower. This will allow the oils to more easily be drawn into the feet during the shower and also allow the aroma to be inhaled.

Personal Care and Wellbeing

Exercise Tips:

Muscle Soothing: Massage essential oils such as Deep Blue, marjoram, white fir, or eucalyptus into muscles and joints before and/or after exercise to help naturally soothe and
relax tired and sore muscles and joints.

Yoga: Diffuse or inhale oils like sandalwood and frankincense to help enhance focus and
meditation.

Home Atmosphere Tips:

The aroma of essential oils can be a major contributor to helping create the right atmosphere at home. Studies have shown that certain aromas can help a space feel warm and
inviting, while other aromas, like orange, can help relax and reduce anxiety. Below are a
couple of ideas to get you started, but try experimenting with other oils to see what kind of
mood they contribute to.

Calming/Relaxing: Diffuse oils such as lavender, Serenity, ylang ylang, Roman chamomile,
orange, sandalwood, or rose to help calm and relax (useful for de-stressing after a long day
or for helping children feel calm).

Uplifting/Inviting: Diffuse lemon, grapefruit, or other citrus scents to promote a comfort-
able, refreshing atmosphere (useful for parties or other social gatherings).

Office/School Tips:

Memory/Concentration: The part of the brain responsible for interpreting aromas is closely
tied to the part of the brain responsible for long-term memory and emotions. Studies have
demonstrated the ability of essential oil aromas such as rose-
mary and peppermint (as well as aromas in general) to help
enhance memory and alertness in human trials. Try inhaling
rosemary, peppermint, or frankincense when studying or
learning; then inhale the same aroma when you need to recall
the information. Try diffusing oils such as lavender, lemon, or
rosemary to help aid concentration.

Tired Eye Spray: Add six drops lavender, Roman chamomile, or
melaleuca to 1 oz. water in a small misting spray bottle, and
mist onto face Note: Be certain to keep your eyes closed.
Never spray essential oils directly into eyes.

Refreshing: Inhale lemon, peppermint, Elevation, eucalyptus, or
white fir oil as needed during the day to help invigorate and
refresh.

Kitchen and Bathroom Cleaning and Disinfecting

Many essential oils have demonstrated the ability to inhibit or kill various types of bacteria, mold, spores, and even viruses. These disinfectant properties of essential oils make them a natural substitute for the harsh chemicals used in many commercial cleaners. Essential oils can also work as natural deodorizers, without the artificial fragrances used in some products.

Essential Oils Recommended for Cleaning:

Disinfecting Oils: On Guard, lemon, Purify, melaleuca, lime, cinnamon, thyme, peppermint.

Deodorizing Oils: Purify, peppermint, clary sage, melaleuca, lavender, geranium, eucalyptus.

Kitchen Cleaning Tips:

Disinfecting Spray: Make a disinfecting spray by mixing 5–6 drops of a disinfecting essential oil or blend with 1 oz. water in a small misting spray bottle. Shake, and spray on counters, cutting boards, microwave, refrigerator, garbage cans, or other desired surfaces. (Note: Since some essential oils can clog spray bottles, it may help to dissolve the essential oil in 1 tsp. of grain alcohol before adding water to the spray bottle.).

Counter Cleaning: Add 1–2 drops of lemon, On Guard, or another disinfecting oil to a damp rag, and use to wipe down counters, tables, or stoves.

Trash Can Deodorizer: Add 3–5 drops of a deodorizing essential oil or blend to 1 Tbs. baking powder. Sprinkle into trash can.

Dishes: Add a few drops of lemon to dishwater for sparkling dishes and a great smelling kitchen. You can add the essential oil to a dishwasher as well.

Bathroom Cleaning Tips:

Mildew Spray: Mix 5 drops lemon and 5 drops white fir with 2 oz. water in a small spray bottle. Spray on areas with mildew.

Deodorizing Spray: Place 5–8 drops of a deodorizing essential oil (try 5 drops grapefruit and 1 drop peppermint) in a 1 oz. spray bottle, and fill the remainder of the bottle with water. Shake well, and spray into the air.

Mirror Cleaner: Place 1–2 drops of a disinfecting oil (try lemon) with 1 tsp. vinegar in a 1 oz. spray bottle. Fill the remainder of the bottle with water. Shake well, and spray on mirrors. Use a dry rag or newspapers to wipe off.

Mold: Diffuse On Guard into the air to help eliminate mold.

Other Daily Household Tips

Laundry Tips:

Gum/Grease: Use lemon or Citrus Bliss to help take gum or grease out of clothes (test in a small, inconspicuous area first to ensure that the oil won't affect delicate dyes or fabrics).

Washing: A few drops of Purify in the wash water will help kill bacteria and germs in clothes.

Drying: Put Purify, Elevation, lemongrass, or another favorite oil or blend on a wet rag, and then place rag in the dryer with clothing. Or mist oils from a spray bottle directly into the dryer to keep clothes smelling great—without artificial perfumes or fragrances.

Furniture Tips:

Polish: For a simple furniture polish, put a few drops of lemon, Purify, or white fir oil on a dust cloth and use to wipe down wood.

Clothes/Closets:

Clothing Deodorizer: Place a tissue or cotton ball with several drops of Purify, lavender, lemongrass, melaleuca, peppermint, Citrus Bliss, or another favorite oil in a perforated wood, glass, or stone container. Place container in a closet, shoe cupboard, or drawer to help naturally keep clothes smelling great.

Painting Tips:

Paint Fumes: To effectively remove paint fumes and after smell, add one 15 ml bottle of oil to any 5 gallon bucket of paint. The Purify blend and citrus single oils have been favorites, while Citrus Bliss and Elevation would work just as well. Either a paint sprayer or brush and roller may be used to apply the paint after mixing the oils into the paint by stirring vigorously. Oils may eventually rise to the top if using a water-based paint. Occasional stirring may be necessary to keep the oils mixed.

Carpet Care Tips:

Carpet Cleaner/Deodorizer: Mix 1 cup baking soda and 20–50 drops melaleuca, lemon, Purify, or another favorite oil in a glass jar. Close jar, shake together, and let stand overnight. Sprinkle lightly over carpets, let sit for 15 minutes, and then vacuum.

Grease/Gum Remover: Try lemon or lime oil on stubborn, greasy stains or to help dissolve gum stuck to carpet (be certain to test oil in a small, inconspicuous area of the carpet first to ensure it won't affect any delicate dyes in the carpet).

Bug/Pest Repellent Tips:

Bug Repelling Oils: TerraShield, lavender, lemongrass, patchouli, basil, Purify.

Mice Repelling Oil: Purify.

Personal Bug Repellent: Apply repelling oils directly on the skin (dilute with fractionated coconut oil if you are covering a large area).

Bug Spray: Add 10–15 drops of repelling oil to 1 oz. water in a small misting spray bottle. Shake well, and mist over exposed skin and clothing.

Diffusion: Diffuse repelling oils in a room.

Pest Repellent: Place repelling oils on a string, ribbon, or cotton ball, and hang near air vents or windows, or place in cracks and other areas where bugs or pests come through.

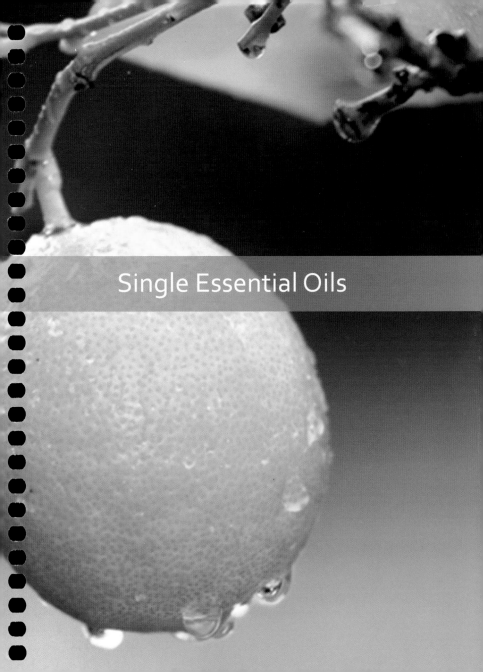

Single Essential Oils

Single Oils

This section is an abbreviated version of the full Single Oils section found in the book Modern Essentials. For much more detailed information on constituents, properties, additional uses, and safety information for each of these oils, please refer to that section.

Arborvitae *Thuja plicata*

Common Primary Uses: ᶜᵉAntibacterial, ᶜᵉAntifungal, ᵉCalming, ᶜᵉCancer, ᵉRepellent

Common Application Methods‡: 🝙: Dilute, and apply to reflex points or to area of concern. 🝙: Diffuse or inhale the aroma directly.

Basil *Ocimum basilicum*

Common Primary Uses: ᶜAmenorrhea, ᶜAutism, ᶜBee/Hornet Stings, ᶜBites/Stings, ᶜᵉBronchitis, ᶜBursitis, ᶜCarpal Tunnel Syndrome, ᶜᵉChronic Fatigue, ᴼᶜCramps (Abdominal), ᶜCuts, ᶜEarache, ᶜFrozen Shoulder, ᶜGreasy/Oily Hair, ᶜHealing, ᶜHiatal Hernia, ᶜIncisional Hernia, ᶜInduce Sweating, ᶜᵉInfertility, ᶜLactation (Increase Milk Production), ᵉᶜMental Fatigue, ᶜᵉMigraines, ᶜMouth Ulcers, ᶜMuscle Spasms, ᶜMuscular Dystrophy, ᵉᶜOlfactory Loss (Sense of Smell), ᶜᵉOvarian Cyst, ᶜSchmidt's Syndrome, ᶜSnake Bites, ᶜSpider Bites, ᶜTransition (Labor), ᶜᵉViral Hepatitis, ᶜWounds

Common Application Methods‡: 🝙: Can be applied neat (with no dilution) when used topically. Dilute with carrier oil for sensitive skin and for children over six. Apply to temples, tip of nose, reflex points, and/or directly on area of concern. 🝙: Diffuse or inhale the aroma directly. 🝙: Take in capsules, or use as a flavoring in cooking.

Bergamot *Citrus bergamia*

Common Primary Uses*: ᵉᶜAgitation (Calms), ᵉᶜBrain Injury, ᶜColic, ᵉᶜDepression, ᵉᶜEmotional Stress, ᵉᶜEnvironmental Stress, ᶜᵉInfection, ᵉᶜMental Stress, ᵉᶜPerformance Stress, ᵉPhysical Energy, ᵉᶜPhysical Stress, ᶜᵉPMS, ᶜRheumatoid Arthritis, ᵉᶜSedative, ᵉᶜStress

Common Application Methods‡: 🝙: Can be applied neat (with no dilution) when used topically. Apply to forehead, temples, reflex points, and/or directly on area of concern. May also be applied as a deodorant. Avoid direct sunlight or UV light for 72 hours after use. 🝙: Diffuse or inhale the aroma directly. 🝙: Use as a flavoring in food and beverages.

Black Pepper *Piper nigrum*

Common Primary Uses*: ᵉAddictions (Tobacco)

Common Application Methods‡: 🝙: Dilute with a carrier oil for children and for those with sensitive skin. Apply to reflex points and/or directly on area of concern. Mix very sparingly with juniper and lavender in a bath to help with chills or to warm one up in the winter. 🝙: Diffuse or inhale the aroma directly. 🝙: Use as a flavoring in cooking.

Cardamom *Elettaria cardamomum*

Common Primary Uses: ⊘Coughs, ⊘Headaches, ⊘⊘Inflammation, ⊘Muscle Aches, ⊘○Nausea, ⊘⊘Respiratory Ailments

Common Application Methods‡: ⊜: Apply to reflex points and/or directly on area of concern. Dilute with base oil, and massage over the stomach, solar plexus, and thighs. This oil is excellent as a bath oil. ⊘: Diffuse or inhale the aroma directly. ○: Place 1 drop under the tongue, or take oil in capsules. Use as a flavoring in cooking or in beverages.

Cassia *Cinnamomum cassia*

Common Primary Uses*: ⊘Antiseptic, ⊘Cooking

Common Application Methods‡: ⊜: Dilute heavily with a carrier oil or blend with milder essential oils before applying on the skin. Apply to forehead, muscles, reflex points, and/or directly on area of concern. ⊘: Diffuse with caution: it will irritate the nasal membranes if it is inhaled directly from the diffuser. ○: Use as a flavoring in cooking (similar to cinnamon but has a stronger, more intense flavor).

Cedarwood *Juniperus virginiana*

Common Primary Uses*: ⊘⊘Calming, ⊘⊘Tension, ⊘⊘Tuberculosis, ⊘Urinary Infection, ⊘Yoga

Common Application Methods‡: ⊜: Dilute with a carrier oil for children and for those with sensitive skin. Apply to reflex points and/or directly on area of concern. ⊘: Diffuse, or inhale the aroma directly.

Cilantro *Coriandrum sativum L.*

Common Primary Uses*: ⊘Anxiety, ○Cooking

Common Application Methods‡: ⊜: Can be applied neat (with no dilution) when used topically. Apply to reflex points and directly on area of concern. ⊘: Diffuse or inhale the aroma directly. ○: Use as a flavoring in cooking.

Cinnamon *Cinnamomum zeylanicum*

Common Primary Uses*: ⊘Airborne Bacteria, ⊘⊘Bacterial Infections, ⊘Bites/Stings, ⊘⊘Breathing, ○⊘Diabetes , ⊘Diverticulitis, ⊘⊘Fungal Infections, ⊘⊘General Tonic, ⊘Immune System (Stimulates), ⊘⊘Infection, ⊘⊘Libido (Low), ⊘⊘Mold, ⊘⊘Pancreas Support, ⊘Physical Fatigue, ⊘Pneumonia, ⊘⊘Typhoid, ⊘Vaginal Infection, ⊘Vaginitis, ⊘Viral Infections, ⊘Warming (Body)

Common Application Methods‡: ⊜: Dilute 1:3 (1 drop essential oil to at least 3 drops carrier oil) before using topically. Apply directly on area of concern or on reflex points. ⊘: Diffuse with caution; it may irritate the nasal membranes if it is inhaled directly from a diffuser. ○: Use as a flavoring in cooking.

Single Oils

Clary Sage *Salvia sclarea*

Common Primary Uses*: ⊘⊘Aneurysm, ⊘Breast Enlargement, ⊘Cholesterol, ⊘Convulsions, ⊘Cramps (Abdominal), ⊘Dysmenorrhea, ⊘⊘Emotional Stress, ⊘Endometriosis, ⊘Epilepsy, ⊘Estrogen Balance, ⊘⊘Frigidity, ⊘Hair (Fragile), ⊘⊘Hormonal Balance, ⊘Hot Flashes, ⊘⊘Impotence, ⊘⊘Infection, ⊘⊘Infertility, ⊘⊘Insomnia (Older Children), ⊘Lactation (Start Milk Production), ⊘Mood Swings, ⊘Muscle Fatigue, ⊘Parkinson's Disease, ⊘⊘PMS, ⊘⊘Postpartum Depression, ⊘Premenopause, ⊘Seizure

Common Application Methods‡: ⊘: Can be applied neat (with no dilution) when used topically. Apply to reflex points and/or directly on area of concern. ⊘: Diffuse, or inhale the aroma directly. ⊘: Take in capsules, or use as a flavoring in cooking.

Clove *Eugenia caryophyllata*

Common Primary Uses*: ⊘Addictions (Tobacco), OAntioxidant, O⊘Blood Clots, O⊘Candida, ⊘Cataracts, ⊘Corns, ⊘Disinfectant, OFever, ⊘⊘Fungal Infections, ⊘Herpes Simplex, ⊘Hodgkin's Disease, ⊘Hormonal Balance, ⊘⊘Hypothyroidism, ⊘⊘Liver Cleansing, ⊘Lupus, ⊘Macular Degeneration, ⊘⊘Memory, ⊘Metabolism Balance, ⊘⊘Mold, ⊘Muscle Aches, ⊘Muscle Pain, ⊘Osteoporosis, ⊘⊘Plague, ⊘Rheumatoid Arthritis, ⊘⊘Termites, ⊘⊘Thyroid Dysfunction, ⊘Toothache (Pain), ⊘⊘Tumor (Lipoma), ⊘⊘Viral Infections, ⊘Warts, ⊘Wounds

Common Application Methods‡: ⊘: Dilute 1:1 (1 drop essential oil to 1 drop carrier oil) before topical use. Apply to reflex points and/or directly on area of concern. Rub directly on the gums surrounding an infected tooth. Place on tongue with finger to remove desire to smoke, or place on back of tongue to fight against tickling cough. ⊘: Diffuse with caution; it may irritate the nasal membranes if it is inhaled directly from a diffuser. ⊘: Place 1 drop under the tongue, or take in capsules. Use as a flavoring in cooking.

Coriander *Coriandrum sativum L*

Common Primary Uses*: ⊘Cartilage Injury, ⊘Muscle Aches, ⊘Muscle Development, ⊘Muscle Tone, ⊘Whiplash

Common Application Methods‡: ⊘: Can be applied neat (with no dilution) when used topically. Apply directly on area of concern or to reflex points. ⊘: Diffuse or inhale the aroma directly. ⊘: Use as a flavoring in cooking.

Cypress *Cupressus sempervirens*

Common Primary Uses*: ⊘⊘Aneurysm, ⊘Bone Spurs, ⊘Bunions, ⊘Bursitis, ⊘Carpal Tunnel Syndrome, ⊘⊘Catarrh, ⊘⊘Circulation, ⊘Concussion, ⊘Dysmenorrhea, ⊘Edema, ⊘Endometriosis, ⊘⊘Environmental Stress, ⊘⊘Flu (Influenza), ⊘Greasy/Oily Hair, ⊘Hemorrhoids, ⊘Hernia (Hiatal), ⊘Incontinence, ⊘Lou Gehrig's Disease, ⊘⊘Lympha tic Decongestant, ⊘Menopause, ⊘Menorrhagia, ⊘Muscle Fatigue, ◐Muscle Tone, ◐Pain (Chronic), ◐◗Pleurisy, ◐◗Preeclampsia, ◐Prostatitis, ◐◗Raynaud's Disease, ◐Retina (Strengthen), ◐Rheumatoid Arthritis, ◐Skin (Revitalizing), ◐◗Stroke, ◐Swollen Eyes, ◐◗Toxemia, ◐◗Tuberculosis, ◐Varicose Veins

Common Application Methods‡: 🝙: Can be applied neat (with no dilution) when used topically. Apply to reflex points and directly on area of concern. 🝚: Diffuse or inhale the aroma directly.

Eucalyptus *Eucalyptus radiata*

Common Primary Uses*: ◐Arterial Vasodilator, ◐◗Asthma, ◗Brain Blood Flow, ◐◗Bronchitis , ◐◗Congestion, ◐◗Cooling (Body), ◐◗Coughs, ◐◗Diabetes, ◗Disinfectant, ◐Dysentery, ◐Ear Inflammation, ◐◗Emphysema, ◐◗Expectorant, ◐Fever, ◐◗Flu (Influenza), ◐Hypoglycemia, ◐Inflammation, ◐Iris Inflammation, ◐Jet Lag, ◐Kidney Stones, ◐Lice, ◐◗Measles, ◐Neuralgia, ◐Neuritis, ◐Overexercised Muscles, ◐Pain, ◐◗Pneumonia, ◗Respiratory Viruses, ◐◗Rhinitis, ◐Shingles, ◐◗Sinusitis, ◐Tennis Elbow, ◐◗Tuberculosis

Common Application Methods‡: 🝙: Can be applied neat (with no dilution), or dilute 1:1 (1 drop essential oil to at least 1 drop carrier oil) for children and for those with sensitive skin when using topically. Apply to reflex points and/or directly on area of concern. 🝚: Diffuse, or inhale the aroma directly.

Fennel (Sweet) *Foeniculum vulgare*

Common Primary Uses*: ◐Benign Prostatic Hyperplasia, ◐◐◗Blood Clots, ◐Bruises, ◐◐◗Digestive System Support, ◐◗Gastritis, ◐Kidney Stones, ◐Lactation (Increase Milk Production), ◐◗Pancreas Support, ◐◗Parasites, ◐Skin (Revitalizing), ◐Tissue (Toxin Cleansing), ◐Wrinkles

Common Application Methods‡: 🝙: Can be applied neat (with no dilution), or dilute 1:1 (1 drop essential oil to at least 1 drop carrier oil) for children and for those with sensitive skin when using topically. Apply directly on area of concern or to reflex points. 🝚: Diffuse, or inhale the aroma directly. 🝗: Place 1–2 drops under the tongue, or take in a capsule. Use as a flavoring in cooking.

Frankincense *Boswellia frereana*

Common Primary Uses*: ◐◗Alzheimer's Disease, ◐◗Aneurysm, ◐◗Arthritis, ◐◗Asthma, ◐◗Balance, ◐◗Brain (Aging), ◐◗Brain Injury, ◐◗Breathing, ◗◐◗Cancer, ◐Coma, ◐◗Concussion, ◗Confusion, ◐◗Coughs, ◐◗Depression, ◐Fibroids, ◐Genital Warts, ◐◗Hepatitis, ◐◗Immune System Support, ◐Improve Vision, ◐◗Infected Wounds, ◐◗Inflammation, ◐◗Liver Cirrhosis, ◐◗Lou Gehrig's Disease, ◐◗Memory, ◐◗Mental Fatigue, ◐Miscarriage (After), ◐Moles, ◐MRSA, ◐◗Multiple Sclerosis, ◐◗Nasal Polyp, ◐◗Parkinson's Disease, ◐◗Plague, ◐◗Postpartum Depression, ◐Scarring (Prevention), ◐◗Tumor (Lipoma), ◐◗Ulcers, ◐Uterus Tissue Regeneration, ◐Virus of Nerves, ◐Warts, ◐Wrinkles

Common Application Methods‡: 🌢: Can be applied neat (with no dilution) when used topically. Apply directly on area of concern or to reflex points. 🗗: Diffuse, or inhale the aroma directly. 🌢: Place 1–2 drops under the tongue, or take in a capsule.

Geranium *Pelargonium graveolens*

Common Primary Uses*: 🗗🌢Agitation (Calms), 🗗Airborne Bacteria, 🌢Autism, 🌢Bleeding, 🌢Breasts (Soothes), 🌢Bruises, 🌢Calcified Spine, 🗗🌢Cancer, 🌢Capillaries (Broken), 🗗🌢Diabetes, 🌢Diarrhea, 🌢Dysmenorrhea, 🌢Endometriosis, 🗗🌢Environmental Stress, 🌢Gallbladder Stones, 🌢Hair (Dry), 🌢Hernia (Incisional), 🌢Impetigo, 🗗🌢Insomnia (Older Children), 🗗🌢Jaundice, 🌢Jet Lag, 🌢Libido (Low), 🌢Menorrhagia, 🌢Miscarriage (After), 🌢MRSA, 🌢Osteoarthritis, 🌢Osteoporosis, 🗗🌢Pancreas Support, 🗗🌢Paralysis, 🌢Pelvic Pain Syndrome, 🗗🌢Physical Stress, 🗗🌢PMS, 🌢Post Labor, 🌢Rheumatoid Arthritis, 🌢Skin (Dry), 🌢Skin (Sensitive), 🌢🗢Ulcer (Gastric), 🌢Varicose Ulcer, 🌢Vertigo, 🌢Wrinkles

Common Application Methods‡: 🌢: Can be applied neat (with no dilution) when used topically. Apply directly on area of concern or to reflex points. 🗗: Diffuse, or inhale the aroma directly. 🌢: Take in capsules.

Ginger *Zingiber officinale*

Common Primary Uses*: 🗗🌢Angina, 🌢Club Foot, 🌢🗢Diarrhea, 🌢🗢Gas/Flatulence, 🌢🗢Indigestion, 🗗🌢Libido (Low), 🌢🗢🗗Morning Sickness, 🌢🗢Nausea , 🌢Pelvic Pain Syndrome, 🌢Rheumatic Fever (Pain), 🌢Rheumatoid Arthritis, 🌢🗢Scurvy, 🗗🌢Vertigo, 🌢🗢Vomiting

Common Application Methods‡: 🌢: Can be applied neat (with no dilution), or dilute 1:1 (1 drop essential oil to 1 drop carrier oil) for children and for those with sensitive skin when using topically. Apply directly on area of concern or to reflex points. 🗗: Diffuse, or inhale the aroma directly. 🌢: Take in capsules. Use as a flavoring in cooking.

Grapefruit *Citrus x paradisi*

Common Primary Uses*: 🗗🌢Addictions (Drugs), 🗗Anorexia, 🗗Appetite Suppressant, 🗗Bulimia, 🌢Cellulite, 🌢🗢Dry Throat, 🌢🗢Edema, 🌢Gallbladder Stones, 🗗🌢Hangovers, 🗗🌢Lymphatic Decongestant, 🗗🌢Mental Stress, 🌢Miscarriage (After), 🗗🌢Obesity, 🗗Overeating, 🗗🌢Performance Stress, 🗗🌢PMS, 🗗🌢Slimming/Toning, 🗗🌢Stress, 🗗🌢Withdrawal

Common Application Methods‡: 🌢: Can be applied neat (with no dilution) when used topically. Apply directly on area of concern or to reflex points. Because grapefruit oil has many of the same uses as other citrus oils, it can be used in their place when immediate exposure to the sun is unavoidable. This is because grapefruit oil does not cause as much photosensitivity as the other citrus oils.
🗗: Diffuse, or inhale the aroma directly. 🌢: Take 1–2 drops in a beverage or in capsules. Use as a flavoring in cooking.

Hawaiian Sandalwood *Santalum paniculatum*

Common Primary Uses*: ⚭Alzheimer's Disease, ⚭Aphrodisiac, ☁Back Pain, ☁Cancer, ☁Cartilage Repair, ⊘Confusion, ☁Exhaustion, ⚭Fear, ☁Hair (Dry), ⚭Hiccups, ⚭Laryngitis, ⚭Lou Gehrig's Disease, ⊘Meditation, ☁Moles, ⚭Multiple Sclerosis, ☁Rashes, ☁Skin (Dry), ☁Ultraviolet Radiation, ☁Vitiligo, ⊘Yoga

Common Application Methods‡: ☁: Can be applied neat (with no dilution) when used topically. Apply directly on area of concern or to reflex points. ⊘: Diffuse, or inhale the aroma directly. ◯: Take in capsules.

Helichrysum *Helichrysum italicum*

Common Primary Uses*: ☁Abscess (Tooth), ⚭AIDS/HIV, ⚭Aneurysm, ⚭Bleeding, ☁Bone Bruise, ☁Broken Blood Vessels, ☁Bruises, ⚭Catarrh, ☁Cholesterol, ☁Cleansing, ⚭Colitis, ☁Cuts, ☁Dermatitis/Eczema, ☁Detoxification, ⚭Earache, ☁Fibroids, ☁Gallbladder Infection, ☁Hematoma, ☁Hemorrhaging, ☁Herpes Simplex, ☁Incisional Hernia, ⚭Liver Stimulant, ☁Lymphatic Drainage, ☁Nose Bleed, ☁Pancreas Stimulant, ⚭Phlebitis, ☁Psoriasis, ☁Sciatica, ☁Shock, ☁Staph Infection, ⚭Stroke, ☁Sunscreen, ☁Swollen Eyes, ☁Taste (Impaired), ☁Tennis Elbow, ☁Tinnitus, ☁Tissue Pain, ☁Tissue Repair, ☁Vertigo, ⚭Viral Infections, ☁Wounds

Common Application Methods‡: ☁: Can be applied neat (with no dilution) when used topically. Apply directly on area of concern or to reflex points. ⊘: Diffuse, or inhale the aroma directly. ◯: Take in capsules.

Juniper Berry *Juniperus communis*

Common Primary Uses*: ☁Acne, ⊘Alcoholism, ☁Dermatitis/Eczema, ☁Kidney Stones, ☁Tinnitus

Common Application Methods‡: ☁: Can be applied neat (with no dilution) when used topically. Apply directly on area of concern or to reflex points. ⊘: Diffuse, or inhale the aroma directly. ◯: Place 1 drop under the tongue, or take in capsules. Use with caution if pregnant or nursing.

Lavender *Lavandula angustifolia*

Common Primary Uses*: ☁Abuse (Healing From), ⚭Agitation (Calms), ☁Allergies, ⚭Anxiety, ⊘Appetite Loss, ⚭Arrhythmia, ⊘Atherosclerosis, ☁Bites/Stings, ☁Blisters, ☁Boils, ☁Breasts (Soothes), ☁Burns, ⚭Calming, ⚭Cancer, ☁Chicken Pox, ☁Club Foot, ⊘Concentration, ☁Convulsions, ⚭Crying, ☁Cuts, ☁Dandruff, ⚭◯Depression, ☁Diabetic Sores, ☁Diaper Rash, ☁Diuretic, ☁Dysmenorrhea, ☁Exhaustion, ☁Fever, ☁Gangrene, ◯☁Gas/Flatulence, ◯☁Giardia, ☁Gnats and Midges (Repellent), ⚭Grief/Sorrow, ☁Hair (Dry), ☁Hair (Fragile), ☁Hair (Loss), ☁Hay Fever, ☁Hernia (Inguinal), ☁Herpes Simplex, ⚭Hyperactivity, ☁Impetigo, ☁Inflammation, ⚭Insomnia, ☁Itching, ☁Jet Lag, ☁Lips (Dry), ☁Mastitis, ☁Menopause, ⚭Mental Stress, ⊘Mood Swings, ☁Mosquito Repellent, ☁Muscular Paralysis, ⚭Pain, ⚭Parasympathetic Nervous System Stimulation, ᴄParkinson's Disease, ᴄᴄPhlebitis, ᴄᴄPhysical Stress, ᴄPoison Ivy/Oak, ᴄPost Labor, ᴄᴄPostpartum Depression, ᴄRashes, ᴄᴄRelaxation, ᴄᴄRheumatoid Arthritis, ᴄᴄSedative, ᴄSeizure, ᴄSkin (Dry), ᴄSkin (Sensitive), ᴄSkin Ulcers, ᴄᴄSleep, ᴄᴄStress, ᴄStretch Marks, ᴄSunburn, ᴄᴄTachycardia, ᴄTeeth Grinding, ᴄTeething Pain, ᴄᴄTension, ᴄThrush, ᴄTicks, ᴄUlcers (Leg), ᴄVaricose Ulcer, ᴄVertigo, ᴄᴄWithdrawal, ᴼᴄWorms, ᴄWounds, ᴄWrinkles

Common Application Methods‡: 🖐: Can be applied neat (with no dilution) when used topically. Apply directly on area of concern or to reflex points. 👃: Diffuse, or inhale the aroma directly. 💧: Place 1–2 drops under the tongue, or take in capsules. Can also be used in beverages or as a flavoring in cooking.

Lemon *Citrus limon*

Common Primary Uses*: ᴬAir Pollution, ᴬAnxiety, ᴄᴄAtherosclerosis, ᴄBites/Stings, ᴼBlood Pressure (Regulation), ᴄᴄBrain Injury, ᴄCold Sores, ᴬᴄColds (Common), ᴬConcentration, ᴄConstipation, ᴬᴄᴼDepression, ᴄDigestion (Sluggish), ᴄᴬDisinfectant, ᴼᴄDry Throat, ᴄDysentery, ᴄEnergizing, ᴄExhaustion, ᴼᴄFever, ᴄᴬFlu (Influenza), ᴄFurniture Polish, ᴼᴄGout, ᴄGreasy/Oily Hair, ᴬᴄGrief/Sorrow, ᴄGum/Grease Removal, ᴄᴬHangovers, ᴄHeartburn, ᴼᴄIntestinal Parasites, ᴼKidney Stones, ᴬᴄLymphatic Cleansing, ᴄMRSA, ᴬOvereating, ᴄᴬPancreatitis, ᴬPhysical Energy, ᴬᴄPostpartum Depression, ᴬPurification, ᴬRelaxation, ᴄSkin (Tones), ᴬᴄStress, ᴄᴬᴼThroat Infection, ᴄTonsillitis, ᴬUplifting, ᴄVaricose Veins, ᴼᴄWater Purification

Common Application Methods‡: 🖐: Can be applied neat (with no dilution) when used topically. Apply directly on area of concern or to reflex points. Avoid direct sunlight or UV light for up to 12 hours after using on the skin. 👃: Diffuse, or inhale the aroma directly. 💧: Place 1–2 drops under the tongue, or drink with a beverage. Take in capsules. Use as a flavoring in cooking.

Lemongrass *Cymbopogon flexuosis*

Common Primary Uses*: ᴬAir Pollution, ᴬAirborne Bacteria, ᴄCarpal Tunnel Syndrome, ᴼCholesterol, ᴄCramps/Charley Horses, ᴄCystitis/Bladder Infection, ᴄDiuretic, ᴄEdema, ᴄFleas, ᴄFrozen Shoulder, ᴼGastritis, ᴄᴄGrave's Disease, ᴄᴄHashimoto's Disease, ᴄHernia (Incisional), ᴄHernia (Inguinal), ᴄImprove Vision, ᴼᴄLactose Intolerance, ᴄᴄLymphatic Drainage, ᴬᴄMental Fatigue, ᴄMuscular Dystrophy, ᴄᴄParalysis, ᴬPurification, ᴄRetina (Strengthen), ᴄSprains, ᴄStrain (Muscle), ᴄTissue Repair, ᴄᴬUrinary Tract Infection, ᴄVaricose Veins, ᴄWhiplash (Ligaments), ᴄWounds

Common Application Methods‡: 🖐: Can be applied neat (with no dilution), or dilute 1:1 (1 drop essential oil to 1 drop carrier oil) for children and for those with sensitive skin when using topically. Apply directly on area of concern or to reflex points. 👃: Diffuse, or inhale the aroma directly. 💧: Take in capsules. Use as a flavoring in cooking.

Lime *Citrus aurantifolia*

Common Primary Uses*: ⊘⊘Bacterial Infections, O⊘⊘Fever, ⊘Gum/Grease Removal, ⊘Skin

Common Application Methods‡: ⊘: Can be applied neat (with no dilution) when used topically. Apply directly on area of concern or to reflex points. It makes an excellent addition to bath and shower gels, body lotions, and deodorants. ⊘: Diffuse, or inhale the aroma directly. O: Place 1–2 drops under the tongue, or drink with a beverage. Take in capsules. Use as a flavoring in cooking.

Marjoram *Origanum majorana*

Common Primary Uses*: ⊘Arterial Vasodilator, ⊘⊘Arthritis, ⊘Bone Spurs, ⊘Carpal Tunnel Syndrome, ⊘Cartilage Injury, ⊘Colic, ⊘Constipation, ⊘Cramps/Charley Horses, ⊘⊘Croup, ⊘⊘Expectorant, ⊘⊘High Blood Pressure, ⊘Muscle Aches, ⊘Muscle Fatigue, ⊘Muscle Spasms, ⊘Muscle Tone, ⊘Muscular Dystrophy, ⊘Neuralgia, ⊘Osteoarthritis, ⊘⊘Pancreatitis, ⊘Parkinson's Disease, ⊘⊘Physical Stress, ⊘⊘Prolapsed Mitral Valve, ⊘Rheumatoid Arthritis, ⊘Sprains, ⊘Stiffness, ⊘Tendinitis, ⊘Tension (Muscle), ⊘Whiplash (Muscles)

Common Application Methods‡: ⊘: Can be applied neat (with no dilution) when used topically. Apply directly on area of concern or to reflex points. Use with caution during pregnancy. ⊘: Diffuse, or inhale the aroma directly. O: Place 1–2 drops under the tongue, or take in a capsule. Use as a flavoring in cooking.

Melaleuca *Melaleuca alternifolia*

Common Primary Uses*: ⊘Acne , ⊘Allergies, ⊘⊘Aneurysm, ⊘Athlete's Foot, ⊘Bacterial Infections, ⊘Boils, ⊘⊘Bronchitis, ⊘Candida, ⊘Canker Sores, ⊘Cavities, ⊘⊘Chicken Pox, ⊘Cleansing, ⊘Cold Sores, ⊘⊘Colds (Common), ⊘⊘Coughs, ⊘Cuts, ⊘Dermatitis/Eczema, ⊘Dry/Itchy Eyes, ⊘Ear Infection, ⊘Earache, ⊘⊘Flu (Influenza), ⊘Fungal Infections, ⊘Gum Disease, ⊘⊘Hepatitis, ⊘Herpes Simplex, ⊘Hives, ⊘⊘Immune System (Stimulates), ⊘⊘Infected Wounds, ⊘Infection, ⊘⊘Inflammation, ⊘Jock Itch, ⊘Lice, ⊘MRSA, ⊘⊘Mumps, ⊘Nail Infection, ⊘⊘Pink Eye, ⊘Rashes, ⊘Ringworm, ⊘Rubella, ⊘Scabies, ⊘Shingles, ⊘Shock, ⊘⊘Sore Throat, ⊘Staph Infection, ⊘Sunburn, ⊘Thrush, ⊘⊘Tonsillitis, ⊘Vaginal Infection, ⊘Varicose Ulcer, ⊘⊘Viral Infections, ⊘Warts, ⊘Wounds

Common Application Methods‡: ⊘: Can be applied neat (with no dilution) when used topically. Apply directly on area of concern or to reflex points. ⊘: Diffuse, or inhale the aroma directly. O: Take in capsules.

Melissa (Lemon Balm) *Melissa officinalis*

Common Primary Uses*: ⊘⊘Calming, ⊘Cold Sores, ⊘⊘Viral Infections

Common Application Methods‡: ⊘: Can be applied neat (with no dilution) when used topically. Apply directly on area of concern or to reflex points. ⊘: Diffuse, or inhale the aroma directly. O: Take in capsules. Use as a flavoring in cooking.

Myrrh *Commiphora myrrha*

Common Primary Uses*: ⊘⊘Cancer, ⊘Chapped/Cracked Skin, ⊘⊘Congestion, ⊘Dysentery, ⊘Gum Disease, ⊘⊘Hashimoto's Disease, ⊘⊘Hepatitis, ⊘⊘Hyperthyroidism, ⊘⊘Infection, ⊘⊘Liver Cirrhosis, ⊘Skin Ulcers, ⊘Stretch Marks, O⊘Ulcers (Duodenal), ⊘Weeping Wounds

Common Application Methods‡: ◐: Can be applied neat (with no dilution) when used topically. Apply directly on area of concern or to reflex points. ◐: Diffuse, or inhale the aroma directly. ◯: Place 1–2 drops under the tongue, or take in capsules.

Orange *Citrus sinensis*

Common Primary Uses*: ⊘Anxiety, ⊘Digestion (Sluggish), ⊘Fear, ⊘⊘Heart Palpitations, ⊘⊘Insomnia, ⊘Menopause, ⊘Nervousness, ⊘Uplifting, ⊘⊘Withdrawal

Common Application Methods‡: ◐: Can be applied neat (with no dilution) when used topically. Apply directly on area of concern or to reflex points. Avoid direct sunlight for up to 12 hours after using on skin. ◐: Diffuse, or inhale the aroma directly. ◯: Place 1–2 drops under the tongue, or take in a beverage. Take in capsules. Use as a flavoring in cooking.

Oregano *Origanum vulgare*

Common Primary Uses*: ⊘⊘Athlete's Foot, ⊘Calluses, ⊘OCandida, ⊘Canker Sores, ⊘Carpal Tunnel Syndrome, ⊘Ebola Virus, ⊘⊘OFungal Infections, ⊘⊘OImmune System (Stimulates), ⊘Inflammation, O⊘Intestinal Parasites, ⊘MRSA, ⊘Muscle Aches, ⊘⊘Nasal Polyp, O⊘Parasites, ⊘⊘Plague, ⊘⊘Pneumonia, ⊘⊘Ringworm, ⊘OStaph Infection, ⊘OVaginal Candida, ⊘Viral Infections, ⊘Warming (Body), ⊘Warts, ⊘Whooping Cough

Common Application Methods‡: ◐: Dilute 1:3 (1 drop essential oil to at least 3 drops carrier oil) when used topically. Dilute more heavily for children over 6 or for those with sensitive skin. Apply directly on area of concern or to reflex points. ◐: Diffuse, or inhale the aroma directly. ◯: Place 1–2 drops under the tongue, or take in capsules. Use as a flavoring in cooking.

Patchouli (or Patchouly) *Pogostemon cablin*

Common Primary Uses*: ⊘Diuretic, O⊘⊘Fever, ⊘⊘Mosquito Repellent, ⊘⊘Termite Repellent

Common Application Methods‡: ◐: Can be applied neat (with no dilution) when used topically. Apply directly on area of concern or to reflex points. ◐: Diffuse, or inhale the aroma directly. ◯: Take in capsules.

Peppermint *Mentha piperita*

Common Primary Uses*: ⊘⊘Alertness, O⊘⊘Antioxidant, ⊘⊘Asthma, ⊘Autism, ⊘Bacterial Infections, ⊘⊘Bell's Palsy, ⊘⊘Brain Injury, ⊘⊘Chronic Fatigue, ⊘Cold Sores, O⊘Colon Polyps, ᶜᵉCongestion, ᶜConstipation, ᶜᵉCooling (Body), ᶜCramps/Charley Horses, ᶜᴼCrohn's Disease, ᴼᶜDiarrhea, ᶜDysmenorrhea, ᵉEndurance, ᵉFainting, ᴼᶜᵉFever, ᶜᵉᴼFlu (Influenza), ᴼᶜGamma Radiation Exposure , ᶜᴼGastritis, ᶜHalitosis, ᶜᵉHeadaches , ᶜHeartburn, ᶜHeatstroke, ᶜHernia (Hiatal), ᶜHerpes Simplex, ᶜHives, ᶜHot Flashes, ᶜᵉHuntington's Disease, ᶜᵉHypothyroidism, ᴼᶜᵉIndigestion, ᴼᶜIrritable Bowel Syndrome , ᶜItching, ᶜJet Lag, ᶜLactation (Decrease Milk Production), ᵉᶜMemory , ᶜᵉMigraines, ᵉMotion Sickness, ᶜMRSA, ᶜᵉMultiple Sclerosis, ᶜMuscle Aches, ᶜMuscle Fatigue, ᵉᶜMyelin Sheath, ᵉNausea, ᵉᶜOlfactory Loss (Sense of Smell), ᶜOsteoporosis, ᶜᵉParalysis, ᵉᶜRhinitis, ᶜScabies, ᶜSciatica, ᶜᵉShock, ᵉᶜSinusitis, ᶜSurgical Wounds, ᶜSwollen Eyes, ᶜTennis Elbow, ᶜᵉᴼThroat Infection, ᶜᵉTyphoid, ᴼᶜUlcer (Gastric), ᶜVaricose Veins, ᴼᵉVomiting

Common Application Methods‡: 🖐: Can be applied neat (with no dilution), or dilute 1:1 (1 drop essential oil to 1 drop carrier oil) for children and for those with sensitive skin when using topically. Apply directly on area of concern or to reflex points. 💧: Diffuse, or inhale the aroma directly. ⬤: Place 1–2 drops under the tongue or in a beverage. Take in capsules. Use as a flavoring in cooking.

Roman Chamomile *Chamaemelum nobile*

Common Primary Uses*: ᶜBee/Hornet Stings, ᵉᶜCalming, ᶜClub Foot, ᶜDysentery, ᵉᶜHyperactivity, ᵉᶜInsomnia, ᶜMenopause, ᶜMuscle Spasms, ᶜNeuralgia, ᶜNeuritis, ᴼᶜParasites, ᶜRashes, ᶜSciatica, ᶜShock, ᶜSkin (Dry), ᶜSore Nipples

Common Application Methods‡: 🖐: Can be applied neat (with no dilution), or dilute 1:1 (1 drop essential oil to 1 drop carrier oil) for children and for those with sensitive skin when using topically. 💧: Diffuse, or inhale the aroma directly. ⬤: Take in capsules.

Rose *Rosa damascena*

Common Primary Uses*: ᵉᶜAphrodisiac, ᶜPoison Ivy/Oak, ᶜScarring (Prevention)

Common Application Methods‡: 🖐: Can be applied neat (with no dilution) when used topically. Apply directly on area of concern or to reflex points. 💧: Diffuse, or inhale the aroma directly. ⬤: Take in capsules. Use as a flavoring in cooking.

Rosemary *Rosmarinus officinalis CT 1,8 Cineol*

Common Primary Uses*: ᶜᵉAddictions (Alcohol), ᶜAdenitis, ᴼᶜᵉAntioxidant, ᶜArterial Vasodilator, ᶜᵉArthritis, ᶜᵉBell's Palsy, ᶜᵉCancer, ᶜCellulite, ᵉᶜChemical Stress, ᶜCholera, ᶜClub Foot, ᶜConstipation, ᶜDetoxification, ᶜᵉDiabetes, ᶜDiuretic, ᵉFainting, ᶜᵉFatigue, ᵉᶜFlu (Influenza), ᶜGreasy/Oily Hair, ᶜHair (Loss), ᶜᵉHeadaches, ᶜInflammation, ᶜKidney Infection, ᶜLice, ᵉᶜLow Blood Pressure, ᵉᶜMemory, ᶜMuscular Dystrophy, ᶜOsteoarthritis, ᶜSchmidt's Syndrome, ᵉᶜSinusitis, ᶜVaginal Infection, ᶜVaginitis, ᶜᵉViral Hepatitis, ᶜᴼWorms

---

🖐=Topical, 💧=Aromatic, ⬤=Internal *(See page 33 for further details.)*

Common Application Methods‡: ◐: Can be applied neat (with no dilution), or dilute 1:1 (1 drop essential oil to 1 drop carrier oil) for children and for those with sensitive skin when used topically. Apply directly on area of concern or to reflex points. Avoid use during pregnancy. ◐: Diffuse, or inhale the aroma directly. ◐: Take in capsules, or place 1–2 drops under the tongue. Use as a flavoring in cooking.

Sandalwood *Santalum album*

Common Primary Uses*: ◑◐Alzheimer's Disease, ◑◐Aphrodisiac, ◐Back Pain, ◐Cancer, ◐Cartilage Repair, ◐Coma, ◐Confusion, ◐Exhaustion, ◑◐Fear, ◐Hair (Dry), ◑◐Hiccups, ◑◐Laryngitis, ◑◐Lou Gehrig's Disease, ◐Meditation, ◐Moles, ◑◐Multiple Sclerosis, ◐Rashes, ◐Skin (Dry), ◐Ultraviolet Radiation, ◐Vitiligo, ◐Yoga

Common Application Methods‡: ◐: Can be applied neat (with no dilution) when used topically. Apply directly on area of concern or to reflex points. ◐: Diffuse, or inhale the aroma directly. ◐: Take in capsules.

Thyme *Thymus vulgaris CT Thymol*

Common Primary Uses*: ○◑◐Antioxidant, ◑◐Asthma, ◑◐Bacterial Infections, ◐Bites/Stings, ○◑◐Blood Clots, ○◐Brain (Aging), ◑◐Bronchitis, ◑◐Colds (Common), ◑◐Croup, ◐Dermatitis/Eczema, ◑◐Fatigue, ◐Fungal Infections, ◐Greasy/Oily Hair, ◐Hair (Fragile), ◐Hair (Loss), ◑◐Mold, ◐MRSA, ○◐Parasites, ◑◐Pleurisy, ◑◐Pneumonia, ◐Prostatitis, ◐Psoriasis, ◐Radiation Wounds, ◐Sciatica, ◑◐Tuberculosis

Common Application Methods‡: ◐: Dilute 1:4 (1 drop essential oil to at least 4 drops carrier oil) when used topically. Dilute heavily for children and for those with sensitive skin. Apply directly on area of concern or to reflex points. ◐: Diffuse, or inhale the aroma directly. ◐: Place 1–2 drops under the tongue, or take in capsules. Use as a flavoring in cooking.

Vetiver *Vetiveria zizanioides*

Common Primary Uses*: ◑◐ADD/ADHD, ◑◐Balance, ◑◐Termite Repellent, ◐Vitiligo

Common Application Methods‡: ◐: Can be applied neat (with no dilution) when used topically. Apply directly on area of concern or to reflex points. Also excellent in baths or in massage blends. A very small amount of vetiver oil is all that is needed in most applications. ◐: Diffuse, or inhale the aroma directly. ◐: Take in capsules.

White Fir *Abies alba*

Common Primary Uses*: ◑◐Bronchitis, ◐Bursitis, ◐Cartilage Inflammation, ◑◐Energizing, ◐Frozen Shoulder, ◐Furniture Polish, ◐Muscle Fatigue, ◐Muscle Pain, ◐Overexercised Muscles, ◐Sprains

Common Application Methods‡: ◐: Can be applied neat (with no dilution) when used topically. Dilute 1:1 (1 drop essential oil to at least 1 drop carrier oil) for children and for those with sensitive skin. Apply directly on area of concern or to reflex points. **📀**: Diffuse, or inhale the aroma directly. **⭘**: Take in capsules.

Wintergreen *Gaultheria procumbens*

Common Primary Uses*: ⚬Arthritic Pain, ⚬Bone Pain, ⚬Bone Spurs, ⚬Cartilage Injury, ⚬Dandruff, ⚬Frozen Shoulder, ⚬Joint Pain, ⚬Muscle Development, ⚬Muscle Tone, ⚬Pain, ⚬Rotator Cuff (Sore)

Common Application Methods‡: **📀**: Can be applied neat (with no dilution), or dilute 1:1 (1 drop essential oil to 1 drop carrier oil) for children and for those with sensitive skin when using topically. Apply directly on area of concern or to reflex points. Apply topically on location, and use only small amounts (dilute with fractionated coconut oil for application on larger areas).**📀**: Diffuse, or inhale the aroma directly.

Ylang Ylang *Cananga odorata*

Common Primary Uses*: ⚬⚬Aphrodisiac, ⚬⚬Arrhythmia, ⚬⚬Calming, ⚬Colic, ⚬⚬Crying, ⚬⚬Diabetes, ⚬Exhaustion, ⚬⚬Fear, ⚬Hair (Loss), ⚬⚬High Blood Pressure , ⚬⚬Hormonal Balance, ⚬⚬Hyperpnea, ⚬⚬Libido (Low), ⚬⚬Palpitations, ⚬⚬Relaxation, ⚬⚬Sedative, ⚬⚬Stress, ⚬⚬Tachycardia, ⚬⚬Tension

Common Application Methods‡: **📀**: Can be applied neat (with no dilution) when used topically. Apply directly on area of concern or to reflex points. It may be beneficial when applied over the thymus (to help stimulate the immune system). **📀**: Diffuse, or inhale the aroma directly. **⭘**: Take in capsules.

●=Neat, ●=Dilute for Children/Sensitive Skin, ●=Dilute

Personal Usage Guide

How to Use This Section

This section is a compilation of many different
health conditions and the various essential oils,
blends, and supplements that are commonly used
and recommended for each condition.

Example Entry:

Fear

see also **Anxiety, Calming**

Fear causes the blood vessels to tighten, restricting the amount of
oxygen and nutrients that can reach the cells.

Oils: Grounding Blend, ylang ylang, orange,
sandalwood, clary sage, geranium, juniper
berry, myrrh, bergamot, white fir, cypress,
marjoram

- Diffuse into the air. Inhale directly from bottle. Apply oil to
  hands, tissue, or cotton wick, and inhale.

- Dilute as recommended, and apply 1–2 drops to temples,
  back of neck, or bottoms of feet.

- **Additional Research:**

  Ylang ylang: Subjects who had ylang ylang oil applied to their skin had decreased
  blood pressure, increased skin temperature, and reported feeling more calm and
  relaxed compared to subjects in a control group (Hongratanaworakit et al., 2006).

  Orange: Female patients waiting for dental treatment were found to be less
  anxious, more positive, and more calm when exposed to orange oil odor than were
  patients who were not exposed to the orange oil odor (Lehrner et al., 2000).

Under each **condition**, the oils, blends, and
supplements have been grouped as:

- Primary Recommendations: Try these oils,
blends, or supplements first.

- Secondary Recommendations: Try these oils or
blends second. Supplements listed as secondary
recommendations may be useful for general nutritional support of the body systems involved in
prevention or healing from a specific condition.

- Other Recommendations : Oils, blends, and
supplements that may also help, depending on
the underlying cause.

The criteria for grouping within these categories
include the recommendations of experts within
the field of essential oils, supporting scientific
research studies, historical uses of the oils and
the herbs and plants they are derived from, and
more recent French medicinal uses for the oils.
However, since each individual may have different underlying causes for his or her specific condition, what may work for one individual may be
different than what works for another.

Also listed under each condition are recommendations for how to use or apply these oils or supplements for that particular condition. The three main application and usage methods are aromatic, topical, and internal. The recommended methods are indicated next to each oil as a small 𝒪 for Aromatic, ⬤ for Topical, and 𝐎 for Internal.

𝒪: Aromatic means that the oils are breathed or inhaled through the mouth and nose. This could include breathing the aroma of the oil directly from the bottle or breathing in oil that has been applied to the hands or to another material such as a tissue or cotton wick. It could also mean breathing the vapor or mist of an oil that has been diffused or sprayed into the surrounding air.

⬤: Topical means that the oils are applied directly onto the skin, hair, or other surface of the body. This can be through direct application of the oils to the skin or by using the oils in massages, baths, or within a cream, lotion, or soap. While some oils can be applied neat (without dilution), others may need to be diluted before topical application, especially for young or sensitive skin. Refer to the Single Essential Oils section of this book or the Dilution Reference Chart (following these notes) for recommended dilutions for the oils listed in this book.

𝐎: Internal means that the oils or supplements are taken orally. This can be done either by adding the oil to a food or beverage that is then consumed, placing a drop of oil under the tongue, or by swallowing a capsule that has the essential oil or supplement inside.

For more information on specific ways essential oils can be applied or used, see the Science and Application of Essential Oils section in this book.

The large 𝒪, ⬤, or 𝐎 listed near the bottom of each entry refers to recommended application methods specific for that condition.

⬜: For many conditions listed in this section there is also additional supporting research.

Many entries also include **definitions** of conditions and terms (listed directly underneath the topic), **subtopics** related to that condition, and even **recipes or blends** that can be used for that condition.

Example Entry:

Below are some additional things to keep in mind as you use and apply the essential oils, blends, and supplements listed in this section.

Oils: melaleuca, oregano, peppermint, thyme, geranium, lavender

Blend 1: Combine 2 drops lavender, 2 drops melaleuca, and 2 drops thyme. Apply 1–2 drops on ringworm three times a day for 10 days. Then mix 30 drops melaleuca with 2 Tbs. fractionated coconut oil, and use daily until ringworm is gone.

—Thrush:

Thrush is another name for oral candidiasis (*see Candida above*). Thrush results in uncomfortable or painful white or yellow patches in the mouth.

Oils: melaleuca, lavender, eucalyptus, marjoram, thyme

Modern Essentials Usage Guide

Additional Notes on Using Essential Oils

Below are some additional things to keep in mind as you use and apply the essential oils, blends, and supplements listed in this section.

— If essential oils get into your eyes by accident or if they burn the skin a little, do not try to remove the oils with water. This will only drive the oils deeper into the tissue. It is best to dilute the essential oils on location with a pure vegetable oil (such as fractionated coconut oil).

— The FDA has approved some essential oils generically for internal use and given them the following designations: GRAS (Generally Recognized As Safe for human consumption), FA (Food Additive), or FL (Flavoring agent). *These designations are listed under Oral Use As Dietary Supplement for each single oil in the Single Essential Oils section of* Modern Essentials.

— Using some oils such as lemon, orange, grapefruit, bergamot, etc., before or during exposure to direct sunlight or UV rays (tanning beds, for example) may cause a rash, pigmentation, or even severe burns. Please see the safety information under each oil in the Single Essential Oil chapter of this book for further information; then either dilute these oils and test a small area, or avoid their use altogether.

— Caution should be used with oils such as clary sage and fennel during pregnancy. These oils contain active constituents with hormone-like activity and could possibly stimulate adverse reactions in the mother, although there are no recorded cases in humans.

— Particular care should be taken when using cassia, cinnamon, lemongrass, oregano, and thyme, as they are some of the strongest and most caustic oils. It is best to dilute them with a pure vegetable oil.

— When a blend or recipe is listed in this section, rather than mix the oils together, it may be more beneficial to layer the oils: that is, apply a drop or two of one oil, rub it in, and then apply another oil. If dilution is necessary, a pure vegetable oil can be applied on top. *Effectiveness is in the layering.*

— Less is often better: use one to three drops of oil and no more than six drops at a time. Stir, and rub on in a clockwise direction.

— When applying oils to infants and small children, dilute one to two drops pure essential oil with 1–3 teaspoon (tsp.) of a pure vegetable oil (such as fractionated coconut oil). If the oils are used in the bath, always use a bath gel base as a dispersing agent for the oils. See CHILDREN AND INFANTS in this section for more information about the recommended list of oils for babies and children.

— The body absorbs oils the fastest through inhalation (breathing) and second fastest through application to the feet or ears. Layering oils can increase the rate of absorption.

— The life expectancy of a cell is 120 days (4 months). When cells divide, they makeduplicate cells. If the cell is diseased, new diseased cells will be made. When we stop the mutation of the diseased cells (create healthy cells), we stop the disease. Essential oils have the ability to penetrate and carry nutrients through the cell membrane to the nucleus and improve the health of the cell.

— *Use extreme caution when diffusing cassia or cinnamon* as they may burn the nostrils if you put your nose directly next to the nebulizer of the diffuser where the mist is coming out.

— When traveling by air, you should always have your oils hand-checked. X-ray machines may interfere with the frequency of the oils.

— Keep oils away from the light and heat—although they seem to do fine in temperatures up to 90 degrees. If stored properly in a cool, dark environment, they can maintain their maximum potency for many years.

Primary Recommendations • Secondary Recommendations • Other Recommendations

Personal Usage Guide

ADD/ADHD

Attention deficit disorder or attention deficit/hyperactivity disorder is a psychological condition characterized by inattentiveness, restlessness, and difficulty concentrating. Although most individuals exhibit all of these symptoms at some point, ADD is characterized by a frequency and duration of these symptoms that are inappropriate to an individual's age.

Oils: ☺☺Focus Blend, ☺☺Calming Blend, ☺vetiver, ☺☺lavender

Blend 1: Combine equal parts lavender and basil. Diffuse, or apply 1–3 drops on the crown of the head.

☺: Diffuse into the air. Inhale oil directly from the bottle, or applied to a tissue or cotton wick.

☺: Dilute as recommended, and apply 1–3 drops on the bottoms of the feet and/or on the spine.

AIDS/HIV

see also **Antiviral**

Acquired immune deficiency syndrome (AIDS) is a disease of the human immune system. AIDS progressively inhibits the effectiveness of the immune system, leaving the human body susceptible to both infections and tumors. AIDS is caused by the human immunodeficiency virus (HIV), which is acquired by direct contact of the bloodstream or mucous membrane with a bodily fluid (such as blood, breast milk, vaginal fluid, semen, and preseminal fluid) containing HIV.

Oils: ☺☺helichrysum☺, ☺Protective Blend, ☺☺lemon, ☺☺bergamot☺, ☺Grounding Blend

☺: Diffuse into the air. Inhale oil applied to a tissue or cotton wick.

☺: Dilute as recommended, and apply 1–3 drops on the bottoms of the feet and/or on the spine.

☺: **Additional Research:**

Helichrysum: Arzanol, extracted from helichrysum, inhibited HIV-1 replication in T cells and also inhibited the release of pro-inflammatory cytokines (chemical messengers) in monocytes (Appendino et al., 2007).

Bergamot: Bergamot extract was found to have potent antiretroviral activity towards HTLV-1 (a human retrovirus that causes T-cell leukemia and lymphoma) and HIV-1 expression in infected cells (Balestrieri et al., 2011).

Abscess

see **Oral Conditions:Abscess**

Abuse

Abuse is the harmful treatment or use of something or someone. Abuse has many different forms: physical, sexual, verbal, spiritual, psychological, etc. Abuse in all of its forms often has long-lasting negative effects on the person or thing abused.

Oils: ☺Joyful Blend, ☺lavender, ☺melissa, ☺sandalwood

☺: Apply oil topically over the heart, rub on each ear, and then cup hands and inhale deeply to help release negative emotions associated with abuse.

Acne

Acne is a skin condition, generally of the face, commonly found in adolescents and young adults. Acne is characterized by red, irritating blemishes (pimples) on the skin. Most commonly, acne is found on the oil-producing parts of the body such as the face, chest, back, upper arms, and back of neck. Acne is a blockage of a skin pore by dead skin cells, tiny hairs, and oil secreted by the sebaceous glands located near the hair follicles in the face, neck, and back. This blockage occurs deep within the skin. Acne is not currently believed to be caused by dirt on the face or by eating certain foods, and research has indicated that over-scrubbing the face may actually make acne worse.

Oils: ⊙Topical Blend, ⊙melaleuca⊙, ⊙juniper berry, ⊙lavender, ⊙cedarwood, ⊙geranium, ⊙sandalwood, ⊙thyme, ⊙vetiver, ⊙lemon, ⊙lemongrass, ⊙marjoram, ⊙patchouli

Other Products: ⊙Face Wash

—Infectious:

Oils: ⊙Topical Blend, ⊙melaleuca⊙, ⊙clove

Other Products: ⊙Face Wash

⊜: Dilute as recommended, and apply one of the above oils on location. Place about 10 drops of an oil in a 1–2 ounce spray bottle filled with water, and mist your face several times per day.

⊡: **Additional Research:**

Melaleuca: Tea tree oil and several of its main components were found to be active against Propionibacterium acnes, a bacteria involved in the formation of acne. This oil was also found to be active against two types of staphylococcus bacteria (Raman et al., 1995).

Melaleuca: A topical gel containing 5% tea tree oil was found to be more effective than a placebo at preventing acne lesions and severity in patients suffering from acne vulgaris (Enshaieh et al., 2007).

Melaleuca: A gel with 5% tea tree oil was found to be as effective as a 5% benzoyl peroxide (a common chemical used to treat acne) lotion, with fewer side effects (Bassett et al., 1990).

Addictions

Addiction is an obsession, compulsion, or extreme psychological dependence that interferes with an individual's ability or desire to function normally. Common addictions include drugs, alcohol, coffee, tobacco, sugar, video games, work, gambling, money, explicit images, compulsive overeating, etc.

—Alcohol:

Oils: ⊙⊘rosemary, ⊙⊘Cleansing Blend, ⊙⊘Calming Blend, ⊙⊘juniper berry, ⊙⊘helichrysum, ⊙⊘lavender, ⊙⊘orange

—Drugs:

Oils: ⊙⊘Cleansing Blend, ⊙⊘Calming Blend, ⊙⊘grapefruit (withdrawal)⊙, ⊙⊘lavender, ⊙⊘basil, ⊙⊘eucalyptus, ⊙⊘marjoram, ⊙orange, ⊙sandalwood, ⊙Roman chamomile, ⊙wintergreen

—Smoking:

Oils: ⊘black pepper, ⊙clove or ⊙Protective Blend on tongue

—Sugar:

> **Oils:** ◎Cleansing Blend, ◎Calming Blend

—Withdrawal:

> **Oils:** ◎⊘lavender, ◎⊘grapefruit, ◎⊘orange, ◎⊘sandalwood, ◎⊘marjoram

—Work:

> **Oils:** ⊘lavender, ⊘basil, ⊘marjoram, ⊘geranium

⊘: Diffuse into the air. Inhale the aroma of the oil directly.

◎: Dilute as recommended, and apply to temples or to reflex points.

▭: Additional Research:

> **Grapefruit and orange:** Injection of limonene, a common terpene found in many citrus essential oils, inhibited behavioral manifestations of drug use on rats administered methamphetamine (METH). Examination of the nucleus accumbens of the rats revealed that limonene may produce its effects by regulating dopamine levels and serotonin receptor function (Yun, 2014).
>
> **Black pepper:** Inhaled vapor of black pepper oil was found to reduce cravings for cigarettes and symptoms of anxiety in smokers deprived from smoking, compared to a control (Rose et al., 1994).

Addison's Disease

see **Adrenal Glands:Addison's Disease**

Adenitis

Adenitis is an acute or chronic inflammation of the lymph glands or lymph nodes.

Oils: ◎rosemary

◎: Dilute as recommended, and apply on location.

Adrenal Glands

The adrenal glands are two small glands located on top of the kidneys. The inner part of the adrenal gland, called the medulla, is responsible for producing adrenalin, a hormone that helps control blood pressure, heart rate, and sweating. The outer part of the adrenal gland, called the cortex, is responsible for producing corticosteroids, hormones that help control metabolism and help regulate inflammation, water levels, and levels of electrolytes such as sodium and potassium. An imbalance in adrenal function can lead to problems such as Addison's disease (a lack of adrenal hormones in the body due to suppressed adrenal functioning) or Cushing's syndrome (an over-abundance of corticosteroids, typically due to over-active adrenal functioning).

Oils: ◎basil, ◎rosemary, ◎clove, ◎Joyful Blend

Other Products: ○Cellular Vitality Complex, ○Food Nutrient Complex, ○Chewable Multivitamin, ○Essential Oil Omega Complex or Vegan Essential Oil Omega Complex, ○Omega-3 Fish Oil

—Addison's Disease:

> Addison's disease is a condition where the function of the adrenal glands is either severely limited or completely shut down in their ability to produce hormones. This is most often caused by an autoimmune disorder where the body's own immune system attacks the cells in the adrenal glands, but it can also be caused by cancer, tuberculosis, or other diseases. The loss of hormones from the adrenal cortex can cause extreme dehydration due to fluid

loss and low levels of sodium. Early symptoms can include tiredness, dizziness when standing up, thirst, weight loss, and dark patches of pigmentation appearing on the skin. If untreated, this disease can eventually lead to kidney failure, shock, and death.

Oils: ☺Joyful Blend

Other Products: OFood Nutrient Complex , OCellular Vitality Complex (for cellular support), OChewable Multivitamin, OEssential Oil Omega Complex or Vegan Essential Oil Omega Complex, OOmega-3 Fish Oil

—Cushing's Syndrome:

Cushing's syndrome is a condition where there is an over-abundance of corticosteroids (such as cortisol) in the body, typically caused by an over-production of these steroids by the adrenal glands. This over-production in the adrenal glands can be caused by a growth in the adrenal glands or by a tumor in the thyroid leading to the production of too much corticotropin (the hormone that stimulates production of corticosteroids in the adrenal gland). This syndrome can also be caused by taking artificial cortisone or cortisone-like substances. Symptoms of excessive corticosteroids include weight gain, muscle loss, and weakness, bruising, and osteoporosis.

Oils: ☺Joyful Blend, ☺lemon, ☺basil, ☺Protective Blend

Other Products: OFood Nutrient Complex , OCellular Vitality Complex (for cellular support), OChewable Multivitamin, OEssential Oil Omega Complex or Vegan Essential Oil Omega Complex, OOmega-3 Fish Oil

—Schmidt's Syndrome *(Polyglandular Deficiency Syndrome (or Autoimmune Polyendocrine Syndrome) Type 2):*

This syndrome refers specifically to an autoimmune disorder that causes Addison's disease as well as decreased thyroid function. See *Addison's Disease* (above) and *Thyroid: Hypothyroidism* for oils and products to help support the adrenal glands and thyroid.

Stimulate glands: ☺basil, ☺rosemary, ☺clove, ☺geranium

Strengthen glands: ☺peppermint

☻: Apply as a warm compress over kidney area. Dilute as recommended, and apply on location or on reflex points on the feet.

◔: Take capsules as directed on package.

Aging

*See also **Alzheimer's Disease, Antioxidant, Cells, Female-Specific Conditions:Menopause, Hair:Loss,** and **Skin:Wrinkles** for other age-related issues.*

Oils: OCellular Complex, ☺Anti-Aging Blend, Olemon☺, ☺frankincense, ☺sandalwood

Other Products: ☺Anti-Aging Moisturizer, ☺Facial Cleanser, ☺Ingivorating Scrub, ☺Skin Toner, ☺Skin Serum. OEnergy & Stamina Complex, OCellular Vitality Complex, OEssential Oil Omega Complex or Vegan Essential Oil Omega Complex, OOmega-3 Fish Oil, OFood Nutrient Complex, OProbiotic Defense Formula

◔: Take oil with food, or take capsules as directed on package.

☻: Dilute as recommended, and apply to skin. Combine with carrier oil, and massage into skin.

⊘: Diffuse, or inhale from a tissue or cotton wick.

▭: **Additional Research:**

Lemon: Based on lemon essential oil's acetylcholinesterase inhibitory activity, butyrylcholinesterase inhibitiory activity, and antioxidant power, this essential oil could be used in the management and/or prevention of neurodegenerative conditions like Alzheimer's disease (Oboh et al., 2014).

Lemon: A study using mice demonstrated that pretreatment with lemon essential oil causes an increase in antioxidant enzymatic activities and decreased lipid degradation in the hippocampus (Campelo et al., 2011). Antioxidant and bioprotective activities, like that of lemon essential oil, can reduce damage to neurons produced by neurodegenerative disease (Campelo et al., 2011).

Agitation
see **Calming**

Airborne Bacteria
see **Antibacterial**

Air Pollution

Air Pollution is the presence in the atmosphere of chemicals, biological material, or other matter that can potentially harm humans, the environment, or other living organisms.

Oils: ⊘Cleansing Blend, ⊘Protective Blend, ⊘lemon, ⊘lemongrass, ⊘peppermint, ⊘rosemary, ⊘eucalyptus, ⊘cypress, ⊘grapefruit

—**Disinfectants:**

Oils: ⊘Cleansing Blend, ⊘lemon, ⊘eucalyptus, ⊘clove, ⊘grapefruit, ⊘peppermint, ⊘wintergreen

Blend 1: Combine lemongrass and geranium oil, and diffuse into the air⊘.

⊘: Diffuse into the air.

▭: **Additional Research:**

Blend 1: A formulation of lemongrass and geranium oil was found to reduce airborne bacteria by 89% in an office environment after diffusion for 15 hours (Doran et al., 2009).

Alcoholism
see **Addictions:Alcohol**

Alertness

Alertness is the state of being watchful or paying close attention. It includes being prepared to react quickly to danger, emergencies, or any other situation.

Oils: ⊘peppermint⊘, ⊘ylang ylang⊘, ⊘lemon, ⊘basil, ⊘rosemary

⊘: Diffuse into the air. Inhale oil applied to a tissue or cotton wick.

◉: Dilute as recommended, and apply to the temples and bottoms of the feet.

▭: **Additional Research:**

Peppermint: In human trials, the aroma of peppermint was found to enhance memory and increase alertness (Moss et al., 2008).

Ylang ylang: Inhaled ylang ylang oil was found to decrease blood pressure and pulse rate and to enhance attentiveness and alertness in volunteers compared to an odorless control (Hongratanaworakit et al., 2004).

Allergies

An allergy is a damaging immune system response to a substance that does not bother most other people. Common allergies are to food, insect bites, pollen, dust, medicine, pets, and mold. Allergy symptoms vary greatly, but common allergic responses include itching, swelling, runny nose, asthma, and sneezing. Both host factors (gender, race, heredity) and environmental factors can cause allergies.

Oils: ⊘melaleuca⊘, O⊘lavender⊘, O⊘lemon⊘, O⊘peppermint⊘, ⊘Roman chamomile, ⊘⊘melissa, ⊘⊘patchouli, ⊘eucalyptus

Other Products: OSeasonal Blend Softgels, ORespiratory Lozenge Drops, OFood Nutrient Complex , OCellular Vitality Complex, OChewable Multivitamin

—Coughing:

Oils: ⊘⊘Cleansing Blend

—Hay Fever

Oils: ⊘lavender⊘, ⊘eucalyptus, ⊘rose, ⊘peppermint

Recipe 1: Apply 1 drop of peppermint on the base of the neck two times a day. Tap the thymus (located just below the notch in the neck) with pointer fingers. Diffuse peppermint.

Recipe 2: For allergy rashes and skin sensitivity, apply 3 drops lavender, 6 drops Roman chamomile, 2 drops myrrh, and 1 drop peppermint on location.

⊜: Dilute as recommended, and apply to sinuses and to bottoms of feet.

⊘: Diffuse into the air. Inhale oil applied to a tissue or cotton wick.

⊙: **Additional Research:**

Melaleuca: Tea tree oil was found to reduce swelling during a contact hypersensitivity response in the skin of mice sensitized to the chemical hapten (Brand et al., 2002).

Melaleuca: Tea tree oil applied to histamine-induced edema (swelling) in mice ears was found to significantly reduce swelling (Brand et al., 2002).

Melaleuca: Tea tree oil applied to histamine-induced weal and flare in human volunteers was found to decrease the mean weal volume when compared to a control (Koh et al., 2002).

Lavender: Lavender oil was found to inhibit immediate-type allergic reactions in mice and rats by inhibiting mast cell degranulation (Kim et al., 1999).

Lemon: A study including 100 patients (ages 3 to 79) suffering from vasomotor allergic rhinopathy, showed that topical application of a citrus lemon based spray resulted in a total reduction of eosinophils granulocytes and mast cells. These results suggest that the lemon-based nasal spray is a good alternative to conventional medicine for the treatment of perennial and seasonal allergic and vasomotor rhinopathy (Ferrara et al., 2012).

Peppermint: L-menthol (from peppermint) was found to inhibit production of inflammation mediators in human monocytes (a type of white blood cell involved in the immune response) (Juergens et al., 1998).

Alzheimer's Disease

see also **Brain, Memory**

Alzheimer's is a progressive and fatal disease that attacks and kills brain cells, causing a loss of memory and other intellectual capacities. Alzheimer's is most commonly diagnosed in individuals over the age of 65. As the disease progresses, sufferers often experience mood swings, long-term memory loss, confusion, irritability, aggression, and a decreased ability to communicate.

Oils: ⊘coriander⊘, ⊘Olemon⊙

Supplements: ○Energy & Stamina Complex, ○Cellular Vitality Complex☺

—Blood-Brain Barrier:

> Studies have shown that sesquiterpenes can pass the blood-brain barrier. Oils high in sesquiterpenes include sandalwood, ginger, myrrh, vetiver, ylang ylang, and frankincense.

Oils: ✪○frankincense, ✪○sandalwood☺

○: Take oils in capsules. Take supplements as directed on package.

✷: Diffuse oils into the air.

☽: Dilute as recommended, and apply over brain stem area on back of neck.

▭: **Additional Research:**

> **Coriander:** Inhalation of coriander volatile oil was found to possess antianxiety, antidepressant, and antioxidant properties in Alzheimer's disease conditions in a rat model of beta-amyloid Alzheimer's disease (Cioanca et al., 2014).

> **Coriander:** Repeated inhalation of coriander oil was found to prevent memory impairment and oxidative damage in a rat model of beta-amyloid Alzheimer's disease, when compared to control (Cioanca et al., 2013).

> **Lemon:** Based on lemon essential oil's acetylcholinesterase inhibitory activity, butyrylcholinesterase inhibitiory activity, and antioxidant power, this essential oil could be used in the management and/or prevention of neurodegenerative conditions like Alzheimer's disease (Oboh et al., 2014).

> **Cellular Vitality Complex:** In a recent study at UCLA, the polyphenol curcumin was found to inhibit amyloid beta accumulation and to cross the blood-brain barrier of mice and bind amyloid plaques. Amyloid beta plaques are theorized to have a role in the development of Alzheimer's disease (Yang et al., 2005).

> **Cellular Vitality Complex:** Curcumin was found to reduce the effects of amyloid beta-caused oxidative stress and DNA damage in neuronal cells (Park et al., 2008).

> **Sandalwood:** A blend of ethanol extracts from 8 herbs, including sandalwood, orally   administered to a mice model of Alzheimer's disease was shown to improve amyloid β protein-induced memory impairment, suppress amyloid β protein levels, and diminish plaque deposition in the brain as much as that of donepezil treatment. This study suggests that the 8-herb blend may develop as a therapeutic drug for treatment of Alzheimer's disease patients (Jeon et al., 2011).

> **Cinnamon:** An aqueous cinnamon extract was found to inhibit beta-amyloid oligomer and fibril formation and alleviate Alzheimer's disease symptoms in the Drosophila and mouse models of Alzheimer's disease (Frydman-Marom et al., 2011).

Amnesia
see **Memory**

Analgesic
see **Pain**

Aneurysm
see also **Blood**

An Aneurysm is a swelling or dilation of a blood vessel in the area of a weakened blood vessel wall.

Oils: ☽✷cypress, ☽✷melaleuca, ☽✷clary sage, ☽✷helichrysum, ☽✷frankincense

Blend 1: Combine 5 drops frankincense, 1 drop helichrysum, and 1 drop cypress. Diffuse.

Herbs: Cayenne pepper, garlic, hawthorn berry

☽: Dilute as recommended, and apply to temples, heart, and reflex points for heart on the feet.

✷: Diffuse into the air. Inhale oil applied to a tissue or cotton wick.

Anger
see **Calming**

Angina

see **Cardiovascular System:Angina**

Animals

Only 1–2 drops of oil are necessary on most animals, as they respond more quickly to the oils than do humans. Fractionated coconut oil can be added to extend the oil over larger areas and to heavily dilute the essential oil for use on smaller animals, especially cats.

—Bleeding:

Oils: ⊘helichrysum, ⊘geranium

—Bones (Pain):

Oils: ⊘wintergreen, ⊘Soothing Blend, ⊘lemongrass

—Calm:

Oils: ⊘⊘Calming Blend, ⊘⊘lavender, ⊘⊘Invigorating Blend

—Cancer, Skin

Oils: ⊘sandalwood⊕, ⊘frankincense

—Cats:

Valerie Worwood says that you can treat a cat like you would a child (*see* **Children/Infants**). Dilute oils heavily with carrier oil. *Avoid melaleuca, and use oils with extreme caution.*

—Colds and Coughs:

Oils: ⊘eucalyptus, ⊘melaleuca (not for cats). Apply on fur or stomach.

—Cows:

Oils: For scours, use 5 drops ⊘Digestive Blend on stomach (dilute with fractionated coconut oil to cover a larger area). Repeat 2 hours later.

—Dogs:

  –Anxiety/Nervousness

Oils: ⊘Calming Blend, ⊘lavender, ⊘Grounding Blend. Rub 1–2 drops between hands, and apply to muzzle, between toes, on tops of feet for the dog to smell, and on edges of ears.

  –Arthritis:

Oils: ⊘frankincense⊕

Blend 1: Blend equal parts rosemary, lavender, and ginger. Dilute with fractionated coconut oil, and apply topically on affected joints.

  –Bone Injury:

Oils: ⊘wintergreen

  –Dermatitis:

Oils: ⊘melaleuca⊕. Note: Some adverse effects have been reported with the use of larger amounts of melaleuca oil on some species of dogs. Contact a veterinarian before using melaleuca on a dog. For smaller dogs, use only a small amount of oil, heavily diluted.

–Heart Problems:

Oils: ⬭peppermint (on paws), ⬭Protective Blend (apply on back with warm compress)

–Sleep:

Oils: ⬭lavender (on paws), ⬭Calming Blend (on stomach)

–Stroke:

Oils: ⬭frankincense (on brain stem/back of neck), ⬭Grounding Blend (on each paw)

–Ticks and Bug Bites:

Oils: ⬭Cleansing Blend (drop directly on tick, or dilute and apply to wound)

–Travel Sickness:

Oils: ⬭peppermint (dilute, and rub on stomach)

—Earache:

Blend 2: Combine 1 drop melaleuca, 1 drop lavender, and 1 drop Roman chamomile in 1 tsp. fractionated coconut oil. Apply 1–2 drops to inside and outside of ear.

—Ear Infections:

Oils: ⬭Cleansing Blend. Dip cotton swab in oil, and apply to inside and front of ear.

—Fleas:

Oils: ⬭lemongrass, ⬭eucalyptus. Add 1–2 drops of oil to shampoo.

—Horses:

–Anxiety/Nervousness

Oils: ⬭Calming Blend. Rub 1–2 drops between hands, and apply to nose, knees, tongue, and front of chest.

–Hoof Rot:

Blend 3: Combine 1 drop Roman chamomile, 1 drop thyme, and 1 drop melissa in 1 tsp. fractionated coconut oil, and apply on location.

–Infection:

Oils: ⬭Protective Blend

–Leg Fractures:

Oils: ⬭ginger. Dilute oil, and apply oil to leg with a hot compress wrapped around the leg. Massage leg after the fracture is healed with a blend of ⬭rosemary and ⬭thyme diluted with fractionated coconut oil. This may strengthen the ligaments and prevent calcification.

–Muscle Tissue

Oils: Apply equal parts ⬭lemongrass and ⬭lavender on location, and wrap to help regenerate torn muscle tissue.

-Wounds:

Oils: ⊜helichrysum

—Parasites:

Oils: ⊜lavender, ⊜Digestive Blend, ⊜cedarwood. Rub on paws to help release parasites.

⊜: Apply as directed above. Dilute as recommended, and apply on location.

⊘: Diffuse into the air.

⊡: **Additional Research:**

Sandalwood: Sandalwood oil was found to decrease skin papilloma (tumors) in mice (Dwivedi et al., 1997).

Sandalwood: Alpha-santalol, derived from sandalwood EO, was found to delay and decrease the incidence and multiplicity of skin tumor (papilloma) development in mice (Dwivedi et al., 2003).

Sandalwood: Various concentrations of alpha-santalol (from sandalwood) were tested against skin cancer in mice. All concentrations were found to inhibit skin cancer development (Dwivedi et al., 2005).

Sandalwood: A solution of 5% alpha-santalol (from sandalwood) was found to prevent skin-tumor formation caused by ultraviolet-b (UVB) radiation in mice (Dwivedi et al., 2006).

Sandalwood: Oral sandalwood oil use enhanced GST activity (a protein in cell membranes that can help eliminate toxins) and acid-soluble SH levels. This suggests a possible chemopreventive action on carcinogenesis (Banerjee et al., 1993).

Sandalwood: Pre-treatment with alpha-santalol before UVB (ultraviolet-b) radiation significantly reduced skin tumor development and multiplicity and induced proapoptotic and tumor-suppressing proteins (Arasada et al., 2008).

Frankincense: An acetone extract of frankincense was found to decrease arthritic sores, reduce paw edema (swelling), and suppress pro-inflammatory cytokines (cellular messengers) (Fan et al., 2008).

Melaleuca: A cream with 10% tea tree oil was found to be more effective at treating dermatitis in dogs than a commercially-available skin cream (Reichling et al., 2004).

Lime, Lavender, Marjoram, Oregano, Peppermint, Helichrysum: Malacalm®, a commercially available mixture containing lime, lavender, marjoram, oregano, peppermint, and helichrysum essential oils, was clinically successful at treating *Malassezia pachydermatis* (a fungal skin infection) in dogs (Nardoni et al., 2014).

Oregano: Four out of seven cats with the fungus mycoses (*Microsporum canis*) recovered both clinically and culturally with topical application of diluted oregano oil for a month (Mugnaini et al., 2012).

Anorexia
see **Eating Disorders:Anorexia**

Antibacterial
see also **Disinfectant**

The term antibacterial refers to anything that kills bacteria or that limits its ability to grow or reproduce.

Oils: ⊙⊜Protective Blend,⊜melaleuca⊙, ⊜⊘thyme⊙, ⊜⊘cinnamon ⊙, ⊜peppermint⊙, ⊘⊜Cleansing Blend, ⊜⊘lime, ⊜⊘lemongrass⊙, ⊜helichrysum⊙, ⊜⊘geranium⊙, ⊜rosemary⊙, ⊜⊘clove, ⊜oregano⊙, ⊘Respiratory Blend, ⊜cypress⊙, ⊜arborvitae⊙, ⊜cedarwood, ⊜basil, ⊜cassia⊙, ⊜⊘lemon, ⊜eucalyptus, ⊜grapefruit, ⊜marjoram, ⊜clary sage, ⊜lavender⊙, ⊜frankincense, ⊜juniper berry

Blend 1: For an antibiotic blend, place 12 drops of Protective Blend, 6 drops oregano, and 2 drops frankincense in a size "00" capsule, and ingest every 4–8 hours.

Other Products: ⊙Protective Softgels, ⊜Protective Hand Wash & ⊜Soothing Skin Ointment to help eliminate bacteria on the skin, ⊜Protective Cleaner to help eliminate bacteria from household surfaces, ⊙Probiotic Defense Formula, ⊙GI Cleansing Formula to help support the intestinal tract against harmful bacteria.

—Airborne Bacteria:

Oils: 🖐cinnamon👄, 🖐lemongrass👄, 🖐geranium👄, 🖐Protective Blend, 🖐Cleansing Blend, 🖐oregano

—Cleansing:

Oils: Cleansing Blend

—MRSA (Methicillin Resistant *Staphylococcus aureus*):

Oils: 👄melaleuca👄, 👄oregano👄, 👄geranium👄, 👄Protective Blend, 👄frankincense, 👄peppermint👄, 👄lemon, 👄thyme, 👄cinnamon, 👄clove, 👄eucalyptus, 👄lemongrass, 👄orange, 👄grapefruit, 👄lavender

Recipe 1: Place 2–5 drops each of oregano, Protective Blend, and frankincense (followed by lemon and peppermint) on bottoms of feet every 2 hours.

—Staph (*Staphylococcus aureus*) Infection:

Oils: ◯👄Protective Blend,◯👄melaleuca👄, 👄oregano👄, 👄helichrysum👄, 👄thyme👄, 👄geranium👄, 👄Cleansing Blend, 👄lavender Note: peppermint may make a staph infection more painful.

Other Products: ◯Protective Softgels

👄: Dilute as recommended, and apply on location. Dilute and apply to liver area and bottoms of the feet. Use hand wash as directed on packaging.

◯: Place 1–2 drops of oil under the tongue, or place oils in empty capsules and swallow. Take supplements as directed.

🖐: Diffuse into the air. Combine a few drops in a small spray bottle with distilled water, and spray into the air.

⊕ Additional Research:

Melaleuca: Tea tree oil was found to disrupt the cellular membrane and inhibited respiration in Candida albicans, Gram-negative E. coli, and Gram-positive Staphylococcus aureus (Staph) (Cox et al., 2000).

Melaleuca: In a human trial, most patients receiving treatment with Melaleuca alternifolia oil placed topically on boils experienced healing or reduction of symptoms; while of those receiving no treatment (control), half required surgical intervention, and all still demonstrated signs of the infection (Feinblatt et al., 1960).

Melaleuca: Gram-positive strains of Staphylococcus aureus and Enterococcus faecalis were shown to have very low frequencies of resistance to tea tree oil (Hammer et al., 2008).

Melaleuca: Tea tree, peppermint, and sage oils were found to inhibit oral bacteria, with thymol and eugenol being the most active components of these oils (Shapiro et al., 1994).

Melaleuca: Cinnamon oil exhibited a strong antimicrobial activity against two detrimental oral bacteria. Manuka, tea tree, and the component thymol also exhibited antimicrobial potency (Filoche et al., 2005).

Melaleuca: MRSA (methicillin-resistant staph) and MSSA (methicillin-sensitive staph) in biofilms (plaque/microcolonies) were eradicated by a 5% solution of tea tree oil, as were 5 of 9 CoNS (coagulase-negative staph) (Brady et al., 2006).

Melaleuca: 66 isolates of Staphylococcus aureus (Staph), including 64 methicillin-resistant (MRSA) and 33 mupirocin-resistant strains, were inhibited by tea tree essential oil (Carson et al., 1995).

Melaleuca: A combination of Citricidal and geranium oil demonstrated strong antibacterial effects on MRSA. Geranium and tea tree demonstrated strong antibacterial effects on Staphylococcus aureus (Edwards-Jones et al., 2004).

Melaleuca: Tea tree oil and its component terpinen-4-ol demonstrated antibacterial activity against Staphylococcus aureus (Staph) bacteria, superior to the activities of several antibiotic drugs—even against antibiotic-resistant strains (Ferrini et al., 2006).

Melaleuca: Tea tree oil demonstrated ability to kill Staphylococcus aureus (Staph) bacteria both within biofilms and in the stationary growth phase at concentrations below 1% (Kwieciński et al., 2009).

Melaleuca: Turpin-4-ol, found in tea tree oil, was found to effectively inhibit MRSA and CoNS, while not exhibiting toxicity to human fibroblast cells (Loughlin et al., 2008).

Thyme: Tea tree, peppermint, and sage oils were found to inhibit oral bacteria, with thymol and eugenol being the most active components of these oils (Shapiro et al., 1994).

Thyme: Cinnamon oil exhibited a strong antimicrobial activity against two detrimental oral bacteria. Manuka, tea tree, and the component thymol also exhibited antimicrobial potency (Filoche et al., 2005).

Thyme: Cinnamon bark, lemongrass, and thyme oils were found to have the highest level of activity against common respiratory pathogens among 14 essential oils tested (Inouye et al., 2001).

Thyme: Thyme oil demonstrated a strong antibacterial effect against Staph and E. coli bacteria (Mohsenzadeh et al., 2007).

Thyme: Oils with aldehydes or phenols as major components demonstrated a high level of antibacterial activity (Inouye et al., 2001).

Cinnamon: Cinnamon oil exhibited a strong antimicrobial activity against two detrimental oral bacteria. Manuka, tea tree, and the component thymol also exhibited antimicrobial potency (Filoche et al., 2005).

Cinnamon: Cinnamon bark, lemongrass, and thyme oils were found to have the highest level of activity against common respiratory pathogens among 14 essential oils tested (Inouye et al., 2001).

Peppermint: Tea tree, peppermint, and sage oils were found to inhibit oral bacteria, with thymol and eugenol being the most active components of these oils (Shapiro et al., 1994).

Peppermint: Peppermint and spearmint oil inhibited resistant strains of Staphylococcus, E. coli, Salmonella, and Helicobacter pylori (Imai et al., 2001).

Peppermint: Peppermint and rosemary oils were each found to be more effective at preventing dental biofilm (plaque) formation than chlorhexidine (an antiseptic) (Rasooli et al., 2008).

Lemongrass: Cinnamon bark, lemongrass, and thyme oils were found to have the highest level of activity against common respiratory pathogens among 14 essential oils tested (Inouye et al., 2001).

Lemongrass: A formulation of lemongrass and geranium oil was found to reduce airborne bacteria by 89% in an office environment after diffusion for 15 hours (Doran et al., 2009).

Lemongrass: Lemongrass and lemon verbena oil were found to be bactericidal to Helicobacter pylori at very low concentrations. Additionally, it was found that this bacteria did not develop a resistance to lemongrass oil after 10 passages, while this bacteria did develop resistance to clarithromycin (an antibiotic) under the same conditions (Ohno et al., 2003).

Helichrysum: Helichrysum oil was found to exhibit definite antibacterial activity against six tested Gram (+/-) bacteria (Chinou et al., 1996).

Helichrysum: Helichrysum was found to inhibit both the growth and some of the enzymes of the Staphylococcus aureus (staph) bacteria (Nostro et al., 2001).

Geranium: A combination of Citricidal and geranium oil demonstrated strong antibacterial effects on MRSA. Geranium and tea tree demonstrated strong antibacterial effects on Staphylococcus aureus (Edwards-Jones et al., 2004).

Geranium: A formulation of lemongrass and geranium oil was found to reduce airborne bacteria by 89% in an office environment after diffusion for 15 hours (Doran et al., 2009).

Rosemary: Peppermint and rosemary oils were each found to be more effective at preventing dental biofilm (plaque) formation than chlorhexidine (an antiseptic) (Rasooli et al., 2008).

Oregano: Oregano oil was found to inhibit MRSA (Nostro et al., 2004).

Cypress: Cypress essential oil was found to possess antibacterial activity against *Staphlococcus aureus*, *Klebsiella pneumoniae*, and *Salmonella indica* when tested for antimicrobial properties against 13 microorganisms (Selim et al., 2014).

Cassia: Cinnamaldehyde, the main constituent of cassia oil, showed strong growth inhibiting activity toward five human intestinal bacteria in vitro (Lee et al., 1998).

Arborvitae: Arborvitae essential oil vapor and liquid displayed bactericidal activity against seven bacteria (including three Gram-positive organisms, Bacillus subtilis, Streptococcus pyogenes, and Enterococcus fecalis, and four Gram-negative organisms, Acinetobacter baumannii, Hemophilus influenzae, Salmonella enteritidis, and Escherichia coli) as well as the bacterial spores of Bacillus subtilis (Hudson et al., 2011).

Lavender: Scanning electron microscopy analysis and zeta potential measurement revealed that lavender essential oil's antibacterial action against multi-drug-resistant *Escherichia coli* occurs via two mechanisms: alteration of outer membrane permeability and possible inhibition of bacterial quorum sensing (Yap et al., 2014).

Anticatarrhal
see **Congestion:Catarrh**

Anticoagulant
see **Blood:Clots**

Antidepressant
see **Depression**

Antifungal

Fungi are a broad range of organisms such as yeast, mold, and mushrooms. While many fungi are safe and beneficial, some create mycotoxins, which are chemicals that can be toxic to plants, animals, and humans. Examples of fungi that can be detrimental to humans include black mold, *Candida*, and ringworm.

Oils: ⊜melaleuca⊙, ⊜⊘⊙oregano⊙, ⊜thyme⊙, ⊜⊘cinnamon⊙, ⊜clove⊙, ⊜⊘Protective Blend, ⊜arborvitae⊙, ⊜lavender⊙, ⊜peppermint⊙, ⊜rosemary⊙, ⊜lemon⊙, ⊘Cleansing Blend, ⊜⊘patchouli, ⊜lemongrass, ⊜juniper berry ⊜geranium

Other Products: ⊜Protective Hand Wash, ⊜Protective Cleaner, ⊙Probiotic Defense Formula, ⊙GI Cleansing Formula

—Athlete's Foot:

Athlete's foot (tinea pedis) is a fungal infection that develops on the skin of the feet. This infection causes itching, redness, and scaling of the skin, and in severe cases it can cause painful blistering or cracking of the skin.

Oils: ⊜melaleuca⊙, ⊘⊘oregano⊙, ⊜cypress, ⊜thyme, ⊜geranium, ⊜lavender

—Candida:

Candida refers to a genus of yeast that are normally found in the digestive tract and on the skin of humans. These yeast are typically symbiotically beneficial to humans. However, several species of *Candida*, most commonly *Candida albicans*, can cause infections such as vaginal candidiasis or thrush (oral candidiasis) that cause localized itching, soreness, and redness *(see* **Vaginal:Candida** *for further application methods)*. In immune-system compromised individuals, these infection-causing species of *Candida* can spread further, leading to serious, life-threatening complications.

Oils: ⊜melaleuca⊙, ⊜⊙oregano⊙, ⊜clove⊙, ⊜Protective Blend, ⊜⊘peppermint⊙, ⊜thyme⊙, ⊜dill⊙, ⊜cilantro⊙, ⊜lavender⊙, ⊜eucalyptus, ⊜rosemary, ⊜⊙Digestive Blend

—Mold:

Mold are a type of microscopic multi-cellular fungi that grow together to form filaments. Mold is found throughout the world and can survive in extreme conditions. While most mold does not adversely affect humans, an over-abundance of mold spores can cause allergies or other problems within the respiratory system. Additionally, some types of mold produce toxins that can be harmful to humans or to animals.

Oils: ⊘Protective Blend, ⊘⊙clove⊙, ⊘⊙thyme⊙, ⊘⊙cinnamon⊙, ⊘⊙oregano⊙, ⊘⊙rose-
mary⊙, ⊘Cleansing Blend

—Ringworm:

Ringworm (or tinea) is a fungal infection of the skin that can cause itching, redness,
and scaling of the skin. The name comes from the ring-shaped patches that often form
on the skin.

Oils: ⊙melaleuca, ⊘⊙oregano⊙, ⊙peppermint, ⊙thyme, ⊙bergamot⊙, ⊙geranium,
⊙lavender

Blend 1: Combine 2 drops lavender, 2 drops melaleuca, and 2 drops thyme. Apply 1–2
drops on ringworm three times a day for 10 days. Then mix 30 drops melaleuca with
2 Tbs. fractionated coconut oil, and use daily until ringworm is gone.

—Thrush:

Thrush is another name for oral candidiasis (*see **Candida** above*). Thrush results in
uncomfortable or painful white or yellow patches in the mouth.

Oils: ⊙melaleuca⊙, ⊙lavender, ⊙eucalyptus, ⊙marjoram, ⊙thyme

⊙: Dilute as recommended, and apply on location. Apply as a warm compress over affected area.

⊘: Diffuse into the air.

◐: Take capsules as directed on package.

▢: **Additional Research:**

Melaleuca: Tea tree oil was found to inhibit 301 different types of yeasts isolated from the mouths of cancer patients suffering from advanced cancer, including 41 strains that are known to be resistant to antifungal drugs (Bagg et al., 2006).

Melaleuca: Eleven types of Candida were found to be highly inhibited by tea tree oil (Banes-Marshall et al., 2001).

Melaleuca: Tea tree oil was found to disrupt the cellular membrane and to inhibit respiration in Candida albicans (Cox et al.,
2000).

Melaleuca: Melaleuca oil at concentrations of .16% was found to inhibit the transformation of C. albicans from single-cell
yeast to the pathogenic mycelial (multi-cellular strands) form (D'Auria et al., 2001).

Melaleuca: Tea Tree oil was found to alter the membrane properties and functions of Candida albicans cells, leading to cell
inhibition or death (Hammer et al., 2004).

Melaleuca: Terpinen-4-ol, a constituent of tea tree oil, and tea tree oil were found to be effective against several forms of
vaginal Candida infections in rats, including azole-resistant forms (Mondello et al., 2006).

Melaleuca: Melaleuca oil inhibited several Candida species in vitro (Vazquez et al., 2000).

Melaleuca: Patients with tinea pedis (athlete's foot) were found to have a higher rate of cure and a higher clinical response
when treated topically with 25 or 50% tea tree oil solution compared to control (Satchell et al., 2002).

Melaleuca: When applied as a coating to protect oranges after harvest, a mixture containing chitosan and melaleuca essential
oil was found to reduce fungal growth by 50% (Cháfer et al., 2012).

Oregano: In a test of nine oils, clove, followed by cinnamon, oregano, and mace oil, was found to be inhibitory to two
toxin-producing fungi. It was also shown that whole and ground cloves stored with grain reduced the amount of aflatoxin
contamination (Juglal et al., 2002).

Oregano: The vapor of oregano oil was found to be fungicidal against the Trichophyton mentagrophytes fungi (a fungi that
causes a skin infection known as Malabar itch) (Inouye et al., 2006).

Oregano: Mice infected with Candida albicans who were fed origanum oil or carvacrol diluted in olive oil had an 80%
survival rate after 30 days, while infected mice fed olive oil alone all died after 10 days (Manohar et al., 2001).

Oregano: Cinnamon, thyme, oregano, and cumin oils inhibited the production of aflatoxin by aspergillus fungus (Tantaoui-
Elaraki et al., 1994).

Thyme: Cinnamon, thyme, oregano, and cumin oils inhibited the production of aflatoxin by aspergillus fungus (Tantaoui-
Elaraki et al., 1994).

Thyme: Thyme oil was found to inhibit Candida species by causing lesions in the cell membrane, as well as inhibiting germ tube (an outgrowth that develops when the fungi is preparing to replicate) formation (Pina-Vaz et al., 2004).

Thyme: Eugenol from clove and thymol from thyme were found to inhibit the growth of Aspergillus flavus and Aspergillus versicolor at concentrations of .4 mg/ml or less (Hitokoto et al., 1980).

Cinnamon: In a test of nine oils, clove, followed by cinnamon, oregano, and mace oil, was found to be inhibitory to two toxin-producing fungi. It was also shown that whole and ground cloves stored with grain reduced the amount of aflatoxin contamination (Juglal et al., 2002).

Cinnamon: Cinnamon, thyme, oregano, and cumin oils inhibited the production of aflatoxin by aspergillus fungus (Tantaoui-Elaraki et al., 1994).

Cinnamon: Vapor of cinnamon bark oil and cinnamic aldehyde was found to be effective against fungi involved in respiratory tract mycoses (fungal infections) (Singh et al., 1995).

Clove: In a test of nine oils, clove, followed by cinnamon, oregano, and mace oil, was found to be inhibitory to two toxin-producing fungi. It was also shown that whole and ground cloves stored with grain reduced the amount of aflatoxin contamination (Juglal et al., 2002).

Clove: Eugenol from clove and thymol from thyme were found to inhibit the growth of Aspergillus flavus and Aspergillus versicolor at concentrations of .4 mg/ml or less (Hitokoto et al., 1980).

Clove: Clove oil was found to have very strong radical scavenging activity (antioxidant). It was also found to display an antifungal effect against tested Candida strains (Chaieb et al., 2007).

Arborvitae: Arborvitae essential oil and liquid displayed antifungal activity against two commonly encountered fungi (the medically important yeast Candida albicans, and the filamentous mold Aspergillus niger)(Hudson et al., 2011).

Lavender: Lavandula oil demonstrated antifungal activity against three pathogenic fungi (Behnam et al., 2006).

Lavender: Lavender oil demonstrated both fungistatic (stopped growth) and fungicidal (killed) activity against Candida albicans (D'Auria et al., 2005).

Dill: Dill essential oil was demonstrated to induce apoptosis (cell death) in *Candida albicans* in a metacaspase-dependent manner (Chen et al., 2014).

Cilantro: Cilantro essential oil was found to have fungicidal effect against *Candida albicans* and other yeasts. The oil appeared to act by binding to membrane ergosterol, rendering the cell membrane more permeable and ultimately causing cell death (Freires Ide et al., 2014).

Peppermint: Peppermint oil was found to have a higher fungistatic and fungicidal activity against various fungi (including Candida) than the commercial fungicide bifonazole (Mimica-Dukić et al., 2003).

Bergamot: Bergamot essential oil is active in vitro against several common species of ringworm (Sanguinetti et al., 2007).

Rosemary: Rosemary oil was found to inhibit aflatoxin production by aspergillus fungi (a highly toxic and carcinogenic substance produced by these fungi) (Rasooli et al., 2008).

Lemon: Lemon oil was found to be an effective antifungal agent against two bread-mold species (Caccioni et al., 1998).

Cassia: Cassia essential oil was found to have a strong inhibitory effect against *Aspergillus* mold in vitro and in grapes (Kocevski et al., 2013).

Antihemorrhaging
see **Blood:Hemorrhaging**

Antihistamine
see **Allergies**

Anti-Infectious
see **Infection, Antibacterial, Antiviral, Antifungal**

Anti-Inflammatory
see **Inflammation**

Antimicrobial
see **Antibacterial, Antifungal, Antiviral**

Antioxidant

As part of its normal metabolic processes, the body uses and creates oxidative molecules, each capable of transferring electrons to itself from other molecules or substances. This type of reaction can create molecules known as free radicals (Davies, 1995). If left unchecked in the body, these free radicals can bind or react with different molecular structures, altering their abilities to function normally. Under normal, healthy conditions, the body's own systems are able to create or metabolize enough antioxidant materials to neutralize the ability of these oxidative molecules to create free radicals. But when the body comes under stress—including physical stress, psychological stress, poor nutrition, or disease—the amount of oxidative molecules being produced can increase, and the delicate balance between oxidative molecules and antioxidants can be thrown off, potentially overwhelming the body's own antioxidant mechanisms. This "oxidative stress" (Sies, 1997) creates a condition optimal for the formation of many free radicals, which in turn can potentially cause enough damage to the cell's normal structures to cause cell death, mutation, or loss of its ability to function normally within the body (Rhee, 2006; Vertuani et al., 2004).

Oils: ○Cellular Complex, ©©clove©, ○©©thyme©, ©©rosemary©, ©©peppermint©, ©©melaleuca©, ©©helichrysum©, ©©Cleansing Blend, ©©Protective Blend, ©©Respiratory Blend, ©©Soothing Blend, ©cinnamon, ©©frankincense, ©©oregano©, ©©Roman chamomile

> **Other Products:** ○Cellular Vitality Complex or ○Chewable Multivitamin, which contains polyphenols that act as powerful antioxidants, such as quercetin©, epigallocatechin gallate©, ellagic acid©, resveratrol©, baicalin©, and others©. ○Energy & Stamina Complex. ○Fruit & Veggie Drink Mix for a whole food source of essential nutrients and antioxidants.

○: Take capsules as directed. Use oils recommended as flavoring agents in cooking. Place 1–3 drops of oil in an empty capsule, and ingest it as a dietary supplement.

⊘: Diffuse into the air. Inhale directly from bottle. Apply oil to hands, tissue, or cotton wick, and inhale.

⊜: Dilute as recommended, and apply on the skin and reflex points on the feet. Dilute in a carrier oil, and massage into the skin. Apply as a hot compress.

▭: **Additional Research:**

> **Clove:** Clove oil was found to have very strong radical scavenging activity (antioxidant). It was also found to display an antifungal effect against tested Candida strains (Chaieb et al., 2007).
>
> **Clove:** Various essential oils demonstrated an antioxidant effect toward skin lipid squalene oxidized by UV irraditation, with a blend of thyme and clove oil demonstrating the highest inhibitory effect (Wei et al., 2007).
>
> **Thyme:** Extracts from eucalyptus and thyme were found to have high nitrous oxide scavenging abilities and inhibited nitrous oxide production in macrophage cells. This could possibly explain their role in aiding respiratory inflammatory diseases (Vigo et al., 2004).
>
> **Thyme:** Older rats whose diets were supplemented with thyme oil were found to have a higher level of the antioxidant enzymes superoxide dismutase and glutathione peroxidase in the heart, liver, and kidneys than older rats without this supplementation (Youdim et al., 1999).
>
> **Thyme:** Aging rats fed thyme oil or the constituent thymol were found to have higher levels of the antioxidant enzymes superoxide dismutase and glutathione peroxidase in the brain than aging rats not fed the oil or constituent (Youdim et al., 2000).
>
> **Rosemary:** Extracts from rosemary were found to have high antioxidant properties. Rosmarinic acid and carnosic acid from rosemary were found to have the highest antioxidant activities of studied components of rosemary (Almela et al., 2006).

Rosemary: An ethanol extract of rosemary was found to have an antiproliferative effect on human leukemia and breast carcinoma cells, as well as an antioxidant effect (Cheung et al., 2007).

Rosemary: Extracts from rosemary were found to have high antioxidant levels. Additionally, a methanol extract with 30% carnosic acid, 16% carnosol, and 5% rosmarinic acid were found to be effective against gram-positive and negative bacteria, and yeast (Moreno et al., 2006).

Rosemary: In patients with chronic bronchitis, rosemary, basil, fir, and eucalyptus oils were found to demonstrate an antioxidant effect. Lavender was found to promote normalization of lipid levels (Siurin, 1997).

Peppermint: Peppermint oil was found to be an effective antibacterial and antioxidant agent (Mimica-Dukić et al., 2003).

Peppermint: Peppermint oil fed to mice prior to exposure to gamma radiation was found to decrease levels of damage from oxidation when compared to mice not pretreated with peppermint (Samarth et al., 2006).

Peppermint: Peppermint extract fed orally to mice demonstrated the ability to protect the testis from gamma radiation damage (Samarth et al., 2009).

Melaleuca: Melaleuca alternifolia oil was found to reduce reactive oxygen species (ROS) production in neutrophils (a type of white blood cell), indicating an antioxidant effect and decreased Interleukin 2 (a chemical messenger that helps trigger an inflammatory response) secretion, while increasing the secretion of Interleukin 4 (a chemical messenger involved in turning off the inflammatory response) (Caldefie-Chézet et al., 2006).

Melaleuca: Melaleuca alternifolia oil was found to mediate the Reactive Oxygen Species (ROS) production of leukocytes (white blood cells), indicating a possible anti-inflammatory activity (Caldefie-Chézet et al., 2004).

Helichrysum: Arzanol (extracted from helichrysum), at non-cytotoxic concentrations, showed a strong inhibition of TBH-induced oxidative stress in VERO cells (Rosa et al., 2007).

Oregano: The antioxidant activity of oregano essential oil added to extra virgin olive oil at 0.05% was found to retard the lipid oxidation process in olive oil and prolong the olive oil's shelf life (Asensio et al., 2011).

Quercetin: Quercetin was found to increase plasma antioxidant status in healthy volunteers who took it as a supplement over four weeks (Boots et al., 2008).

Epigallocatechin gallate: Epigallocatechin-3-gallate (EGCG) supplementation was found to improve the antioxidant status of heat-stressed Japanese quail (Tuzcu et al., 2008).

Epigallocatechin gallate: Epigallocatechin-3-gallate (EGCG) was found to improve body weight and increase enzymatic and non-enzymatic antioxidants in bleomycin-induced pulmonary fibrosis in rats (Sriram et al., 2008).

Ellagic acid: Ellagic acid supplementation was found to significantly decrease mitochondrial and microsomal lipid peroxidation in endrin-induced hepatic lipid peroxidation (Bagchi et al., 1993).

Resveratrol: Resveratrol was found to act as an antioxidant and to reverse the anti-apoptotic effects of repetitive oxidative stress on lung fibroblasts in vitro (Chakraborty et al., 2008).

Baicalin: Baicalin was found to be an effective antioxidant, and to counteract oxidative stress induced to retinal cells and brain membranes of rats (Jung et al., 2008).

Other Polyphenols: Extracts from bilberry and blueberry were found to have higher ORAC values than strawberry, cranberry, elderberry, or raspberry and were found to significantly inhibit both H2O2 and TNF alpha induced VEGF expression by human keratinocytes (Roy et al., 2002).

Other Polyphenols: Catechins and procyanidins extracted from various berries were found to provide substantial antioxidant protection (Maatta-Riihinet et al., 2005).

Other Polyphenols: Oral supplementation of bilberry extract was found to reduce the degree of oxidative stress and kidney damage by potassium bromate oxidization in mice (Bao et al., 2008).

Antiparasitic

see **Parasites**

Antirheumatic

see **Arthritis:Rheumatoid Arthritis**

Antiseptic

see **Antibacterial, Antifungal, Antiviral**

Antiviral

The term "antiviral" refers to something that is able to inhibit or stop the development, function, or replication of an infection-causing virus.

Oils: ☺⊘helichrysum⊙, ☺⊘melaleuca⊙, ☺⊘clove⊙, ☺⊘Protective Blend, ☺⊘melissa⊙, ⊘Respiratory Blend, ☺⊘lime, ☺cinnamon, ⊘lemon, ☺⊘oregano, ☺⊘peppermint⊙, ⊘⊘eucalyptus⊙, ☺thyme, ⊘orange, ⊘grapefruit, ☺⊘clary sage, ☺⊘juniper berry, ☺⊘myrrh, ☺⊘geranium, ☺⊘lavender, ☺⊘sandalwood, ☺rosemary, ☺⊘cypress

Other Products: OProtective Softgels, ⊘Protective Hand Wash to help protect against skin-borne microorganisms, ⊘Protective Cleaner to help eliminate microorganisms from household surfaces. OProtective Throat Drops to soothe irritated and sore throats. OCellular Vitality Complex, OChewable Multivitamin, OEssential Oil Omega Complex or Vegan Essential Oil Omega Complex, OOmega-3 Fish Oil, OFood Nutrient Complex to help support the immune system.

—Airborne Viruses:

  Oils: ⊘Protective Blend

—Ebola Virus:

  Oils: ☺cinnamon, ☺oregano

—Epstein-Barr Virus:

  Oils: ☺Protective Blend

—Herpes Simplex:

  Oils: ☺peppermint⊙, ☺clove⊙, ☺helichrysum⊙, ☺melaleuca⊙, ☺lavender, ☺eucalyptus, ☺cypress, ☺lemon

—HIV: *see also AIDS*

  Oils: ☺⊘helichrysum, ☺Protective Blend, ☺⊘lemon, ☺Grounding Blend

—Respiratory:

  Oils: ⊘eucalyptus, ⊘Protective Blend

—Spine:

  Blend 1: 5 drops oregano and 5 drops thyme. Apply to bottoms of feet and along the spine.

☻: Dilute as recommended, and apply on location or to reflex points on the bottoms of the feet. Use hand wash as directed on packaging.

⊘: Diffuse into the air. Inhale oil applied to a tissue or cotton wick.

◯: Take capsules as directed on package.

▣: **Additional Research:**

  Helichrysum: Arzanol, extracted from helichrysum, inhibited HIV-1 replication in T cells and also inhibited the release of pro-inflammatory cytokines (chemical messengers) in monocytes (Appendino et al., 2007).

  Helichrysum: Helichrysum was found to have significant antiviral activity against the herpes virus at non-cytotoxic concentrations (Nostro et al., 2003).

  Melaleuca: Tea tree and eucalyptus oil demonstrated an ability to inhibit the Herpes simplex virus (Schnitzler et al., 2001).

  Clove: Eugenol (found in clove oil) was found to be virucidal to Herpes simplex and to delay the development of herpes-induced keratitis (inflammation of the cornea) in mice (Benencia et al., 2000).

Melissa: Melissa oil demonstrated inhibition of Herpes simplex type 1 and 2 viruses (Schnitzler et al., 2008).

Peppermint: Peppermint oil demonstrated a direct virucidal activity against herpes type 1 and 2 viruses (Schuhmacher et al., 2003).

Eucalyptus: Tea tree and eucalyptus oil demonstrated an ability to inhibit the Herpes simplex virus (Schnitzler et al., 2001).

Menthol, thymol, methyl salicylate, and eucalyptol: A trial including 80 subjects with *Herpes labialis* showed that rinsing with an essential oil containing mouthrinse resulted in effectively zero recoverable virions at 30 seconds post rinse and a significant reduction in saliva viral presence 30 minutes post rinse, suggesting that an essential oil mouthrinse can reduce viral contamination of saliva (Meiller et al., 2005).

Anxiety

Anxiety is the body's way of preparing itself to deal with a threat or to deal with future stressful events. While this response is normal and happens as part of the body's natural response to stress, this response can also happen at inappropriate times or too frequently, as in the case of anxiety disorders. Anxiety can include both physical and mental symptoms such as fear, nervousness, nausea, sweating, increased blood pressure and heart rate, feelings of apprehension or dread, difficulty concentrating, irritability, restlessness, panic attacks, and many others.

Oils: lavender, orange, lemon, Focus Blend, Calming Blend, Massage Blend, Joyful Blend, Grounding Blend (on back of neck) and Respiratory Blend (on chest), ylang ylang, melissa, frankincense, sandalwood, cedarwood, juniper berry Invigorating Blend, bergamot, geranium, lime, clary sage, rose, basil, cypress, marjoram

Other Products: Therapeutic Bath Salts. Add 1–2 drops of essential oil to 1/4 cup bath salts, and dissolve in warm bathwater for an anxiety-relieving bath.

⟳: Diffuse into the air. Inhale directly from bottle. Apply oil to hands, tissue, or cotton wick, and inhale.

◠: Place 1–2 drops in 1 Tbs. fractionated coconut oil and massage into the skin. Dilute as recommended, and apply to back of neck, temples, or reflex points on feet. Add 1–2 drops to 1/4 cup bath salts, and dissolve in warm bathwater.

◌: **Additional Research:**

Lavender: Exposure to lavender odor was found to decrease anxiety in gerbils in the elevated plus maze, with a further decrease in anxiety in females after prolonged (2 week) exposure (Bradley et al., 2007).

Lavender: Subjects receiving a lozenge containing lavender oil, hops extract, lemon balm, and oat were found to have increases in alpha 1, alpha 2, and beta 1 electrical output (Dimpfel et al., 2004).

Lavender: In patients admitted to an intensive care unit, those receiving lavender aromatherapy reported a greater improvement in mood and perceived levels of anxiety compared to those receiving massage or a period of rest (Dunn et al., 1995).

Lavender: Female patients being treated for chronic hemodialysis demonstrated less anxiety when exposed to lavender aroma compared to control (Itai et al., 2000).

Lavender: Lavender oil was found to demonstrate anticonflict effects in mice similar to the anxiolytic (antianxiety) drug diazepam (Umezu, 2000).

Lavender: Patients waiting for dental treatment were found to be less anxious and to have a better mood when exposed to the odor of lavender or orange oil as compared to control (Lehrner et al., 2005).

Lavender and Roman Chamomile: A study with 56 percutaneous coronary intervention patients in an intensive care unit found that an aromatherapy blend of lavender, Roman chamomile, and neroli decreased anxiety and improved sleep quality when compared to conventional nursing intervention (Cho et al., 2013).

Orange: Patients waiting for dental treatment were found to be less anxious and to have a better mood when exposed to the odor of lavender or orange oil as compared to control (Lehrner et al., 2005).

Orange: Bitter orange peel oil taken orally by mice was found to reduce anxiety, increase sleeping time, and increase the time before a chemically-induced seizure started (Carvalho-Freitas et al., 2002).

Orange: Female patients waiting for dental treatment were found to be less anxious, more positive, and more calm when exposed to orange oil odor than patients who were not exposed to the orange oil odor (Lehrner et al., 2000).

Orange: Dental patients (aged 6-9 years) displayed reduce salivary cortisol, pulse rate, and anxiety while undergoing dental treatments when inhaling wild orange essential oil, compared to no aroma (Jafarzadeh et al., 2013).

Orange: Healthy male subjects displayed reduced anxiety after five minutes of inhalation of orange essential oil compared to the inhalation of melaleuca essential oil or distilled water when submitted to an anxiety inducing situation (Goes et al., 2012).

Orange: Rats subjected to the elevated plus-maze following exposure to the aroma of orange essential oil for five minutes displayed reduced anxiety as compared to exposure to melaleuca essential oil (Faturi et al., 2010).

Lemon: Rats exposed long-term to lemon essential oil were found to demonstrate different anxiety and pain threshold levels than untreated rats. It was also found that exposure to lemon oil induced chemical changes in the neuronal circuits involved in anxiety and pain (Ceccarelli et al., 2004).

Lemon: Lemon oil was found to have an antistress effect on mice involved in several behavioral tasks (Komiya et al., 2006).

Melissa: Results of a clinical trial indicate that a combination of melissa and valerian oils may have anxiety-reducing properties at some doses (Kennedy et al., 2006).

Bergamot: Inhalation of bergamot essential oil produced similar anxiolytic results as acute injection of an antianxiety drug, diazepam, administered to mice subjected to two behavioral measurements of anxiety (the elevated plus maze test and the hole-board test) (Saiyudthong et al., 2011). Bergamot essential oil also reduced the corticosterone response to stress exposure of the mice (Saiyudthong et al., 2011).

Clary Sage: Dietary administration of clary sage oil (from conception) was found to have an anti-anxiety and submissive effect on mice, when compared to administration of sunflower oil (from conception and weaning) and clary sage (from weaning) (Gross et al., 2013).

Cassia: A single treatment of cassia extract decreased anxiety in mice by causing a change of serotonin receptors in the dorsal raphe nucleus (Jung et al., 2012).

Cypress: In rats, *Chamaecyparis obtusa* essential oil (a Japanese plant belonging to the same botanical family as cypress essential oil) decreased anxiety-related behaviors caused by the early life stress of maternal separation. This decrease in anxiety was comparable to the effects of fluoxetine, a drug commonly used to treat depression and anxiety disorders. The same study found that cytokine gene expression in the hippocampus was altered by the inhalation of *Chamaecyparis obtusa* (Park et al., 2014).

Aromatherapy Massage: Results from a randomized, controlled trial suggest that aromatherapy massage can be an effective therapeutic option for the short-term management of mild to moderate anxiety and depression in patients with cancer (Wilkinson et al., 2007).

Carvacrol in thyme and oregano: Carvacrol is a monoterpenic phenol found in thyme and oregano. Oral administration of carvacrol produced antianxiety-like effects in mice (Melo et al., 2010).

Apathy
see **Depression**

Aphrodisiac

An Aphrodisiac is a substance used to stimulate feelings of love or sexual desire. Many books of aromatherapy tout the aphrodisiac qualities of a number of oils. Perhaps an aphrodisiac to one individual may not be to another. The most important factor is to find an oil that brings balance to the mind and body. A balanced individual is more likely to extend love.

Oils: ⊘◯sandalwood, ⊘◯ylang ylang, ⊘◯rose, ⊘◯jasmine, ⊘◯Women's Blend, ⊘cinnamon, ⊘◯ginger, ⊘◯clary sage

🕭: Diffuse into the air. Dissolve 2–3 drops in 2 tsp. pure grain or perfumers alcohol, combine with distilled water in a 1 or 2 oz. spray bottle, and spray into the air or on clothes or bed linens.

🖐: Dilute as recommended and wear on temples, neck, or wrists as a perfume or cologne. Combine 3–5 drops of your desired essential oil with 1 Tbs. fractionated coconut oil to use as a massage oil. Combine 1–2 drops with 1/4 cup Therapeutic Bath Salts, and dissolve in warm bathwater for a romantic bath.

Appetite

Appetite is the body's desire to eat, expressed as hunger. Appetite is important in regulating food intake to provide the body with the necessary nutrients to sustain life and maintain energy.

—Loss of Appetite:

   Oils: ⊘lavender◌, ⊘ginger, ⊘lemon, ⊘orange

—Suppressant:

   Oils: O⊘Metabolic Blend, ⊘grapefruit◌

   Other Products: OTrim Shakes

○: Add 8 drops of Metabolic Blend to 16 oz. of water, and drink throughout the day between meals. Drink Trim or V Shake 1–2 times a day as a meal alternative.

⊘: Diffuse into the air. Inhale oil applied to a tissue or cotton wick.

⊡: **Additional Research:**

   Lavender: Lavender oil was found to inhibit sympathetic nerve activity while exciting parasympathetic nerve activity and increasing appetite and weight gain in rats. Linalool, a component of lavender, was shown to have similar effects (Shen et al., 2005).

   Grapefruit: The scent of grapefruit oil and its component, limonene, was found to affect the autonomic nerves by exciting sympathetic nerve activity and inhibiting parasympathetic nerve activity. It was also found to reduce appetite and body weight in rats exposed to the oil for 15 minutes three times per week (Shen et al., 2005).

Arteries

See also **Blood, Cardiovascular System**

Arteries are the vessels of the circulatory system that function to carry blood away from the heart.

—Arterial Vasodilator:

   A vasodilator is a substance that causes a blood vessel to dilate (increase in diameter) through the relaxation of the endothelial cells lining the vessel walls. This gives the blood more room to flow and lowers blood pressure.

   Oils: ⊙eucalyptus◌, ⊙rosemary◌, ⊙marjoram

—Atherosclerosis:

   Atherosclerosis is a hardening of the arteries due to a build-up of plaques along the arterial wall.

   Oils: ⊙⊘lemon◌,⊘lavender◌, ⊙rosemary, ⊙ginger, ⊙cedarwood, ⊙thyme, ⊙juniper berry, ⊙wintergreen

⊜: Dilute as recommended, and apply to carotid arteries in neck, over heart, and reflex points on the feet.

⊘: Diffuse into the air. Inhale directly from bottle. Apply oil to hands, tissue, or cotton wick, and inhale.

⊡: **Additional Research:**

   Eucalyptus: Treatment of rats with 1,8-cineole (or eucalyptol found in eucalyptus and rosemary) demonstrated an ability to lower mean aortic pressure (blood pressure), without decreasing heart rate, through vascular wall relaxation (Lahlou et al., 2002).

Rosemary: Treatment of rats with 1,8-cineole (or eucalyptol found in eucalyptus and rosemary) demonstrated an ability to lower mean aortic pressure (blood pressure), without decreasing heart rate, through vascular wall relaxation (Lahlou et al., 2002).

Lemon: Lemon oil and one of its components, gamma-terpinene, were found to inhibit oxidation of low-density lipoprotein (LDL). Oxidation of LDL has been found to increase the risk of atherosclerosis and cardiac disease (Grassmann et al., 2001).

Lavender: Inhalation of lavender and monarda oils was found to reduce cholesterol content and atherosclerotic plaques in the aorta (Nikolaevskiĭ et al., 1990).

Arthritis

see also **Inflammation, Joints**

Arthritis is the painful swelling, inflammation, and stiffness of the joints.

Oils: ⊜❷frankincense⊡, ⊜❷rosemary⊡, ⊜❷marjoram⊡, ⊜Soothing Blend, ⊜❷eucalyptus⊡, ⊜❷white fir, ⊜❷peppermint⊡, ⊜❷lavender⊡, ⊜❷cypress, ⊜❷juniper berry, ⊜❷ginger, ⊜❷Roman chamomile, ⊜❷helichrysum, ⊜❷cedarwood, ⊜❷wintergreen, ⊜❷basil, ⊜❷clove⊡

Blend 1: Combine equal parts wintergreen and Soothing Blend. Apply on location.

Other Products: ⊙Cellular Vitality Complex⊡

—Arthritic Pain:

Oils: ⊜Soothing Blend, ⊜wintergreen, ⊜ginger

—Osteoarthritis:

Osteoarthritis is a degenerative arthritis where the cartilage that provides lubrication between the bones in a joint begins to break down, becoming rough and uneven. This causes the bones in the joint to wear and create rough deposits that can become extremely painful.

Oils: ⊜rosemary, ⊜marjoram, ⊜Soothing Blend, ⊜geranium, ⊜wintergreen, ⊜thyme, ⊜basil, ⊜lavender, ⊜eucalyptus

Other Products: ⊙Cellular Vitality Complex

—Rheumatoid Arthritis:

Rheumatoid arthritis is arthritis caused by inflammation within the joint, causing pain and possibly causing the joint to degenerate.

Oils: ⊜marjoram, ⊜lavender, ⊜cypress, ⊜Soothing Blend, ⊜geranium, ⊜bergamot, ⊜clove⊡, ⊜ginger⊡, ⊜lemon, ⊜rosemary, ⊜wintergreen, ⊜cinnamon⊡, ⊜eucalyptus, ⊜oregano (chronic), ⊜peppermint, ⊜❷Roman chamomile, ⊜thyme

Other Products: ⊙Cellular Vitality Complex⊡

🜄: Dilute as recommended, and apply on location. Apply as a warm compress over affected area. Dilute 1–2 drops in 1 Tbs. fractionated coconut oil, and use as a massage oil. Add 1–2 drops to 1/4 cup Therapeutic Bath Salts, and dissolve in warm bathwater for a soaking bath.

🜁: Diffuse into the air.

🜂: **Additional Research:**

Frankincense: An acetone extract of frankincense was found to decrease arthritic scores, reduce paw edema (swelling) and suppress pro-inflammatory cytokines (cellular messengers) (Fan et al., 2005).

Rosemary: In patients suffering from arthritis, it was found that a blend of lavender, marjoram, eucalyptus, rosemary, and peppermint blended with carrier oils reduced perceived pain and depression compared to control (Kim et al., 2005).

Marjoram: In patients suffering from arthritis, it was found that a blend of lavender, marjoram, eucalyptus, rosemary, and peppermint blended with carrier oils reduced perceived pain and depression compared to control (Kim et al., 2005).

Eucalyptus: In patients suffering from arthritis, it was found that a blend of lavender, marjoram, euca-lyptus, rosemary, and peppermint blended with carrier oils reduced perceived pain and depression compared to control (Kim et al., 2005).

Peppermint: In patients suffering from arthritis, it was found that a blend of lavender, marjoram, euca-lyptus, rosemary, and peppermint blended with carrier oils reduced perceived pain and depression compared to control (Kim et al., 2005).

Lavender: In patients suffering from arthritis, it was found that a blend of lavender, marjoram, euca-lyptus, rosemary, and peppermint blended with carrier oils reduced perceived pain and depression compared to control (Kim et al., 2005).

Cellular Vitality Complex: Epigallocatechin-3-gallate was found to ameliorate experimental rheumatoid arthritis in the short term (Morinobu et al., 2008).

Clove: Eugenol and ginger oil taken orally were found to reduce paw and joint swelling in rats with induced severe arthritis (Sharma et al., 1994).

Ginger: Eugenol and ginger oil taken orally were found to reduce paw and joint swelling in rats with induced severe arthritis (Sharma et al., 1994).

Eugenol (found in cassia, cinnamon, and clove): Eugenol was found to ameliorate experimental arthritis in mice by inhibit-ing mononuclear cell infiltration into the knee joints and lowering cytokine levels (Grespan et al., 2012).

Cinnamon: The polyphenol fraction from cinnamon bark was found to improve inflammation and pain in animal models of inflammation and rheumatoid arthritis (Rathi et al., 2013).

Coriander: Coriander extract produced a dose dependent inhibition of joint swelling in two mice models of induced arthritis (Nair et al., 2012).

Asthma

Asthma is a disease that causes the lung's airways to narrow, making it difficult to breathe. Episodes (or attacks) of asthma can be triggered by any number of things, including smoke, pollution, dust mites, and other allergens. Asthma causes reoccurring periods of tightness in the chest, coughing, shortness of breath, and wheezing.

Oils: eucalyptus, frankincense, peppermint, thyme, Respiratory Blend, oregano, lemon, myrrh, lavender, geranium, cy-press, clary sage, ylang ylang, rose, helichrysum, marjoram, rosemary

—Attack

Oils: Respiratory Blend, eucalyptus, frankincense (calming), lavender, marjoram

: Diffuse into the air. Inhale directly from bottle. Apply oil to hands, tissue, or cotton wick, and inhale.

: Dilute as recommended and apply to the chest, throat, or back. Add 2–3 drops to 1 Tbs. fractionated coconut oil, and massage onto chest, shoulders, and back.

: **Additional Research:**

Eucalyptus: Extracts from eucalyptus and thyme were found to have high nitrous oxide (NO) scavenging abilities and in-hibited NO production in macrophage cells. This could possibly explain their role in aiding respiratory inflammatory diseases (Vigo et al., 2004).

Eucalyptus: Therapy with 1,8 cineole (eucalyptol, found in eucalyptus) in both healthy and bronchitis-afflicted humans was shown to reduce production of LTB4 and PGE2, both metabolites of arachidonic acid (a known chemical messenger involved in inflammation), in white blood cells (Juergens et al., 1998).

Peppermint: L-menthol (found in peppermint) was found to inhibit production of inflammation mediators in human monocytes (a type of white blood cell involved in the immune response) (Juergens et al., 1998).

Lavender: Long-term inhalation of lavender oil was found to suppress allergic airway inflammation and mucous cell hyperplasia in a mouse model of acute asthma (Ueno-Iio et al., 2014).

Laurel Leaf (Bay) in Respiratory Blend: Magnolialide, extracted from laurel leaf, was found to inhibit key factors in the development and amplification of type I hypersensitivity responses (implicated in the cause of allergic asthma)(Lee, T. et al., 2013).

Athlete's Foot
see **Antifungal:Athlete's Foot**

Attention Deficit Disorder
see **ADD/ADHD**

Autism

Autism is a developmental disorder that impairs the normal development of communication, sociality, and human interaction.

—**Reduce Anxiety/Fear:** *see also* **Anxiety**

Oils: ⬭geranium, ⬭clary sage, ⬭bergamot

—**Stimulate the Senses:** *see also* **Stimulating**

Oils: ⬭peppermint, ⬭basil, ⬭lemon, ⬭rosemary

⬭: Add 1–2 drops to 1 Tbs. fractionated coconut oil, and massage into skin.

Comments: Only apply these oils when the autistic child is willing and open to receive them. If the experience is forced or negative, the autistic child will associate these oils with a negative experience when used again.

Auto-Immune Diseases
see **Grave's Disease, Hashimoto's Disease, Lupus**

Awake
see **Alertness, Jet Lag**

Babies
see **Children and Infants**

Back

Oils: ⬭Soothing Blend, ⬭Grounding Blend, ⬭cypress, ⬭eucalyptus, ⬭geranium, ⬭lavender, ⬭Roman chamomile, ⬭oregano, ⬭peppermint, ⬭rosemary, ⬭juniper berry, ⬭thyme

—**Calcified Spine**

Calcification occurs when calcium builds up in tissue and causes the tissue to harden. As people age, calcification can cause the ligaments of the spine to thicken and harden, making the spinal canal narrow and create pressure on the spinal nerve.

Oils: ⬭Soothing Blend, ⬭geranium, ⬭rosemary

—**Deteriorating Spine:**

Deteriorating disc disease occurs as people age and their spinal discs begin to deteriorate. As deterioration progresses, movement becomes restricted and pain in the neck and back increases. Although most commonly associated with aging, disc deterioration can be caused by back injuries as well.

Oils: ⚬Soothing Blend

—Herniated Discs:

In between the bones of the spine are cushioning discs that keep the spine flexible and act as shock absorbers. A herniated disc is caused when one of the discs of the spine is damaged and either bulges or breaks open. When the herniated disc presses on a nerve, it causes pain in the buttock, thigh, and calf. Herniated discs can be caused by spinal injuries or by the wear and tear that come with age as the discs begin to dry out

Oils: ⚬Soothing Blend, ⚬Grounding Blend (3 drops on location), ⚬peppermint, ⚬cypress (strengthens blood capillary walls, improves circulation, anti-inflammatory)

—Lumbago/Lower Back Pain:

Oils: ⚬sandalwood, ⚬Soothing Blend

—Muscular Fatigue:

Oils: ⚬clary sage, ⚬marjoram, ⚬lavender, ⚬rosemary

—Pain:

Oils: ⚬Grounding Blend, ⚬Soothing Blend

Blend 1: Combine 5–10 drops each of lavender, eucalyptus, and ginger, and apply 2–3 drops on location or as a warm compress.

Blend 2: Combine 5–10 drops each of peppermint, rosemary, and basil, and apply 2–3 drops on location or as a warm compress.

—Stiffness:

Oils: ⚬marjoram, ⚬Grounding Blend

—Viruses Along Spine:

Oils: ⚬oregano, ⚬eucalyptus

⚬: Dilute as recommended, and apply along the spine, on affected muscles, or on reflex points on the feet. Dilute 1–3 drops in 1 Tbs. fractionated coconut oil, and massage into muscles on the back or along the spine. Apply as a warm compress over affected area.

Bacteria

see Antibacterial

Balance

Oils: ⚬⚭Grounding Blend, ⚬⚭frankincense, ⚬⚭vetiver, ⚬⚭ylang ylang, ⚭cedarwood

—Electrical Energies:

Oils: ⚬Grounding Blend, ⚬frankincense

Application Methods:

⚬: Dilute as recommended, and apply on location. Apply 3–6 drops of Grounding Blend to the bottom of each foot, and, if desired, apply some to the neck and shoulders. Hold the palm of each hand to the bottom of each corresponding foot (left to left and right to right) for 5–15 minutes to help balance electrical energies.

❷: Diffuse into the air.

Baldness
see Hair:Loss

Bath

Using essential oils in the bath can be a wonderful way to receive and possibly enhance the benefits of the oils.

Oils: ⊙lavender, ⊙geranium, ⊙Roman chamomile, ⊙ylang ylang

Some common ways to use essential oils in the bath include the following:

Direct: Add 1–3 drops of oil directly to bathwater while the bath is filling. Oils will be drawn to your skin quickly from the top of the water, so use non-irritating oils such as lavender, ylang ylang, etc., or dilute the oil with fractionated coconut oil to safe topical application dilutions.

Bath Gel: To disperse the oil throughout the bathwater, add 5–10 drops of your favorite essential oil to one-half ounce of unscented bath and shower gel.

Bath Salts: For a relaxing mineral bath, add 1–5 drops of your desired essential oil to 1/4–1/2 cup of Therapeutic Bath Salts or Epsom salts; mix well. Dissolve salts in warm bathwater while the tub is filling.

Bed Wetting
see Bladder:Bed Wetting

Bell's Palsy
see Nervous System:Bell's Palsy

Birthing
see Pregnancy/Motherhood

Bites/Stings
see also Insects/Bugs:Repellent

Oils: ⊙thyme, ⊙basil, ⊙lemon, ⊙cinnamon, ⊙lavender

—Allergic:
   Oils: ⊙Cleansing Blend

—Bees and Hornets
   Oils: ⊙Roman chamomile, ⊙basil, ⊙Cleansing Blend, ⊙lavender, ⊙lemongrass, ⊙lemon, ⊙peppermint, ⊙thyme

   Recipe 1: Remove the stinger, and apply a cold compress of Roman chamomile to the area for several hours or for as long as possible.

—Gnats and Midges:
   Oils: ⊙lavender

Recipe 2: Mix 3 drops thyme in 1 tsp. cider vinegar or lemon juice. Apply to bites to stop irritation.

—Mosquitoes:

Oils: ☺lavender, ☺helichrysum

—Snakes:

Oils: ☺basil

—Spiders:

Oils: ☺basil, ☺Cleansing Blend (with melaleuca), ☺lavender, ☺lemongrass, ☺lemon, ☺peppermint, ☺thyme

Recipe 3: Mix 3 drops lavender and 2 drops Roman chamomile with 1 tsp. alcohol. Apply to area three times per day.

—Ticks:

Oils: After getting the tick out, apply 1 drop lavender every 5 minutes for 30 minutes:

Removing Ticks:

Do not apply mineral oil, Vaseline, or anything else to remove the tick, as this may cause it to inject the spirochetes into the wound.

Be sure to remove the entire tick. Get as close to the mouth as possible, and firmly tug on the tick until it releases its grip. Don't twist. If available, use a magnifying glass to make sure that you have removed the entire tick.

Save the tick in a jar, and label it with the date, where you were bitten on your body, and the location or address where you were bitten for proper identification by your doctor, especially if you develop any symptoms.

Do not handle the tick.

Wash hands immediately.

Check the site of the bite occasionally to see if any rash develops. If it does, seek medical advice promptly.

—Wasps:

Recipe 4: Combine 1 drop basil, 2 drops Roman chamomile, 2 drops lavender, and 1 tsp. apple cider vinegar. Apply to area three times a day.

☺: Dilute as recommended, and apply on location.

Bladder

see also **Urinary Tract**

The Urinary Bladder is a hollow organ that collects urine before it is disposed by urination. The bladder sits on the pelvic floor.

—Bed Wetting and Incontinence:

Oils: ☺cypress (rub on abdomen at bedtime), ☺ylang ylang☺.

—Cystitis/Infection:

Oils: ⊖lemongrass, O⊕Protective Blend, ⊖sandalwood, ⊖juniper berry, ⊖thyme, ⊖cedarwood, ⊖basil, ⊖cinnamon, ⊖clove, ⊖eucalyptus, ⊖frankincense, ⊖lavender, ⊖bergamot, ⊖fennel, ⊖marjoram, ⊖oregano

Other Products: OProtective Softgels

⊖: Dilute as recommended, and apply on abdomen and on reflex points on the feet. Add 1–2 drops to warm bathwater; bathe for 10–15 minutes.

○: Add 1 drop to 8 oz. juice or water; drink three times a day.

⊡: **Additional Research:**

Ylang ylang: Ylang ylang oil induced relaxation in rat (in vitro) and rabbit (in vivo) bladder smooth muscle, suggesting that ylang ylang may be effective at alleviating an overactive bladder (Kim et al., 2003).

Bleeding
see Blood:Bleeding

Blister (on lips from sun)

Oils: ⊖lavender

⊖: Apply oil to blister often to help take the fever out and return the lip to normal.

Bloating
see Digestive System:Bloating

Blood

Blood is the fluid inside the body that transports oxygen and nutrients to the cells and carries waste away from the cells. It also transports cells involved in the immune and inflammatory response, hormones and other chemical messengers that regulate the body's functions, and platelets that help facilitate the blood clotting necessary to repair damaged blood vessels. Blood is primarily composed of plasma (water with dissolved nutrients, minerals, and carbon dioxide) that carries red blood cells (the most numerous type of cells in blood, responsible for transporting oxygen), white blood cells (cells involved in the immune system and immune response), and platelet cells. Blood is circulated in the body by the pumping action of the heart propelling blood through various blood vessels. Proper and healthy circulation and function of blood throughout the body is critical for health and even for the sustaining of life.

—Blood Pressure

Oils: Olemon (will regulate pressure—either raise or lower as necessary), ⊖⊘lime

—High (hypertension)

Oils: ⊘⊘ylang ylang⊡, ⊘⊘marjoram⊡, ⊘⊘eucalyptus⊡, ⊘⊘lavender, ⊘clove, ⊖⊘clary sage, ⊖⊘lemon, ⊖⊘wintergreen **Note:** Avoid rosemary, thyme, and possibly peppermint.

Bath 1: Place 3 drops ylang ylang and 3 drops marjoram in bathwater, and bathe in the evening twice a week.

Blend 1: Combine 10 drops ylang ylang, 5 drops marjoram, and 5 drops cypress in 1 oz. fractionated coconut oil. Rub over heart and reflex points on left foot and hand.

Blend 2: Combine 5 drops geranium, 8 drops lemongrass, and 3 drops lavender in 1 oz. fractionated coconut oil. Rub over heart and reflex points on left foot and hand.

–Low

Oils: ⊘☺rosemary☺

☻: Diffuse into the air. Inhale the aroma directly.

◯: Place 1–2 drops of oil under the tongue or place 1–3 drops of oil in an empty capsule; ingest up to 3 times per day.

☻: Dilute as recommended, and apply on location, on reflex points on feet and hands, and over heart.

—Bleeding (stops):

Oils: ☺helichrysum, ☺geranium, ☺rose

☻: Dilute as recommended, and apply on location.

—Broken Blood Vessels

Oils: ☺helichrysum, ☺grapefruit

☻: Dilute as recommended, and apply on location, on reflex points on feet and hands, and over heart.

—Cholesterol:

Cholesterol is a soft, waxy substance found in the bloodstream and in all of the body's cells. The body requires some cholesterol to function properly, but high levels of cholesterol narrow and block the arteries and increase the risk of heart disease.

Oils: ☺helichrysum

☻: Dilute as recommended, and apply on reflex points on feet and hands, and over heart.

—Circulation: *see Cardiovascular System*

—Cleansing

Oils: ☺helichrysum, ☺geranium, ☺Roman chamomile

☻: Dilute as recommended, and apply on reflex points on feet and hands, and over heart.

—Clots:

Blood Clots occur as a natural bodily defense to repair damaged blood vessels and to keep the body from losing excessive amounts of blood. However, clotting can become dangerous if an internal blood clot breaks lose in the circulatory system and blocks the flow of blood to vital organs.

Oils: ☺◯clove☺, ◯☺⊘fennel☺, ☺⊘thyme, ☺grapefruit

◯: Place 1–2 drops of oil under the tongue or place 1–3 drops of oil in an empty capsule; ingest up to 3 times per day.

☻: Dilute as recommended, and apply on location, on reflex points on feet and hands, and over heart.

☻: Diffuse into the air. Inhale the aroma directly.

—Hemorrhaging:

Hemorrhaging is excessive or uncontrollable blood loss.

Oils: ⊘helichrysum, ⊘ylang ylang, ⊘rose

⊜: Dilute as recommended, and apply on location.

—Low Blood Sugar:

The term "blood sugar" refers to the amount of glucose in the bloodstream. When the blood glucose drops below its normal level, this is called "low blood sugar" or "hypoglycemia." Since glucose is such an important source of energy for the body, low blood sugar can result in light-headedness, hunger, shakiness, weakness, confusion, nervousness, difficulty speaking, and anxiety.

Oils: ⊘Protective Blend, ⊘cinnamon, ⊘clove, ⊘thyme

Other Products: ⊙Protective Softgels

⊜: Dilute as recommended, and apply on location, on reflex points on feet and hands, and over heart.

—Stimulates Blood Cell Production

Oils: ⊙⊘peppermint⊙, ⊙⊘lemon

◯: Place 1–2 drops of oil under the tongue or place 1–3 drops of oil in an empty capsule; ingest up to 3 times per day. Take supplement as directed.

⊜: Dilute as recommended, and apply on location, on reflex points on feet and hands, and over heart.

—Vessels: *see Arteries, Capillaries, Veins*

⬚: **Additional Research:**

Ylang ylang: Subjects who had ylang ylang oil applied to their skin had decreased blood pressure, increased skin temperature, and reported feeling more calm and relaxed than did subjects in a control group (Hongratanaworakit et al., 2006).

Ylang ylang: Inhaled ylang ylang oil was found to decrease blood pressure and pulse rate and to enhance attentiveness and alertness in volunteers compared to an odorless control (Hongratanaworakit et al., 2004).

Ylang ylang, lavender, marjoram: Eighty-three hypertensive or prehypertensive subjects were divided into the following three groups: a study group (exposed to an essential oil blend containing lavender, ylang ylang, marjoram, and neroli), a placebo group (exposed to artificial fragrance), and a control group (no interventions). The study group was found to have an immediate and long-term decrease in home blood pressure (Kim et al., 2012).

Marjoram: Treatment of rats with 1,8-cineole (or eucalyptol, found in eucalyptus, rosemary, and marjoram) demonstrated an ability to lower mean aortic pressure (blood pressure), without decreasing heart rate, through vascular wall relaxation (Lahlou et al., 2002).

Eucalyptus: Treatment of rats with 1,8-cineole (or eucalyptol, found in eucalyptus, rosemary, and marjoram) demonstrated an ability to lower mean aortic pressure (blood pressure), without decreasing heart rate, through vascular wall relaxation (Lahlou et al., 2002).

Rosemary: Oral treatment with rosemary essential oil on primary hypotensive subjects was found to increase blood pressure values when compared to the subjects' placebo treatments before and after rosemary treatment (Fernández et al., 2014).

Clove: Clove oil demonstrated an ability to prevent the aggregation of platelets that can lead to blood clots and thrombosis both in vivo and in vitro (Saeed et al., 1994).

Fennel: Both fennel oil and its constituent, anethole, were found to significantly reduce thrombosis (blood clots) in mice. They were also found to be free from the prohemorrhagic (increased bleeding) side effect that aspirin (acetylsalicylic acid) has (Tognolini et al., 2007).

Peppermint: In mice exposed to whole-body gamma irradiation, only 17% of mice who had been fed peppermint oil died, while 100% of mice who did not receive peppermint oil died. It was also found that the mice pre-fed peppermint oil were able to return blood cell levels to normal after 30 days, while the control mice were not able to (and consequently died), suggesting a protective or stimulating effect of the oil on blood stem cells (Samarth et al., 2004).

Body Systems

see **Cardiovascular System, Digestive System, Endocrine System, Lymphatic System, Muscles/Connective Tissue, Bones, Nervous System, Respiratory System, Skin**

Boils

see also **Antibacterial**

A boil is a skin infection that forms in a hair follicle or oil gland. The boil starts as a red, tender lump that after a few days forms a white or yellow point in the center as it fills with pus. Boils commonly occur on the face, neck, armpits, buttock, and shoulders and can be very painful.

Oils: ⊘melaleuca⊘, ⊘lavender, ⊘Cleansing Blend, ⊘lemongrass, ⊘lemon, ⊘frankincense, ⊘clary sage

⊘: Dilute as recommended, and apply on location.

⊙: **Additional Research:**

> **Melaleuca:** In a human trial, most patients receiving treatment with Melaleuca alternifolia oil placed topically on boils experienced healing or reduction of symptoms; while of those receiving no treatment (control), half required surgical intervention, and all still demonstrated signs of the infection (Feinblatt, 1960).

Bones

Oils: ⊘wintergreen, ⊘white fir, ⊘cypress, ⊘juniper berry, ⊘⊘cedarwood, ⊘lavender, ⊘lemongrass, ⊘marjoram, ⊘peppermint, ⊘sandalwood

Other Products: ⊙Food Nutrient Complex contains nutrients essential for bone development, such as calcium, magnesium, zinc, and vitamin D.

—Bone Spurs:

A bone spur (osteophyte) is a bony projection formed on a normal bone. Bone spurs form as the body tries to repair itself by building extra bone in response to continued pressure, stress, or rubbing. Bone spurs can cause pain if they rub against soft tissues or other bones.

Oils: ⊘wintergreen, ⊘cypress, ⊘marjoram

—Broken:

Oils: ⊘Soothing Blend (for pain), ⊘⊙frankincense

Recipe 1: Apply wintergreen and cypress oils at night before bed. Apply helichrysum, oregano, and Grounding Blend in the morning.

Blend 1: Combine equal parts lemongrass, clove, eucalyptus, and melaleuca. Apply on location.

Other Products: ⊙Food Nutrient Complex contains essential bone nutrients calcium, magnesium, zinc, and vitamin D.

—Bruised

Oils: ⊘Soothing Blend, ⊘helichrysum

—Cartilage:

Cartilage is a type of connective tissue in the body that provides structure and support for other tissues without being hard and rigid like bone. Unlike other connective tissues, cartilage does not have blood vessels. Cartilage is found in many areas of the body, including the joints, ears, nose, bronchial tubes, and intervertebral discs.

Oils: ⊘sandalwood (helps regenerate), ⊘white fir (inflammation)

—Development:

Other Products: Ⓞ Food Nutrient Complex contains essential bone nutrients necessary for development, such as calcium, magnesium, zinc, and vitamin D.

—Osteomyelitis: *see also Antibacterial, Antifungal*

Osteomyelitis is a bone infection that is usually caused by bacteria. The infection often starts in another area of the body and then spreads to the bone. Symptoms include fever, pain, swelling, nausea, drainage of pus, and uneasiness. Diabetes, hemodialysis, recent trauma, and IV drug abuse are risk factors for osteomyelitis.

Recipe 1: Apply equal parts lemongrass, clove, eucalyptus, and melaleuca, either blended together or applied individually on location.

—Osteoporosis:

Osteoporosis is a disease characterized by a loss of bone density, making the bones extremely fragile and susceptible to fractures and breaking. Osteoporosis develops when bone resorption exceeds bone formation. Osteoporosis is significantly more common in women then in men, especially after menopause; but the disease does occur in both genders.

Oils: ⊘clove, ⊘geranium, ⊘peppermint, ⊘wintergreen, ⊘white fir, ⊘Soothing Blend, ⊘thyme, ⊘rosemary⊕, ⊘lemon, ⊘cypress

Other Products: �Ⓞ Bone Nutrient Complex, Ⓞ Phytoestrogen Complex

—Pain:

Oils: ⊘Soothing Blend, ⊘wintergreen, ⊘juniper berry, ⊘white fir

—Rotator Cuff: *see Joints:Rotator Cuff*

⊜: Dilute as recommended, and apply on location or on reflex points on feet.

◐: Take capsules as directed. Place 1–2 drops of oil in an empty capsule; swallow.

⊙: **Additional Research:**

Rosemary and eucalyptus: Oral intake of rosemary or eucalyptus essential oil (as well as several monoterpenes found in other essential oils) was shown to inhibit bone resorption in rats (Mühlbauer et al., 2003).

Bowel

see Digestive System

Brain

The brain is the central part of the nervous system. It is responsible for processing sensory stimuli and for directing appropriate behavioral responses to each stimulus, or set of stimuli. The brain also stores memories and is the center of thought.

Oils: ⊘©lavender©, ⊘©lemon©, ⊘©lemongrass, ⊘©clary sage, ⊘©cypress, ⊘©geranium

Other Products: O Essential Oil Omega Complex or Vegan Essential Oil Omega Complex or O Omega-3 Fish Oil for omega-3 fatty acids essential for proper brain function, O Food Nutrient Complex for vitamins and minerals critical for brain health.

⊘: Diffuse into the air. Inhale directly from bottle. Apply oil to hands, tissue, or cotton wick, and inhale.

©: Dilute as recommended, and rub onto the brain stem area, back of neck, temples, behind ears down to jaw, or on reflex points on the feet. Apply as a cold compress.

O: Take capsules as directed on package. Place 1–2 drops of oil under the tongue; or place 1–2 drops of oil in an empty capsule and swallow the capsule.

—Activates Right Brain

Oils: ⊘©geranium, ⊘©grapefruit, ⊘©helichrysum, ⊘©wintergreen, ⊘©Roman chamomile

⊘: Diffuse into the air. Inhale directly from bottle. Apply oil to hands, tissue, or cotton wick, and inhale.

©: Dilute as recommended, and rub onto the brain stem area, or on reflex points on the feet.

—Aging:

Oils: O©thyme©, ⊘©frankincense, myrrh©, rose©

O: Place 1–2 drops of oil under the tongue or place 1–2 drops of oil in an empty capsule; swallow capsule.

©: Dilute as recommended, and rub onto the brain stem area, back of neck, temples, behind ears down to jaw, or on reflex points on the feet.

—Broken Blood Vessels: *see Blood:Broken Blood Vessels*

—Concentration: *see Concentration*

—Concussion:

A Concussion is a type of brain injury that causes temporary or permanent impairment in the brain's functioning. Concussions most commonly occur as a result of a blow to the head. Concussion symptoms include headaches, dizziness, blurred vision, vomiting, disorientation, difficulty focusing attention, ringing in the ears, selective memory loss, etc.

Oils: ⊘©frankincense©, ©cypress

⊘: Diffuse into the air. Inhale directly from bottle. Apply oil to hands, tissue, or cotton wick, and inhale.

©: Dilute as recommended, and rub onto the brain stem area, back of neck, temples, behind ears down to jaw, or on reflex points on the feet. Apply as a cold compress.

—Injury

Oils: ⊘©frankincense©, ⊘©bergamot©, ⊘©peppermint©, ⊘©lemon©, ⊘©Grounding Blend, ⊘©lemongrass

⊘: Diffuse into the air. Inhale the aroma of the oil directly.

⊘=Aromatic, ©=Topical, O=Internal *(See page 33 for further details.)*   107

: Dilute as recommended, and rub onto the brain stem area, back of neck, temples, behind ears down to jaw, or on reflex points on the feet.

—Integration

Oils: Grounding Blend, helichrysum, geranium, clary sage, cypress, lemongrass

: Diffuse into the air. Inhale the aroma of the oil directly.

: Dilute as recommended, and rub onto the brain stem area, back of neck, temples, behind ears down to jaw, or on reflex points on the feet.

—**Learning and Memory:** *see Memory*

—**Mental Fatigue:**

Oils: frankincense

—**Myelin Sheath:**

The myelin sheath is an insulating layer of protein and fatty substances that forms around nerves (including those in the brain), increasing the speed of nerve impulses. Damage to the myelin sheath interrupts these nerve impulses and can cause diseases such as multiple sclerosis, peripheral neuropathy, central pontine myelinolysis, and other neurological diseases.

Oils: peppermint, frankincense, lemongrass, juniper berry, Grounding Blend, geranium

Other Products: O Essential Oil Omega Complex or Vegan Essential Oil Omega Complex or O Omega-3 Fish Oil, which contains the omega-3 fatty acid DHA that helps support the myelin sheath

: Diffuse into the air. Inhale directly from bottle. Apply oil to hands, tissue, or cotton wick, and inhale.

: Apply as a cool compress over the brain stem area, back of neck, temples, behind ears down to jaw, or on reflex points on the feet.

—**Oxygenate:**

Oils: eucalyptus, rosemary, helichrysum, sandalwood, marjoram

Recipe 1: Place three drops each of helichrysum and sandalwood on the back of the neck, on the temples, and behind the ears down to the jaw once or twice a day.

: Diffuse into the air. Inhale the aroma directly.

: Dilute as recommended, and rub onto the brain stem area, back of neck, temples, behind ears down to jaw, or on reflex points on the feet.

—**Stroke:** *see Stroke*

—**Tumor:** *see Cancer:Brain*

: **Additional Research:**

Lavender: Subjects who smelled a cleansing gel with lavender aroma were more relaxed and able to complete math computations faster (Fielt et al., 2005).

Lavender: Subjects exposed to 3 minutes of lavender aroma were more relaxed and were able to perform math computations faster and more accurately. Subjects exposed to rosemary aroma were more alert and completed math computations faster (but not more accurately) (Diego et al., 1998).

Lemon: Several constituents of lemon oil and their metabolites (chemicals made from these constituents by the body) were found to increase the release of monoamines (various chemicals responsible for neurotransmission and neuromodulation) in rat brain tissue, indicating a possible effect on brain nerve cell behavior (Fukumoto et al., 2006).

Lemon: Pretreatment of human and rat astrocyte cells (cells found in the nerve and brain that support the blood-brain barrier and help repair the brain and spinal cord following injuries) with lemon oil was found to inhibit heat-shock induced apoptosis (Koo et al., 2002.

Thyme: Aging rats fed thyme oil or the constituent thymol were found to have higher levels of the antioxidant enzymes superoxide dismutase and glutathione peroxidase in the brain than did aging rats not fed the oil or constituent (Youdim et al., 2000).

Rose: The chloroform extract of *Rosa damascena* was found to cause neurite outgrowth activity in rat cortical neurons subjected to neurotic atrophy conditions. These findings suggest that Rosa damascena possesses neuronal protective properties that may benefit persons with dementia (Awale et al., 2011).

Myrrh: Three new cadinane sesquiterpenes isolated from myrrh resin were found to have neuroprotective activities against 1-methyl-4-phenylpyridinium induced neuronal cell death in a human derived cell line cells (Xu et al., 2011).

Frankincense: Incensole acetate, isolated from frankincense resin, was found to demonstrate an anti-inflammatory and neuroprotective effect in mice with a closed head injury (Moussaieff et al., 2008).

Bergamot: Bergamot essential oil was found to exert neuroprotective effects against brain injury in rats with induced cerebral ischemia (Amantea et al., 2009).

Bergamot: Bergamot essential oil was found to reduce excitotoxic neuronal damage caused by exposure of human neuroblastoma cells to NMDA in vitro, displaying the neuroprotection capabilities of bergamot oil (Corasaniti et al., 2007).

Peppermint: Pretreatment of human and rat astrocyte cells (cells found in the nerve and brain that support the blood-brain barrier and help repair the brain and spinal cord following injuries) with peppermint oil was found to inhibit heat-shock induced apoptosis of these cells (Koo et al., 2001).

Eucalyptus: Imaging of the brain demonstrated that inhalation of 1,8-cineol (eucalyptol, a constituent of many essential oils, especially eucalyptus, rosemary, and marjoram) increased global cerebral blood flow after an inhalation time of 20 minutes (Nasel et al., 1994).

Rosemary: Imaging of the brain demonstrated that inhalation of 1,8-cineol (eucalyptol, a constituent of many essential oils, especially eucalyptus, rosemary, and marjoram) increased global cerebral blood flow after an inhalation time of 20 minutes (Nasel et al., 1994).

Marjoram: Imaging of the brain demonstrated that inhalation of 1,8-cineol (eucalyptol, a constituent of many essential oils, especially eucalyptus, rosemary, and marjoram) increased global cerebral blood flow after an inhalation time of 20 minutes (Nasel et al., 1994).

(-)-Linalool (found in basil, bergamot, cinnamon, clary sage, coriander, cypress, eucalyptus, fennel (sweet), geranium, ginger, helichrysum, jasmine, lavender, lemon, lemongrass, lime, marjoram, oregano, peppermint, rosemary, tangerine, thyme, wild orange, and ylang ylang essential oils): In two mice models of chronic pain, inflammatory pain and neuropathic pain, (-)-linalool was able to promote marked and long-lasting reduction in sensitivity to pain when compared to the control (Batista et al., 2010).

Bergamot: Using a mouse model of neuropathic pain, researchers discovered that injections of bergamot or linalool (a main chemical constituent of bergamot) provided reduction of pain symptoms by inhibiting phosphorylation of the spinal ERK pathway (Kuwahata et al., 2013).

Breast

see also **Cancer:Breast. For issues related to lactation and motherhood,** *see* **Pregnancy/ Motherhood**

Oils: ⊙clary sage, ⊙geranium, ⊙lemongrass, ⊙fennel, ⊙cypress, ⊙vetiver

—Enlarge and Firm:

Oils: ⊙clary sage

⊙: Dilute as recommended, and apply on location or on reflex points on feet.

Breathing

see **Respiratory System:Breathing**

Bronchitis

see also **Antibacterial, Antifungal, Antiviral, Congestion, Inflammation, Respiratory System**

Bronchitis is the inflammation of the bronchi (the tubes that lead from the trachea to the lungs). Symptoms include coughing, breathlessness, and thick phlegm.

Oils: ⊘⊘eucalyptus☺, ⊘⊘thyme☺, ⊘⊘white fir, ⊘⊘basil, ⊘⊘Respiratory Blend, ⊘⊘Protective Blend, ⊘⊘clary sage, ⊘⊘cypress, ⊘⊘cedarwood, ⊘⊘melaleuca, ⊘⊘marjoram, ⊘⊘peppermint, ⊘⊘rosemary, ⊘⊘wintergreen, ⊘⊘myrrh, ⊘⊘clove, ⊘⊘frankincense, ⊘⊘ginger, ⊘⊘lavender, ⊘⊘lemon, ⊘⊘sandalwood, ⊘⊘bergamot

—Chronic

Oils: ⊘⊘eucalyptus, ⊘⊘oregano, ⊘⊘sandalwood

—Children

Oils: ⊘⊘eucalyptus, ⊘⊘melaleuca, ⊘⊘lavender, ⊘⊘Roman chamomile, ⊘⊘rosemary

—Clear Mucus:

Oils: ⊘⊘sandalwood, ⊘⊘thyme, ⊘⊘bergamot, ⊘⊘Protective Blend,

🕭: Diffuse into the air. Inhale directly from bottle. Apply oil to hands, tissue, or cotton wick, and inhale.

💧: Dilute as recommended, and apply to chest, sinuses, neck, or reflex points on the feet. Add 2–3 drops to water; gargle.

📖: **Additional Research:**

Eucalyptus: Extracts from eucalyptus and thyme were found to have high nitrous oxide scavenging abilities and inhibited nitrous oxide production in macrophage cells. This could possibly explain their role in aiding respiratory inflammatory diseases (Vigo et al., 2004).

Eucalyptus: Eucalyptus oil was found to have an anti-inflammatory and mucin-inhibitory effect in rats with lipopolysaccharide-induced bronchitis (Lu et al., 2004).

Eucalyptus: Therapy with 1,8 cineole (eucalyptol) in both healthy and bronchitis-afflicted humans was shown to reduce production of LTB4 and PGE2 (both metabolites of arachidonic acid, a known chemical messenger involved in inflammation) in white blood cells (Juergens et al., 1998).

Thyme: Extracts from eucalyptus and thyme were found to have high nitrous oxide scavenging abilities and inhibited nitrous oxide production in macrophage cells. This could possibly explain their role in aiding respiratory inflammatory diseases (Vigo et al., 2004).

Bruises

see also **Capillaries**

A bruise is an injury to tissue that results in blood capillaries breaking and spilling blood into the tissue. This can cause swelling, soreness, and a visible discoloration when the bruise is near the skin.

Oils: ⊘helichrysum, ⊘geranium, ⊘fennel, ⊘Soothing Blend (for pain), ⊘Protective Blend, ⊘lavender

💧: Dilute as recommended, and apply 1–2 drops on location.

Bugs

see Insects/Bugs

Bulimia

see Eating Disorders:Bulimia

Bunions

see Bursitis:Bunion

Burns

A burn is an injury to tissue caused by heat, chemicals, or radiation. The tissue most often affected by burns is the skin. Minor burns can cause redness and pain over a small area and do not break the skin. For minor heat burns, immediately immerse the affected skin in cool water to stop the heat from causing more damage to the tissue. More serious burns that involve areas of the body larger than the palm of the hand or that involve blistering, swelling, intense pain that lasts for more than a day, or visible skin damage should be attended to by a medical professional. Skin damaged by burns is more prone to developing infection as it cannot act as a barrier against invading microorganisms.

Oils: ◔lavender, ◔geranium, ◔melaleuca, ◔peppermint, ◔helichrysum, ◔Roman chamomile

Other Products: ○Food Nutrient Complex to help replace minerals depleted from the skin and tissues surrounding a burn.

—**Infected:**

    Oils: ◔Cleansing Blend

—**Pain:**

    Oils: ◔lavender

—**Healing:**

    Oils: ◔lavender

    Blend 1: Blend together 1 drop geranium and 1 drop helichrysum; apply on location.

—**Peeling:**

    Oils: ◔lavender

—**Sunburn:**

    Oils: ◔lavender, ◔melaleuca, ◔Roman chamomile

    Recipe 1: Place 10 drops lavender in a 4 oz. misting spray bottle filled with distilled water. Shake well, and spray on location to aid with pain and healing.

—**Sun Screen:**

    Oils: ◔helichrysum

◔: Dilute as recommended, and apply on location. Add 2–3 drops oil to 1 oz. water in a spray bottle; shake well, and mist on location.

Bursitis

Bursitis is the inflammation of the fluid-filled sack located close to joints that provides lubrication for tendons, skin, and ligaments rubbing against the bone. Bursitis is caused by infection, injury, or diseases such as arthritis and gout. Bursitis causes tenderness and pain which can limit movement.

Oils: ⊙Grounding Blend, ⊙white fir, ⊙basil, ⊙cypress, ⊙Soothing Blend, ⊙ginger, ⊙Roman chamomile, ⊙marjoram, ⊙juniper berry, ⊙wintergreen

Recipe 1: Apply 1–3 drops each of Grounding Blend, white fir, and basil on location. Alternate cold and hot packs (10 min. cold and then 15 min. hot) until pain subsides.

Recipe 2: Apply 6 drops marjoram on shoulders and arms, and wait six minutes. Then apply 3 drops of wintergreen, and wait six minutes. Then apply 3 drops cypress.

—Bunion:

A bunion is bursitis of the big toe. It is often caused by constrictive shoes that force the big toe to point inward and the base of the big toe to jut outward. This misplacement can irritate the bursa at the base of the toe and cause it to become inflamed, causing further irritation.

Oils: ⊙cypress, ⊙juniper berry

🔄: Dilute as recommended, and apply 1–2 drops on location.

Callouses
see **Skin:Callouses**

Calming
see also **Anxiety**

Oils: ⊘⊙lavender⊙, ⊘⊙Focus Blend, ⊘⊙ylang ylang⊙, ⊘⊙melissa⊙, ⊘⊙Calming Blend, ⊘⊙cedarwood, ⊘Invigorating Blend, ⊘⊙myrrh, ⊘⊙juniper berry

—Agitation:

Oils: ⊘⊙lavender⊙, ylang ylang⊙, ⊘⊙geranium⊙, ⊘⊙bergamot, ⊘⊙Calming Blend, ⊘⊙sandalwood, ⊘⊙cedarwood, ⊘⊙cedarwood, ⊘⊙Grounding Blend, ⊘⊙marjoram, ⊘⊙myrrh, ⊘⊙clary sage, ⊘⊙rose, ⊘⊙frankincense, ⊘⊙Joyful Blend

—Anger:

Oils: ⊘⊙Calming Blend, ⊘⊙lavender, ⊘⊙ylang ylang, ⊘⊙Grounding Blend, ⊘⊙Joyful Blend, ⊘⊙bergamot, ⊘⊙geranium, ⊘⊙cedarwood, ⊘⊙frankincense, ⊘⊙sandalwood, ⊘⊙cypress, ⊘⊙lemon, ⊘⊙myrrh, ⊘⊙marjoram, ⊘⊙helichrysum, ⊘⊙rose, ⊘⊙orange

—Hyperactivity:

Oils: ⊙⊘Focus Blend, ⊘⊙lavender⊙, ⊘⊙Calming Blend, ⊘⊙Grounding Blend, ⊘⊙Roman chamomile, ⊘Invigorating Blend

—Sedative:

Oils: ⊘⊙lavender⊙, ⊘⊙Calming Blend, ⊘Invigorating Blend, ⊘⊙bergamot⊙, ⊘⊙ylang ylang⊙, ⊘⊙cedarwood, ⊘⊙geranium, ⊘⊙vetiver, ⊘⊙juniper berry, ⊘⊙frankincense, ⊘⊙sandalwood, ⊘⊙orange, ⊘⊙rose, ⊘⊙lemongrass, ⊘⊙clary sage, ⊘⊙marjoram

🌀: Diffuse into the air. Inhale directly from bottle. Apply oil to hands, tissue, or cotton wick, and inhale.

🜁: Dilute as recommended, and apply 1–2 drops to back of neck, temples, chest, shoulders, back, or reflex points on the feet. Place 1–2 drops in 1 Tbs. fractionated coconut oil, and massage into the back, shoulders, neck, or arms.

📖: **Additional Research:**

Lavender: Lavandula angustifolia essential oil demonstrated ability to inhibit GABA-A receptor channels of rat brain cells (Huang et al., 2008).

Lavender: Inhaling lavender oil was found to be effective at alleviating agitated behaviors in older Chinese patients suffering from dementia (Lin et al., 2007).

Lavender: Female patients waiting for dental treatment were found to be less anxious, more positive, and more calm when exposed to orange oil odor than were patients who were not exposed to the orange oil odor (Lehrner et al., 2000).

Lavender: Exposure to inhaled lavender oil and to its constituents, linalool and linalyl acetate, was found to decrease normal movement in mice as well as to return mice to normal movement rates after caffeine-induced hyperactivity (Buchbauer et al., 1991).

Lavender: Swiss mice fed lavender oil diluted in olive oil were found to be more sedate in several common behavioral tests (Guillemain et al., 1989).

Lavender: Linalool, found in several essential oils, was found to inhibit induced convulsions in rats by directly interacting with the NMDA receptor complex (Brum et al., 2001).

Ylang ylang: In human trials, the aroma of peppermint was found to enhance memory and to increase alertness, while ylang ylang aroma was found to increase calmness (Moss et al., 2008).

Ylang ylang: Subjects who had ylang ylang oil applied to their skin had decreased blood pressure, increased skin temperature, and reported feeling more calm and relaxed, as compared to subjects in a control group (Hongratanaworakit et al., 2006).

Melissa: Melissa (lemon balm) oil applied topically in a lotion was found to reduce agitation and to improve quality of life factors in patients suffering severe dementia, as compared to those receiving a placebo lotion (Ballard et al., 2002).

Geranium: Geraniol and eugenol, two components of rose oil (among others), were found to demonstrate antianxiety effects on mice in several tests (Umezo et al., 2008).

Ylang ylang: In healthy control subjects, inhalation of ylang ylang aroma significantly reduced the P300 (an event-related potential interpreted to reflect attentional allocation and working memory) amplitude when compared to inhalation without aroma. These results suggest that ylang ylang produces a relaxing effect on cognition (Watanabe et al., 2013).

Bergamot: A study using 114 subjects found that listening to soft music and/or inhaling *Citrus bergamia* essential oil were effective methods of relaxation, as indicated by a shift of the autonomic balance toward parasympathetic (Peng et al., 2009).

Cancer

Cancer can be any of many different conditions where the body's cells duplicate and grow uncontrollably, invade healthy tissues, and possibly spread throughout the body. It is estimated that 95% of cancers result from damage to DNA during a person's lifetime rather than from a pre-existing genetic condition (American Cancer Society, 2008). The most important factor leading to this DNA damage is DNA mutation. DNA mutation can be caused by radiation, environmental chemicals we take into our bodies, free radical damage, or DNA copying or division errors. If the body is working properly, it can correct these mutations either by repairing the DNA or by causing the mutated cell to die. When the DNA mutation is severe enough that it allows the cell to bypass these controls, however, the mutated DNA can be copied to new cells that continue to replicate and create more and more new cells uncontrollably, leading to a cancerous growth within an individual.

Oils: 🄰🄾🄲frankincense🄲, 🄲🄾🄲sandalwood🄲, 🄰🄲lavender🄲, 🄾Cellular Complex, 🄲🄰arborvitae🄲, 🄲🄾🄲rosemary🄲, 🄰🄲🄾lemongrass🄲, 🄰🄾🄲clove🄲, 🄰🄲basil🄲, 🄲🄾🄲geranium🄲, 🄰🄾🄲clary sage🄲, 🄲citrus oils🄲, 🄲rose

Other Products: 🄾Cellular Vitality Complex contains multiple nutrients that have been studied for their abilities to combat different types of cancer, including polyphenols (such as resveratrol[⊕], baicalin[⊕], EGCG[⊕], quercetin[⊕], ellagic acid[⊕], and catechin[⊕]) and coenzyme Q10. ^OEssential Oil Omega Complex or Vegan Essential Oil Omega Complex or ^OOmega-3 Fish Oil and ^OFood Nutrient Complex to help support cellular and immune function.

Note: Health care professionals are emphatic about avoiding heavy massage when working with cancer patients. Light massage may be used—but never over the trauma area.

—Bone:

Oils: [☉]frankincense

—Brain:

Oils: ☺☻frankincense[⊕], ☺☻myrrh[⊕], ☺☻clove

Recipe 1: Combine 15 drops frankincense, 6 drops clove, and 1 Tbs. fractionated coconut oil. Massage lightly on spine every day. Diffuse 15 drops frankincense and 6 drops clove for 30 minutes, three times a day.

Recipe 2: Diffuse frankincense, and massage the brain stem area lightly with frankincense neat.

—Breast:

Oils: ☺☻rosemary[⊕], ☺☻lavender[⊕], ☺☻frankincense[⊕], ☺☻arborvitae[⊕], ☺☻clary sage[⊕], ☺☻clove, ☺☻basil[⊕], ☺☻sandalwood, ☺☻oregano, ☺☻lemongrass, ☺☻marjoram

—Cervical:

Oils: ☺☻frankincense, ☺☻geranium, ☺☻white fir, ☺☻cypress, ☺☻clove, ☺☻lavender, ☺☻lemon

—Colon:

Oils: O☺☻lavender[⊕], ☺☻geranium[⊕], ☺☻frankincense , ☺☻arborvitae[⊕], ☺☻lemongrass[⊕]

—Leukemia:

Oils: ☺☻frankincense[⊕] , ☺☻lemongrass[⊕], ☺☻rosemary[⊕], ☺☻clary sage[⊕], ☺☻clove[⊕]

—Liver:

Oils: ☺☻frankincense[⊕], ☺☻lemongrass[⊕], ☺☻lavender[⊕] , ☺☻rosemary[⊕]

—Lung:

Oils: ☺☻frankincense[⊕] (apply to chest, or mix 15 drops with 1 tsp. fractionated coconut oil for nightly rectal retention enema), ☺☻lavender[⊕]

—Prostate

Oils: ☺☻frankincense (blend 15 drops with 1 tsp. fractionated coconut oil for nightly rectal retention enema), ☺☻arborvitae[⊕]

—Skin/Melanoma:

Oils: ☺OHawaiian sandalwood [⊕], ☺☻arborvitae[⊕], ☺frankincense, Ocitrus oils[⊕]

—Throat:

Oils: ☺☻frankincense, ☺☻lavender

— **Uterine:**

Oils: ⚬⚬geranium, ⚬frankincense

⚬: Dilute as recommended, and apply 1–5 drops on location and on reflex points on the feet and hands. Apply as a warm compress over affected area.

⚬: Diffuse into the air. Inhale oil directly or applied to hands, tissue, or a cotton wick.

⚬: Take capsules as recommended on package. Place 1–2 drops of oil under the tongue or add 1–3 drops of oil in an empty capsule; swallow capsule. Repeat up to twice daily as needed.

⚬: **Additional Research:**

Frankincense: An extract from *Boswellia carterii* was found to induce apoptosis (cell death) in 2 leukemia cell lines (Hunan et al., 1999).

Frankincense: An extract from frankincense was found to produce apoptosis in human leukemia cells (Bhushan et al., 2007).

Frankincense: β-elemene—a sesquiterpene found in curcumin and *Boswellia freeana* and black pepper essential oils—is currently being studied for its promising potential to induce apoptosis and inhibit cancer cell proliferation in ovarian (Zou et al, 2013), liver (Dai et al, 2013), breast (Zhang et al., 2013, Ding et al., 2013), bladder (Li et al, 2013), lung (Li et al., 2013, Chen et al., 2012), and brain (Li et al., 2013) cancer cell lines, both on its own, and in combination with cisplatin chemotherapy.

Frankincense: Ethanol extract of Boswellia serrata demonstrated antiproliferative effects on 5 leukemia and two brain tumor cell lines. It was more potent than one type of Boswellic acid (AKBA) on three leukemia cell lines (Hostanska et al., 2002).

Frankincense: β-elemene was found to induce apoptosis in brain tumor cells (Li et al., 2013).

Frankincense: Derivatives of β-elemene were found to induce apoptosis in human leukemia cells (Yu et al., 2011).

Frankincense: Proliferation of human hepatoma cells was found to be inhibited by β-elemene in vitro (Dai et al., 2013).

Frankincense: β-elemene, found in Boswellia frereana and black pepper essential oils, was found to have anti-lung cancer properties (Chen et al., 2012).

Frankincense: Beta-elemene was found to decrease MCF-7 human breast cancer cell migration and invasion (Zhang et al., 2013).

Sandalwood: Oral sandalwood oil use enhanced GST activity (a protein in cell membranes that can help eliminate toxins) and acid-soluble SH levels. This suggests a possible chemopreventive action on carcinogenesis (Banerjee et al., 1993).

Sandalwood: Alpha-santalol was found to induce apoptosis in human skin cancer cells (Kaur et al., 2005).

Sandalwood: A solution of 5% alpha-santalol (from sandalwood) was found to prevent skin-tumor formation caused by ultraviolet-b (UVB) radiation in mice (Dwivedi et al., 2006).

Sandalwood: Various concentrations of alpha-santalol (from sandalwood) were tested against skin cancer in mice. All concentrations were found to inhibit skin cancer development (Dwivedi et al., 2005).

Sandalwood: Alpha-santalol, derived from sandalwood EO, was found to delay and decrease the incidence and multiplicity of skin tumor (papilloma) development in mice (Dwivedi et al., 2003).

Sandalwood: Sandalwood oil was found to decrease skin papilloma (tumors) in mice (Dwivedi et al., 1997).

Sandalwood: Pretreatment with alpha-santalol (found in sandalwood) before UVB (ultraviolet-b) radiation significantly reduced skin tumor development and multiplicity and induced proapoptotic and tumor-suppressing proteins (Arasada et al., 2008).

Lavender: In tests for mutagenicity, both tea tree and lavender oils were found to not be mutagenic. In fact, lavender oil was found to have strong antimutagenic activity, reducing mutations of cells exposed to a known mutagen (Evandri et al., 2005).

Lavender: Perillyl alcohol (found in caraway, lavender, and mint), EGCG (polyphenol from green tea), squalene (a triterpene derived from sharks and other vegetable material), and EPA (an essential fatty acid from fish or microalgae) were found to inhibit hyperproliferation of mammary epithelial cells prior to tumorigenisis (Katdare et al., 1997).

Lavender: Rats fed diets containing perillyl alcohol (derived from lavender plants) were found to have less incidence of colon tumors and less multiplicity of tumors in the colon compared to control. Colon tumors of animals fed perillyl alcohol were found to exhibit increased apoptosis of cells compared to control (Reddy et al., 1997).

Lavender: Mice treated with perillyl alcohol (found in lavender and mint plants) had a 22% reduction in tumor incidence and a 58% reduction in tumor multiplicity during a mouse lung tumor bioassay (Lantry et al., 1997).

Lavender: Rats with liver tumors that were treated with perillyl alcohol had smaller tumor sizes than untreated rats due to apoptosis in cancer cells in treated rats (Mills et al., 1995).

Arborvitae: Hinokitiol was found to induce autophagic signaling in murine breast and colorectal tumor cells in vitro (Wang et al., 2014).

Arborvitae: Mice implanted with human colon cancer tumor cells saw a decrease in tumor size and weight when treated with β-thujaplicin (hinokitiol) (Lee et al., 2013).

Arborvitae: Hinokitiol demonstrated inhibition of cell growth and DNA synthesis in human melanoma cells in vitro (Liu et al., 2009).

Rosemary: Rosemary extract injected in rats was found to decrease mammary adenocarcinomas in rats (Singletary et al., 1996).

Rosemary: An ethanol extract of rosemary was found to have an antiproliferative effect on human leukemia and breast carcinoma cells, as well as an antioxidant effect (Cheung et al., 2007).

Rosemary: Carnosic acid (derived from rosemary) was found to inhibit the proliferation of human leukemia cells in vitro (Steiner et al., 2001).

Rosemary: Rosemary extracts induced CYP (cytochrome 450) activity in liver cells, suggesting a possibility of increased ability to remove toxins (Debersac et al., 2001).

Lemongrass: Citral (found in lemongrass, melissa, and verbena oils) was found to induce apoptosis in several cancer cell lines (hematopoietic cells=stem cells that create blood cells) (Dudai et al., 2005).

Lemongrass: Lemongrass oil was found to inhibit multiple cancer cell lines, both in vitro and in vivo, in mice (Sharma et al., 2009).

Lemongrass: Geraniol (found in geranium and lemongrass oil, among others) was found to inhibit colon cancer cell growth while inhibiting DNA synthesis in these cells (Carnesecchi et al., 2001).

Lemongrass: Lemongrass oil and its constituent, isointermedeol, were found to induce apoptosis in human leukemia cells (Kumar et al., 2008).

Lemongrass: An extract from lemongrass was found to inhibit hepatocarcinogenesis (liver cancer genesis) in rats (Puatanachokchai et al., 2002).

Clove: Beta-caryophyllene (found in clove) was found to increase the anticancer activities of paclitaxel (a chemotherapy drug derived from the yew tree) (Legault et al., 2007).

Clary Sage: Sclareol, a chemical constituent found in clary sage essential oil, was found to reduce regulatory T cells frequency and also tumor size in a mouse model of breast cancer, suggesting that sclareol can enhance the effect of cancer therapy as an immunostiumlant (Noori et al., 2013).

Basil: Basil extract was found to inhibit the growth of MCF-7 breast cancer cells, possess antioxidant activity, and protect against DNA damage (Al-Ali et al., 2013).

Basil: Basil and its component, linalool, were found to reduce spontaneous mutagenesis in bacteria cells (Berić et al., 2008).

Geranium: Geraniol (found in geranium and lemongrass oil, among others) was found to inhibit colon cancer cell growth while inhibiting DNA synthesis in these cells (Carnesecchi et al., 2001).

Clary Sage: Sclareol, from clary sage oil, was found to have a cytostatic effect in human leukemia cell lines (Dimas et al., 1999).

Clove: Eugenol, a major chemical constituent of clove essential oil, was found to induce apoptosis in human leukemia cells via reactive oxygen species generation (Yoo et al., 2005).

Citrus oils: In a study of older individuals, it was found that there was a dose-dependent relationship between citrus peel (which are high in d-limonene) consumption and a lower degree of squamous cell carcinoma (SCC) of the skin (Hakim et al., 2000).

Resveratrol: Resveratrol was found to act as an antioxidant and antimutagen in addition to inhibiting several types of cancer cells (Jang et al., 1997).

Resveratrol: Human leukemia cells were found to be irreversibly inhibited by resveratrol, while the effects of resveratrol on nonmalignant human lymphoblastoid cells was largely reversible, suggesting a selective growth inhibition of leukemia cells (Lee et al., 2008).

Resveratrol: A combination of resveratrol, quercetin, and catechin administered orally was found to reduce primary tumor growth of breast cancer tumors in nude mice (Schlachterman et al., 2008).

Baicalin: Baicalin was found to inhibit cyclobutane pyrimidine dimers (a precursor to skin cancer) in fibroblast cells exposed to UVB radiation (Zhou et al., 2008).

Baicalin: Baicalin was found to inhibit several different breast cancer cell lines (Franek et al., 2005).

Baicalin: Baicalin was found to inhibit two prostate cancer cell lines in vitro (Miocinovic et al., 2005).

EGCG: The polyphenol EGCG from green tea was found to inhibit the ability of bronchial tumor cells to migrate in vitro (Hazgui et al., 2008).

EGCG: EGCG was found to inhibit pancreatic cancer growth, invasion, metastasis and angiogenesis (ability to create blood vessels) in mice (Shankar et al., 2008).

Quercetin: A combination of resveratrol, quercetin, and catechin administered orally was found to reduce primary tumor growth of breast cancer tumors in nude mice (Schlachterman et al., 2008).

Quercetin: A combination of low-frequency ultrasound followed by treatment with quercetin was found to selectively kill cancerous skin and prostate cancer cells, while having no effect on nonmalignant skin cells (Paliwal et al., 2005).

Quercetin: Quercetin was found to inhibit and induce apoptosis in cancerous prostate cells, but not in normal prostate epithelial cells in vitro (Aalinkeel et al., 2008).

Quercetin: In a large human study, it was found that increased flavonoid intake in male smokers was found to decrease the risk of developing pancreatic cancer (Bobe et al., 2008).

Quercetin: Flavonol intake was found to reduce the risk of developing pancreatic cancer among smokers (Nothlings et al., 2007).

Quercetin: Flavonol intake (including flavonols such as epicatechin, catechin, quercetin, and kaempferol) was found to be inversely associated with lung cancer among tobacco smokers (Cui et al., 2008).

Ellagic acid: Oral supplementation with ellagic acid was found to decrease the number of induced esophageal tumors in rats, compared to a control (Mandal et al., 1990).

Catechin: A combination of resveratrol, quercetin, and catechin administered orally was found to reduce primary tumor growth of breast cancer tumors in nude mice (Schlachterman et al., 2008).

Catechin: In a large human study, it was found that increased flavonoid intake in male smokers was found to decrease the risk of developing pancreatic cancer (Bobe et al., 2008).

Catechin: Flavonol intake was found to reduce the risk of developing pancreatic cancer among smokers (Nothlings et al., 2007).

Catechin: Flavonol intake (including flavonols such as epicatechin, catechin, quercetin, and kaempferol) was found to be inversely associated with lung cancer among tobacco smokers (Cui et al., 2008).

Myrrh: Treatment with elemene (found in myrrh oil) was found to increase survival time and to reduce tumor size in patients with malignant brain tumor, as compared to treatment with chemotherapy (Tan et al., 2000).

Geranium: Geraniol (found in geranium and lemongrass oil, among others) was found to inhibit colon cancer cell growth while inhibiting DNA synthesis in these cells (Carnesecchi et al., 2001).

Hawaiian Sandalwood: Alpha-santalol was found to induce apoptosis in human skin cancer cells (Kaur et al., 2005).

Hawaiian Sandalwood: A solution of 5% alpha-santalol (from sandalwood) was found to prevent skin-tumor formation caused by ultraviolet-b (UVB) radiation in mice (Dwivedi et al., 2006).

Hawaiian Sandalwood: Various concentrations of alpha-santalol (from sandalwood) were tested against skin cancer in mice. All concentrations were found to inhibit skin cancer development (Dwivedi et al., 2005).

Hawaiian Sandalwood: Alpha-santalol, derived from sandalwood EO, was found to delay and decrease the incidence and multiplicity of skin tumor (papilloma) development in mice (Dwivedi et al., 2003).

Hawaiian Sandalwood: Sandalwood oil was found to decrease skin papilloma (tumors) in mice (Dwivedi et al., 1997).

Hawaiian Sandalwood: Pretreatment with alpha-santalol (found in sandalwood) before UVB (ultraviolet-b) radiation significantly reduced skin tumor development and multiplicity and induced proapoptotic and tumor-suppressing proteins (Arasada et al., 2008).

Candida

see **Antifungal:Candida**

Canker Sores

Canker sores are small, round sores that develop in the mouth, typically inside the lips and cheeks or on the tongue.

Oils: ◎melaleuca, ◎oregano, ◎Protective Blend, ◎Roman chamomile, ◎myrrh

◎: Dilute as recommended, and apply 1 drop on location.

Capillaries

Capillaries are the small, thin blood vessels that allow the exchange of oxygen and other nutrients from the blood to cells throughout the body and allow the exchange of carbon dioxide and other waste materials from these tissues back to the blood. The capillaries connect the arteries (that carry blood away from the heart) and veins (that carry blood back to the heart).

—**Broken Capillaries**:

Oils: ©geranium, ©cypress, ©oregano, ©thyme, ©Roman chamomile

Blend 1: Apply 1 drop lavender and 1 drop Roman chamomile on location.

©: Dilute as recommended, and apply 1–2 drops on location.

Carbuncles

see **Boils**

Cardiovascular System

The cardiovascular—or circulatory—system is the system responsible for transporting blood to the various tissues throughout the body. It is comprised of the heart and blood vessels such as arteries, veins, and capillaries.

Oils: ©©orange, ©©cypress, ©©cinnamon, ©©sandalwood, ©©thyme©

Other Products: OCellular Vitality Complex and OChewable Multivitamin, contain several polyphenols (including proanthocyanidin polyphenols from grape seed©, the polyphenols EGCG©, and ellagic acid©) and coenzyme Q10©, which have been found to have beneficial cardiovascular effects.

©: Dilute oils as recommended, and apply oils to area: to carotid arteries, heart, feet, under left ring finger, above elbow, behind ring toe on left foot, and to reflex points on the feet. Add 1–2 drops to bathwater for a bath. Add 1–2 drops to 1 Tbs. fractionated coconut oil for massage oil, and massage on location or on chest, neck, or feet.

©: Diffuse into the air. Inhale oil applied to hands, tissue, or cotton wick.

—**Angina**:

Angina is pain in the chest due to a lack of blood flow to the heart. Angina is felt as a squeezing, tightening, aching, or pressure in the chest. The pain can also extend to the arms, back, jaw, neck, and teeth.

Oils: ©©ginger, ©©orange (for false angina)

©: Massage gently onto chest and feet, and apply on carotid artery.

©: Diffuse into the air.

—**Arrhythmia**:

Arrhythmia is any abnormal heart rhythm. *See also Palpitations and Tachycardia below.*

Oils: ©©ylang ylang©, ©©lavender, ©©Soothing Blend

©: Diffuse into the air. Inhale the aroma.

©: Dilute oils as recommended, and apply oils to carotid arteries, heart, feet, under left ring finger, above elbow, behind ring toe on left foot, and to reflex points on the feet.

—Atherosclerosis:

Atherosclerosis is a hardening of the arteries due to a buildup of plaques (called atheromas) along the arterial wall.

Oils: O☺️🌿lemon🍋,🌿lavender🍋, O🌿melissa🍋, O🌿dill🍋, OCellular Complex, 🌿rosemary, 🌿ginger, 🌿thyme, 🌿wintergreen

🌿: Diffuse into the air.

🌿: Take 1–2 drops under the tongue or in a capsule or with water.

🌿: Massage gently onto chest and feet, and apply on carotid artery.

—Blood Pressure: *see Blood:Blood Pressure*

—Cardiotonic:

Oils: 🌿🌿lavender, 🌿🌿thyme

🌿: Dilute oils as recommended, and apply oils to carotid arteries, heart, feet, under left ring finger, above elbow, behind ring toe on left foot, and to reflex points on the feet.

🌿: Diffuse into the air. Inhale the aroma.

—Circulation:

Oils: 🌿🌿cypress, 🌿🌿thyme, 🌿🌿peppermint, 🌿🌿clary sage, 🌿🌿wintergreen, 🌿🌿Invigorating Blend, 🌿🌿rosemary, 🌿🌿geranium, 🌿🌿cinnamon, 🌿🌿helichrysum, 🌿🌿Calming Blend, 🌿🌿basil

🌿: Add 1–2 drops to 1 Tbs. fractionated coconut oil for massage oil, and massage on location or on chest, neck, or feet.

🌿: Diffuse into the air. Inhale the aroma.

—Heart:

Oils: 🌿🌿ylang ylang, 🌿🌿marjoram 🌿🌿geranium, 🌿🌿cypress, 🌿Grounding Blend, 🌿🌿ginger, 🌿🌿lavender, 🌿🌿rosemary, 🌿Soothing Blend

🌿: Dilute oils as recommended, and apply oils to carotid arteries, heart, feet, under left ring finger, above elbow, behind ring toe on left foot, and to reflex points on the feet.

🌿: Diffuse into the air. Inhale the aroma.

—Heart Tissue

Oils: 🌿🌿marjoram, 🌿🌿lavender, 🌿🌿peppermint, 🌿🌿rosemary, 🌿cinnamon, 🌿rose

🌿: Dilute oils as recommended, and apply oils to carotid arteries, heart, feet, under left ring finger, above elbow, behind ring toe on left foot, and to reflex points on the feet.

🌿: Diffuse into the air. Inhale the aroma.

—High Cholesterol: *see Cholesterol*

—Hypertension: *see Blood:Blood Pressure*

—Palpitations:

Palpitations are rapid and forceful contractions of the heart.

Oils: 🌿🌿ylang ylang, 🌿🌿orange, 🌿🌿lavender, 🌿🌿melissa, 🌿🌿peppermint

🌿=Aromatic, 🌿=Topical, 🌿=Internal *(See page 33 for further details.)*   119

◉: Dilute oils as recommended, and apply oils to carotid arteries, heart, feet, under left ring finger, above elbow, behind ring toe on left foot, and to reflex points on the feet.

◐: Diffuse into the air. Inhale the aroma.

—Phlebitis:

Phlebitis is the inflammation of a superficial vein, typically in the legs or groin area. Wearing support hose or a compression bandage over the affected area can help aid in healing.

Oils: ◎◉helichrysum, ◎◉lavender, ◎◉cypress, ◎◉geranium, ◎◉grapefruit, ◎◉Grounding Blend

◉: Add 1–2 drops to 1 Tbs. fractionated coconut oil for massage oil, and gently massage on location or on feet.

◐: Diffuse into the air. Inhale the aroma.

—Prolapsed Mitral Valve:

Oils: ◎◉marjoram

◉: Dilute oils as recommended, and apply oils to carotid arteries, heart, feet, under left ring finger, above elbow, behind ring toe on left foot, and to reflex points on the feet.

◐: Diffuse into the air. Inhale the aroma.

—Tachycardia:

Tachycardia is an abnormally rapid resting heart rate, indicating a possible over-working of the heart.

Oils: ◉◎lavender, ◎◎ylang ylang, ◎◎orange

◉: Dilute oils as recommended, and apply oils to carotid arteries, heart, feet, under left ring finger, above elbow, behind ring toe on left foot, and to reflex points on the feet.

◐: Diffuse into the air. Inhale the aroma.

▣: **Additional Research:**

Thyme: Older rats whose diets were supplemented with thyme oil were found to have a higher level of the antioxidant enzymes superoxide dismutase and glutathione peroxidase in the heart, liver, and kidneys, as compared to older rats without this supplementation (Youdim et al., 1999).

Grape seed: An extract of proanthocyanidin polyphenols from grape seed taken as a supplement was found to significantly oxidize LDL (a risk factor for cardiovascular disease) in people with high cholesterol (Bagchi et al., 2003).

EGCG: People who habitually consumed beverages containing EGCG were found to have significantly lower incidences of cardiovascular events (Basu et al., 2007).

EGCG: Supplementation with EGCG was found to lower blood pressure in humans (Brown et al., 2008).

EGCG: EGCG was found to reduce heart weight and cardiac marker enzyme activities in induced heart attacks in rats (Devika et al., 2008).

Ellegic acid: Ellegic acid was found to reduce induced LDL oxidization in vitro (Anderson et al., 2001).

Ellegic acid: Ellegic acid was found to significantly inhibit oxidized LDL proliferation of rat aortic smooth muscle cells (Chang et al., 2008).

Ellegic acid: Supplementation with ellegic acid was found to significantly reduce the amount of atherosclerotic lesions in rabbits fed a high-cholesterol diet (Yu et al., 2005).

Coenzyme Q10: In patients with coronary artery disease, supplementation with CoQ10 was found to improve extracellular superoxide dismutase activity, endothelium-dependent vasodilation, and peak oxygen volume capacity at a level significantly higher as compared to control (Tiano et al., 2007).

Coenzyme Q10: Oral supplementation with CoQ10 was found to improve endothelial function (cells that line the blood vessels) and aerobic capacity of the cardiovascular system in patients with chronic heart failure (Belardinelli et al., 2006).

Coenzyme Q10: Supplementation with CoQ10 was found to improve endothelial dysfunction of the brachial artery in 25 male patients with manifest endothelial dysfunction (Kuettner et al., 2005).

Coenzyme Q10: Chronic heart failure patients receiving CoQ10 supplementation were found to have an improvement in left-ventricle contractility without any side effects (Belardinelli et al., 2005).

Ylang ylang: Inhaled ylang ylang oil was found to decrease blood pressure and pulse rate and to enhance attentiveness and alertness in volunteers compared to an odorless control (Hongratanaworakit et al., 2004).

Lemon: Lemon oil and one of its components, gamma-terpinene, were found to inhibit oxidation of low-density lipoprotein (LDL). Oxidation of LDL has been found to increase the risk of atherosclerosis and cardiac disease (Grassmann et al., 2001).

Lavender: Inhalation of lavender and monarda oils was found to reduce cholesterol content and atherosclerotic plaques in the aorta (Nikolaevskiĭ et al., 1990).

Melissa: Melissa essential oil was found to have hypolipidemic effects in transgenic mice. Mice orally administered Melissa essential oil for two weeks had lower plasma triglyceride concentrations and altered metabolic pathways. These results indicate that melissa oil could be beneficial in preventing hypertriglyceridemia, one of the main contributors to the development of cardiovascular disease (Jun et al., 2012).

Dill: Different fractions of *Anethum graveolens* extract improved hypercholesterolemia in rats fed a high fat diet. Hypercholesterolemia has been found to be a risk factor for the development of atherosclerosis (Bahramikia et al., 2009).

Basil: Short-term oral administration of the hydroalcoholic extract of basil leaves to rats was found to protect the muscular tissue of the heart against a chemically induced heart attack (Fathiazad et al., 2012).

Carpal Tunnel Syndrome

Carpal tunnel syndrome is a painful condition of the hand, wrist, and fingers. This condition is caused by inflamed carpal ligaments in the wrist causing pressure on the median nerve. The carpal ligaments can become inflamed due to one of many possible factors: wrist trauma or injury, fluid retention, work stress, or certain strenuous wrist activities. Symptoms include tingling or numbness of the fingers and hand, pain starting in the wrist and extending to the arm or shoulder or to the palms or fingers, a general sense of weakness, and difficulty grasping small objects.

Oils: frankincense, basil, marjoram, lemongrass, oregano, cypress, eucalyptus, lavender

Recipe 1: Apply 1 drop basil and 1 drop marjoram on the shoulder, and massage oils into the skin. Then apply 1 drop lemongrass on the wrist and 1 drop oregano on the rotator cuff in the shoulder, and massage into the skin. Next apply 1 drop marjoram and 1 drop cypress on the wrists and 1 drop cypress on the neck down to the shoulder, and massage into the skin. Lastly, apply peppermint from the shoulder down the arm to the wrist and then out to the tips of each finger, and massage into the skin.

Dilute oils as recommended, and apply oils on area of concern Add 1–2 drops to 1 Tbs. fractionated coconut oil for massage oil, and massage on location.

Cartilage
see **Bones:Cartilage, Muscles/Connective Tissue:Cartilage Injury**

Cataracts
see **Eyes:Cataracts**

Catarrh
see **Congestion:Catarrh**

Cavities
see **Oral Conditions:Cavities**

Cells

Oils: ⬤Cellular Complex

Other Products: ⬤Cellular Vitality Complex, ⬤Food Nutrient Complex and ⬤Chewable Multivitamin for antioxidant support to help protect cells and DNA and for necessary nutrients, ⬤Energy & Stamina Complex for cellular energy support, and ⬤Essential Oil Omega Complex or Vegan Essential Oil Omega Complex or ⬤⬤Omega-3 Fish Oil for omega-3 fatty acids necessary for cellular health

—DNA & Mutation:

DNA is the genetic material of the cell, DNA contains all of the codes that enables the cell to build the materials needed for proper cell structure and function. Mutation of DNA can lead to cell death or to cancer.

—Antimutagenic Oils:

Oils: ⬤⬤peppermint, ⬤⬤lavender, ⬤⬤rosemary, ⬤⬤basil, ⬤⬤fennel

⬤: Take 3–5 drops in an empty capsule, or with food and beverage. Take up to twice per day as needed.

⬤: Dilute oils as recommended, and apply oils on area of concern Add 1–2 drops to 1 Tbs. fractionated coconut oil for massage oil, and massage on location.

⬤: Diffuse into the air. Inhale oil applied to hands, tissue, or cotton wick.

⬤: **Additional Research:**

Peppermint: Infusions from peppermint and valerian were shown to have antimutagenic properties on fruit flies exposed to the mutagen hydrogen peroxide (Romero-Jiménez et al., 2005).

Lavender: In tests for mutagenicity, both tea tree and lavender oils were found to not be mutagenic. In fact, lavender oil was found to have strong antimutagenic activity, reducing mutations of cells exposed to a known mutagen (Evandri et al., 2005).

Rosemary: An ethanol extract of rosemary demonstrated a protective effect against the oxidative damage to DNA in cells exposed to H2O2 and light-excited methylene blue (Slamenova et al., 2002).

Basil: Basil and its component, linalool, were found to reduce spontaneous mutagenesis in bacteria cells (Berić et al., 2008).

Fennel: Oral pretreatment with fennel essential oil was found to inhibit in vivo genotoxicity of cyclophosphamide (an important chemotherapy medication with adverse effects) in mouse bone marrow and sperm. These findings suggest that fennel could be used as an adjuvant in chemotherapeutic applications to help diminish adverse effects (Tripathi et al., 2013).

Cellulite
see also **Weight**

Cellulite refers to deposits of fat under the skin of the thighs, abdomen, and buttocks that cause the skin to appear dimpled.

Oils: ⬤⬤Metabolic Blend, ⬤grapefruit, ⬤rosemary, ⬤basil, ⬤orange, ⬤lemon, ⬤lime, ⬤cypress, ⬤juniper berry, ⬤lavender, ⬤oregano, ⬤fennel, ⬤geranium

Recipe 1: Add 5 drops grapefruit and 5 drops lemon to 1 gallon drinking water. Adjust to taste, and drink throughout the day.

⬤: Add 8 drops of Metabolic Blend to 16 oz. of water, and drink throughout the day between meals.

☜: Dilute as recommended, and apply 1–2 drops on location. Add 1–2 drops to 1 Tbs. fractionated coconut oil, and massage on location.

Charley Horse
see **Muscles/Connective Tissue:Cramps/Charley Horses**

Chemicals
see **Detoxification**

Childbirth
see **Pregnancy/Motherhood**

Childhood Diseases
see also **Antiviral, Antibacterial**

—**Chicken Pox:** *see also* **Shingles**

Chicken pox is a common childhood illness caused by the virus varicella zoster. Symptoms of chicken pox include mild fever, weakness, and a rash. The rash appears as red spots that form into blisters that eventually burst and then crust over. Chicken pox can occur between 10 and 21 days after contact with the virus and is contagious up to five days before and five days after the rash appears. Chicken pox is highly contagious and can be contracted by anyone, but it is most common in children under the age of 15.

Oils: ☜lavender, ☜☝melaleuca, ☜Roman chamomile, ☜eucalyptus, ☝lemon, ☝bergamot

Recipe 1: Add 10 drops lavender and 10 drops Roman chamomile to 4 oz. calamine lotion. Mix, and apply twice a day over body.

Recipe 2: Add 2 drops lavender to 1 cup bicarbonate of soda (baking soda). Dissolve in warm bathwater, and bathe to help relieve itching.

—**Measles:**

Measles is a viral infection of the respiratory system that causes coughing, runny nose, red eyes, fever, and a rash on the skin.

Oils: ☝☜eucalyptus○, ☝☜melaleuca, ☝☜lavender

—**Mumps:**

Mumps is a viral infection that causes fever, chills, headache, and painful swelling of the saliva glands.

Oils: ☜☝melaleuca, ☜lavender, ☝lemon

—**Rubella (German Measles):**

Rubella, or German measles, is a viral infection that causes rash, fever, runny nose, and joint pain.

Oils: ☜melaleuca, ☜lavender

—**Whooping Cough:**

Whooping cough, or pertussis, is a bacterial infection that causes cold-like symptoms, followed by severe coughing fits.

☝=Aromatic, ☜=Topical, ○=Internal *(See page 33 for further details.)*   123

Oils: ⚬oregano, ⚬⚬basil, ⚬⚬thyme, ⚬clary sage, ⚬cypress, ⚬lavender, ⚬Roman chamomile, ⚬grapefruit, ⚬eucalyptus, ⚬melaleuca, ⚬peppermint, ⚬rose

☝: Dilute as recommended, and apply on location or on chest, neck, back, or reflex points on the feet. Add 1–2 drops to 1 quart warm water, and use water for a sponge bath.

☝: Diffuse into the air. Diffuse other antiviral oils such as lemon as well. *See Antiviral.*

☐: **Additional Research:**

Eucalyptus: A plaque reduction assay showed that eucalyptus essential oil possessed a mild antiviral activity against mumps virus (Cermelli et al., 2008).

Children and Infants

When using essential oils on children and infants, it is always best to dilute the pure essential oil with a carrier oil. For older children, dilute 1–2 drops essential oil in 1/2–1 tsp. of carrier oil. For newborns and infants, dilute 1–2 drops in 2 Tbs. of carrier oil. If the oils are used in a bath, always use a bath gel base as a dispersing agent for the essential oils.

Keep the oils out of children's reach. If an oil is ever ingested, give the child an oil-soluble liquid such as milk, cream, or half & half. Then call your local poison control center, or seek emergency medical attention. A few drops of pure essential oil shouldn't be life-threatening, but it is best to take these precautions.

Several oils that are generally considered safe for children include cypress, frankincense, geranium, ginger, lavender, lemon*, marjoram, melaleuca, orange*, rosemary▽, sandalwood, thyme, and ylang ylang.

*: These oils are photosensitive; always dilute, and do not use when skin will be exposed soon to direct sunlight.

▽: This oil should never be used undiluted on infants or children

—**Colic:**

Colic is any extended period of crying and fussiness that occurs frequently in an infant. While the exact cause is not known, it has been speculated that the cause may be from indigestion, the build-up of gas, lactose intolerance, or a lack of needed probiotic bacteria in the intestines.

Oils: ⚬fennel⚬, ⚬marjoram, ⚬bergamot, ⚬ylang ylang, ⚬ginger, ⚬Roman chamomile, ⚬rosemary, ⚬melissa

Blend 1: Combine 2 Tbs. almond oil with 1 drop Roman chamomile, 1 drop lavender, and 1 drop geranium. Mix, and apply to stomach and back.

☝: Dilute 1–2 drops of oil in 2 Tbs. fractionated coconut oil, and massage a small amount of this blend gently on stomach and back.

—**Common Cold:** *see Antiviral*

A cold is a viral infection that causes a stuffy or runny nose, congestion, cough, and sneezing.

Oils: ⚬⚬thyme, ⚬⚬lemon, ⚬⚬cedarwood, ⚬⚬sandalwood, ⚬⚬rosemary, ⚬⚬rose

☝: Dilute 1–2 drops of oil in 2 Tbs. fractionated coconut oil, and massage a little on neck and chest.

☝: Diffuse into the air.

—Constipation:

Constipation is when feces becomes too hard and dry to expel easily from the body.

Oils: ○rosemary○, ○ginger, ○orange

○: Dilute 1–2 drops of oil in 2 Tbs. fractionated coconut oil, and massage on stomach and feet.

—Cradle Cap:

Cradle cap is a scaling of the skin on the head that commonly occurs in young infants. The scaling is yellowish in color and often disappears by the time the infant is a few months old.

Recipe 1: Combine 2 Tbs. almond oil with 1 drop lemon and 1 drop geranium. Apply a small amount of this blend on the head.

—Croup:

Croup is a viral respiratory infection that causes inflammation of the area around the larynx (voice box) and a distinctive-sounding cough. Often, taking an infant or child outside to breath cool night air can help open the restricted airways, as can humidity.

Oils: ∅○marjoram, ∅○thyme, ∅○sandalwood

∅: Diffuse into the air.

○: Dilute 1–2 drops in 2 Tbs. fractionated coconut oil, and massage on chest and neck.

—Crying:

Oils: ∅○ylang ylang, ∅○lavender, ∅○Roman chamomile, ∅○geranium, ∅○cypress, ∅○frankincense

∅: Diffuse into the air.

○: Dilute 1–2 drops in 2 Tbs. fractionated coconut oil. Massage.

—Diaper Rash:

Diaper rash is a red rash of the skin in the diaper area caused by prolonged skin exposure to the moisture and different pH of urine and feces. Often, more frequent bathing of the area and diaper changes will help alleviate the rash.

Oils: ○lavender

Blend 2: Combine 1 drop Roman chamomile and 1 drop lavender with 1 tsp. fractionated coconut oil, and apply on location.

○: Dilute 1–2 drops in 2 Tbs. fractionated coconut oil, and apply a small amount of this mixture on location.

—Digestion (sluggish):

Oils: ○lemon, ○orange

○: Dilute 1–2 drops in 2 Tbs. fractionated coconut oil, and massage a small amount on feet and stomach.

—Dry Skin:

Oils: ○sandalwood

  ◯: Dilute 1–2 drops in 2 Tbs. fractionated coconut oil, and apply a small amount on location.

—Earache:

  Oils: ◯melaleuca, ◯Roman chamomile, ◯lavender, ◯thyme

  Blend 3: Combine 2 Tbs. fractionated coconut oil with 2 drops lavender, 1 drop Roman chamomile, and 1 drop melaleuca. Put a drop on a cotton ball or cotton swab, and apply in ear, behind the ear, and on reflex points on the feet.

  ◯: Dilute 1–2 drops in 2 Tbs. fractionated coconut oil, and apply a small amount behind the ear. Place a drop on a cotton ball, and place in the ear.

—Fever:

  Oils: ◯lavender, ◯peppermint

  ◯: Dilute 1–2 drops in 2 Tbs. fractionated coconut oil, and massage a small amount on the neck, feet, behind ears, and on back.

  ◯: Diffuse into the air.

—Flu:

  Flu, or influenza, is a viral infection that affects the respiratory system. Symptoms may include coughing, sneezing, fever, runny nose, congestion, muscle aches, nausea, and vomiting.

  Oils: ◯◯cypress, ◯◯lemon

  ◯: Dilute 1 drop oil in an unscented bath gel, and use for a bath.

  ◯: Diffuse into the air.

—Hyperactive: *see Calming, ADD/ADHD*

—Jaundice:

  Jaundice is a condition where the liver cannot clear the pigment bilirubin quickly enough from the blood, causing the blood to deposit the bilirubin into the skin and whites of the eyes, turning them a yellowish color.

  Oils: ◯geranium, ◯lemon, ◯rosemary

  ◯: Dilute 1–2 drops in 2 Tbs. fractionated coconut oil, and massage a small amount on the liver area and on the reflex points on the feet.

—Premature:

  Since premature babies have very thin and sensitive skin, it is best to avoid the use of essential oils.

—Rashes:

  Oils: ◯lavender, ◯Roman chamomile, ◯sandalwood

  ◯: Dilute 1–2 drops in 2 Tbs. fractionated coconut oil, and apply a small amount on location.

—Teeth Grinding:

  Oils: ◯lavender, ◯◯Calming Blend

🖐: Dilute 1–2 drops in 2 Tbs. fractionated coconut oil, and massage a small amount on the feet.

🌀: Diffuse into the air.

—Tonsillitis:

Tonsillitis is inflammation of the tonsils, two lymph-filled tissues located at the back of the mouth that help provide immune support. These may become inflamed due to a bacterial or viral infection.

Oils: 🖐melaleuca, 🖐lemon, 🖐Roman chamomile, 🖐lavender, 🖐ginger

🖐: Dilute 1–2 drops in 2 Tbs. fractionated coconut oil, and apply a small amount to tonsils and lymph nodes.

—Thrush: *see also Antifungal*

Thrush is an oral fungal infection caused by *Candida albicans*. It causes painful white-colored areas to appear in the mouth.

Oils: 🖐melaleuca⬇, 🖐lavender⬇, 🖐thyme⬇, 🖐lemon, 🖐geranium

🖐: Dilute 1–2 drops in 2 Tbs. fractionated coconut oil, and apply a small amount on location.

🔲: **Additional Research:**

Fennel: Fennel seed oil was found to be superior to a placebo in decreasing intensity of infantile colic in a randomized placebo-controlled trial including 121 infants. The oil was administered four times a day and consumption was limited to a maximum of 12 mg/kg/day of fennel seed oil (Alexandrovich et al., 2003).

Fennel and melissa: Colic improved in breastfed infants within 1 week of administering a phytotherapeutic agent containing *Matricariae recutita, Foeniculum vulgare*, and *Melissa officinalis* when compared to a placebo containing vitamins (Savino et al., 2005).

Rosemary: The use of rosemary, lemon, and peppermint oils in massage demonstrated an ability to reduce constipation and increase bowel movements in elderly subjects, compared to massage without the oils (Kim et al., 2005).

Melaleuca: Tea tree oil was found to inhibit 301 different types of yeasts isolated from the mouths of cancer patients suffering from advanced cancer, including 41 strains that are known to be resistant to antifungal drugs (Bagg et al., 2006).

Melaleuca: Eleven types of Candida were found to be highly inhibited by tea tree oil (Banes-Marshall et al., 2001).

Lavender: Lavender oil demonstrated both fungistatic (stopped growth) and fungicidal (killed) activity against Candida albicans (D'Auria et al., 2005).

Thyme: Thyme oil was found to inhibit Candida species by causing lesions in the cell membrane as well as inhibiting germ tube (an outgrowth that develops when the fungi is preparing to replicate) formation (Pina-Vaz et al., 2004).

Chills

see Fever, Warming Oils

Cholera

Cholera is a potentially severe bacterial infection of the intestines by the *Vibrio cholerae* bacteria. This infection can cause severe diarrhea, leading to dehydration that can cause low blood pressure, shock, or death. Rehydration with an oral rehydration solution is the most effective way to prevent dehydration. If no commercially-prepared oral rehydration solution is available, a solution made from 1 tsp. salt, 8 tsp. sugar, and 1 liter clean water (with some mashed fresh banana, if available, to add potassium) can work in an emergency.

Oils: 🖐rosemary, 🖐clove

🖐: Dilute as recommended, and apply to stomach and on reflex points on the feet.

Cholesterol

Cholesterol is an important lipid that comprises part of the cell membrane and myelin sheath and that plays a role in nerve cell function. It is created by the body and can be found in many foods we eat. An imbalance of certain types of cholesterol in the blood has been theorized to play a role in the formation of plaques in the arteries (atherosclerosis).

Oils: Olemongrass◎, ◎clary sage, ◎helichrysum, ◎lavender◎, O◎juniper berry◎

◉: Dilute as recommended, and apply to liver area and reflex points on the feet.

○: Place 1–2 drops in a capsule, and swallow.

◈: Diffuse into the air.

▣: **Additional Research:**

> **Lemongrass:** Supplementation with lemongrass capsules was found to reduce cholesterol in some subjects (Elson et al., 1989).
>
> **Lavender:** Inhalation of lavender and monarda oils was found to reduce cholesterol content and atherosclerotic plaques in the aorta (Nikolaevski⊠ et al., 1990).
>
> **Juniper Berry:** Oral administration of juniper berry essential oil to rats fed a high cholesterol diet resulted in increased antioxidant enzyme activities in the rat heart tissue (Gumral et al., 2013).
>
> **Camphene (found in coriander, frankincense, ginger, lavender, lime, peppermint, roman chamomile, rose, rosemary, spearmint, white fir):** Injection of camphene, a constituent found in many essential oils, was found to reduce plasma cholesterol and triglycerides in naïve and hyperlipidemic rats. Camphene's mechanism of action was different than that of statins (drugs used to lower cholesterol levels) (Vallianou et al., 2011).

Chronic Fatigue

Chronic fatigue syndrome refers to a set of debilitating symptoms that may include prolonged periods of fatigue that are not alleviated by rest, difficulty concentrating, muscle and joint pain, headaches, and sore throats that cannot be explained by any other known medical condition. While the exact cause of chronic fatigue syndrome is not known, some have theorized that it is caused by a virus (such as the Epstein-Barr virus) left in the body after an illness.

Oils: ○◎Protective Blend, ◎◎peppermint, ◎◎basil, ◎◎lemongrass, O◎Digestive Blend, ◎◎rosemary, ◎◎lavender

Other Products: OEnergy & Stamina Complex, OCellular Vitality Complex or OChewable Multivitamin to help support healthy cellular energy levels. OEssential Oil Omega Complex or Vegan Essential Oil Omega Complex or OOmega-3 Fish Oil, and OFood Nutrient Complex to help supply necessary nutrients to support cell and immune function.

◉: Dilute as recommended, and apply 1–2 drops to sore muscles or joints, to the back, or to the feet. Add 1–2 drops to warm bathwater for a bath.

○: Take capsules as directed on package. Add 1–2 drops of oil to an empty capsule; swallow.

◈: Diffuse into the air. Inhale directly from bottle. Apply oil to hands, tissue, or cotton wick, and inhale.

Cigarettes
see **Addictions:Smoking**

Circulatory System
see **Cardiovascular System**

Cirrhosis

see **Liver:Cirrhosis**

Cleansing

see also **Housecleaning**

Oils: ☁☽Cleansing Blend, ☁☽Protective Blend, ☽melaleuca

Other Products: ☁Protective Hand Wash to cleanse hands and protect against harmful microorganisms.

—**Cuts:**

    Oils: ☁lavender, ☽melaleuca

—**Master Cleanse or Lemonade Diet:**

    Combine 2 Tbs. fresh lemon or lime juice (approximately 1/2 lemon), 2 Tbs. grade B maple syrup, and 1/10 tsp cayenne pepper (or to taste) with 10 oz. distilled water. In case of diabetes, use black strap molasses instead of the maple syrup. Drink 6–12 glasses of this mixture daily, with an herbal laxative tea taken first thing in the morning and just before retiring at night. Refer to the booklet *The Master Cleanser* for more specifics and for suggestions of how to come off of this cleanse.

    ☽: Dilute as recommended, and apply on location. Dilute 1–3 drops in 1 Tbs. fractionated coconut oil, and use as massage oil. Use hand wash as directed on packaging.

    ☽: Diffuse into the air.

Colds

see also **Antiviral, Coughs, Congestion**

A cold is a viral infection that causes a stuffy or runny nose, congestion, cough, sore throat, or sneezing.

Oils: ☽☾thyme, ☽☾lemon, ☽☾Protective Blend, ☽☾melaleuca, ☽☾sandalwood, ☾eucalyptus, ☽☾rosemary, ☁☽lime, ☽☾peppermint (for nasal congestion), ☽☾Respiratory Blend (for respiratory congestion), ☁ginger, ☽☾basil, ☽☾lavender, ☾Oorange, ☽☾oregano

Other Products: ORespiratory Lozenge Drops, OProtective Softgels. OFood Nutrient Complex for nutrients essential to support cellular and immune system health.

Recipe 1: When you first notice a sore throat, apply a tiny amount of melaleuca to the tip of the tongue, and then swallow. Repeat this a few times every 5–10 minutes. Then massage a couple of drops on the back of the neck.

    ☽: Dilute as recommended, and apply 1–2 drops to throat, temples, forehead, back of neck, sinus area, below the nose, chest, or reflex points on the feet.

    ☽: Diffuse into the air. Place 1–2 drops in a bowl of hot water, and inhale the vapors. Inhale directly from bottle. Apply oil to hands, tissue, or cotton wick, and inhale.

    O: Take capsules as directed on package. Place 1–2 drops of oil under the tongue or place 1–2 drops of oil in an empty capsule, and swallow.

Cold Sores

see also **Antiviral, Herpes Simplex**

Cold sores are blisters or sores in the mouth area caused by an infection of the herpes simplex virus.

Oils: ⊘melaleuca⊡, ⊘melissa⊡, ⊘peppermint⊡, ⊘lemon, ⊘Protective Blend, ⊘geranium, ⊘lavender, ⊘bergamot

⊜: Dilute as recommended, and apply 1–2 drops on location.

⊡: **Additional Research:**

> **Melaleuca:** Tea tree and eucalyptus oil demonstrated an ability to inhibit the Herpes simplex virus (Schnitzler et al., 2001).
>
> **Melissa:** Melissa oil demonstrated inhibition of herpes simplex type 1 and type 2 viruses (Schnitzler et al., 2008).
>
> **Peppermint:** Peppermint oil demonstrated a direct virucidal activity against herpes type 1 and type 2 viruses (Schuhmacher et al., 2003).

Colic

see **Children and Infants:Colic**

Colitis

see **Colon:Colitis**

Colon

see also **Cancer:Colon, Digestive System**

The colon, or large intestine, is the last part of the digestive system. Its function is to extract water and vitamins created by friendly bacterial flora from the material moving through the digestive system.

Oils: ⊘ODigestive Blend, ⊘Opeppermint

Other Products: OProbiotic Defense Formula to help restore friendly flora to the intestinal wall. OGI Cleansing Formula to help the digestive system eliminate pathogens. ODigestive Softgels to help support healthy digestion. ODetoxification Complex to help support healthy colon functioning.

—**Cancer:** *see* **Cancer:Colon**

—**Colitis:**

> Colitis is inflammation of the large intestine or colon. The exact cause is not known but may involve an auto-immune response. Symptoms can include abdominal pain, tenderness, frequent need to expel stools, diarrhea, and possibly bloody stools and fever in the case of ulcerative colitis.
>
> **Oils:** ⊘ODigestive Blend, ⊘⊘helichrysum, ⊘⊘peppermint⊡, ⊘⊘Othyme⊡, Ooregano⊡, Orosemary⊡, ⊘⊘clove
>
> **Other Products:** ODigestive Softgels to help support healthy digestion.

—**Diverticulitis:**

> Diverticulitis is the inflammation of a diverticula (a small balloon-like sac that sometimes forms along the wall of the large intestine, especially in older individuals), typically due to infection. It causes pain in the abdomen and tenderness on the lower-left-hand part of the stomach.

Oils: ⚫cinnamon, ⚫lavender

—Polyps: *see also* **Cancer:Colon**

Polyps are tumors that arise from the bowel surface and protrude into the inside of the colon. Most polyps eventually transform into malignant cancer tumors.

Oils: O⚫peppermint

⚫: Dilute as recommended, and apply 1–2 drops on lower abdomen or on reflex points on the feet. Use 1–2 drops in warm bathwater for a bath.

◯: Take capsule as directed on package. Place 1–2 drops in an empty capsule; swallow.

⚫: Diffuse into the air. Inhale directly from bottle. Apply oil to hands, tissue, or cotton wick, and inhale.

⬜: **Additional Research:**

Peppermint: L-menthol was found to inhibit production of inflammation mediators in human monocytes (a type of white blood cell involved in the immune response) (Juergens et al., 1998).

Rosemary: Rosemary essential oil was found to be effective in reducing colon tissue lesions and colitis indices when administered orally or intraperitoneally to rats induced with colitis, suggesting that rosemary has anti-colitic activity (Minaiyan et al., 2011).

Thyme and oregano: Oral administration of thyme and oregano oil at a dose of 0.2% thyme and 0.1% oregano was found to be effective in decreasing the mortality rate, accelerating body weight gain recovery, and significantly reducing the macroscopic damage of colonic tissue of mice with induced colitis (Bukovska et al., 2007).

Coma

Oils: ⚫frankincense, ⚫Grounding Blend, ⚫sandalwood, ⚫cypress, ⚫peppermint

⚫: Dilute as recommended, and massage 1–2 drops on the brain stem area, mastoids (behind ears), temples, and bottoms of feet.

Complexion

see **Skin**

Concentration (Poor)

Oils: ⚫⚫Focus Blend, ⚫lavender◯, ⚫lemon◯, ⚫peppermint, ⚫orange, ⚫cedarwood, ⚫cypress, ⚫juniper berry, ⚫eucalyptus, ⚫rosemary, ⚫sandalwood, ⚫ylang ylang

Other Products: ◯Essential Oil Omega Complex or Vegan Essential Oil Omega Complex or ◯Omega-3 Fish Oil, which contains omega-3 fatty acids necessary for proper brain cell function.

⚫: Apply on back of neck and bottoms of feet.

⚫: Diffuse into the air. Apply, and inhale from hands, tissue, or cotton wick.

◯: Take capsules as directed on package.

⬜: **Additional Research:**

Lavender: Subjects who smelled a cleansing gel with lavender aroma were more relaxed and able to complete math computations faster (Field et al., 2005).

Lavender: Subjects exposed to 3 minutes of lavender aroma were more relaxed and able to perform math computations faster and more accurately. Subjects exposed to rosemary aroma were more alert and completed math computations faster (but not more accurately) (Diego et al., 1998).

Lemon: Daily inhalation of lemon essential oil aroma for five minutes was found to have a positive effect on learning in mice (Ogeturk et al., 2010).

Concussion

see Brain:Concussion

Confusion

Oils: ☺☻Focus Blend, ☻frankincense, ☻sandalwood, ☻Grounding Blend, ☻rosemary, ☻peppermint, ☻juniper berry, ☻marjoram, ☻cedarwood, ☻basil, ☻ylang ylang, ☻white fir, ☻thyme, ☻geranium, ☻rose, ☻ginger

☺: Apply on back of neck and bottoms of feet.

☻: Diffuse into the air. Inhale directly from bottle. Apply oil to hands, tissue, or cotton wick, and inhale.

Congestion

Congestion is the blockage of the nasal passages, sinuses, or upper respiratory tract due to inflamed tissues and blood vessels or to an increased output of mucus. Congestion can make it difficult to breathe freely and can sometimes cause pain.

Oils: ☺☻eucalyptus◌, ☺☻peppermint, ☺☻Respiratory Blend, ☻cinnamon, ☺☻juniper berry, ☺☻cypress, ☺☻melaleuca, ☻◉cedarwood, ☻◉cardamom, ☺☻ginger, ☺☻rosemary, ☺☻fennel, ☺☻citrus oils, ☺☻patchouli

—Catarrh:

Catarrh refers to the secretion of mucus and white blood cells from the mucus membranes in the sinuses and nasal passages in response to an infection.

Oils: ☺☻cypress, ☺☻helichrysum, ☺☻Respiratory Blend, ☺☻Protective Blend, ☺☻eucalyptus ☺☻frankincense, ☺☻myrrh, ☺☻rosemary, ☺☻ginger

—Expectorant:

An expectorant is an agent that helps dissolve thick mucus in the trachea, bronchi, or lungs for easier elimination.

Oils: ☻◉eucalyptus◌, ☻◉marjoram, ☻◉frankincense, ☻◉helichrysum, ☻◉cardamom

—Mucus:

Mucus is the substance produced by epithelial cells to coat the mucous membranes in the respiratory tract, digestive tract, and reproductive system. Mucus plays an important role in helping to protect these surfaces from different substances or from microorganisms they come in contact with. When one of these surfaces becomes infected or inflamed, an excess of mucus is often produced. An excess of mucus can lead to difficulty breathing in the sinuses, nasal passages, or respiratory tract. For oils to help combat an excess of mucus, see the entries above.

Oils: ☺◉Digestive Blend (with ginger - helps digest old mucus)

☺: Dilute as recommended, and rub 1–2 drops on the chest, neck, back, and feet. Dilute 1–2 drops in 1 Tbs. fractionated coconut oil, and massage on chest, neck, back, and feet.

☻: Diffuse into the air. Place 1–2 drops in a bowl of hot water, and inhale the vapor. Inhale directly from bottle. Apply oil to hands, tissue, or cotton wick, and inhale.

◯: Add 1–2 drops of each oil to an empty capsule; swallow.

⊙: **Additional Research:**

Eucalyptus: Eucalyptus oil was found to have an anti-inflammatory and mucin-inhibitory effect in rats with lipopolysaccharide-induced bronchitis (Lu et al., 2004).

Conjunctivitis
see **Eyes:Pink Eye**

Connective Tissue
see **Bones:Cartilage, Muscles/Connective Tissue**

Constipation
see **Digestive System:Constipation**

Convulsions
see **Seizure:Convulsions**

Cooling Oils

Typically, oils that are high in aldehydes and esters can produce a cooling effect when applied topically or diffused.

Oils: ⊜⊘peppermint, ⊜⊘eucalyptus, ⊜⊘melaleuca, ⊜⊘lavender, ⊜⊘Roman chamomile, ⊘⊜citrus oils

⊜: Dilute as recommended, and apply 1–2 drops on location. Add 1–2 drops to bathwater, and bathe. Add 1–2 drops to basin of cool water, and sponge over skin.

⊘: Diffuse into the air.

Corns
see **Foot:Corns**

Coughs

A cough is a sudden explosive release of air from the lungs to help clear an excess of mucus, an irritant, or other materials from the airway. Coughing can be caused by foreign material entering the airway or by an infection, asthma, or other medical problem. Proper hydration or steam inhalation can help loosen thick secretions, making them easier to eliminate.

Oils: ⊘⊜Respiratory Blend, ⊘⊜melaleuca, ⊘⊜eucalyptus, ⊘⊜frankincense, ⊘⊜Protective Blend, ⊘⊜cardamom, ⊘⊜peppermint, ⊘⊜white fir, ⊘⊜juniper berry, ⊘⊜cedarwood, ⊘⊜sandalwood, ⊘⊜thyme, ⊘⊜myrrh, ⊘⊜ginger

Other Products: ○Respiratory Lozenge Drops, ○Protective Softgels. ○Protective Throat Drops to soothe irritated and sore throats.

—**Allergy:**

   Oils: ⊘Cleansing Blend

—**Severe:**

   Oils: ⊘⊜frankincense

⊘: Diffuse into the air. Use throat drops as directed on package.

⊜: Dilute as recommended, and apply 1–2 drops on the throat and chest.

⊘=Aromatic, ⊜=Topical, ○=Internal *(See page 33 for further details.)*   133

◯: Take supplements as directed on packaging.

Cradle Cap
see **Children and Infants:Cradle Cap**

Cramps
see **Digestive System:Cramps, Female Specific Conditions:Menstruation, Muscles/Connective Tissue:Cramps/Charley Horses**

Crohn's Disease

Crohn's disease is a chronic inflammation of part of the intestinal wall, thought to be caused by an over-active immune response. It can cause abdominal pain, diarrhea, nausea, and loss of appetite.

Oils: ◯☻peppermint☺, ◯☻Digestive Blend, ☻basil

◯: Add 1–2 drops of oil to an empty capsule; swallow.

☻: Dilute as recommended and apply on stomach and feet.

▭: **Additional Research:**

> **Peppermint:** A combination of peppermint and caraway oil was found to reduce visceral hyperalgesia (pain hypersensitivity in the gastrointestinal tract) after induced inflammation in rats (Adam et al., 2006).

Cuts
see also **Wounds, Antibacterial, Blood:Bleeding**

Oils: ☻helichrysum, ☻lavender, ☻melaleuca, ☻basil☺, ☻Protective Blend, ☻Roman chamomile ☻cypress

☻: Dilute as recommended, and apply 1–2 drops on location.

▭: **Additional Research:**

> **Basil:** Basil (Ocimum gratissimum) oil was found to facilitate the healing process of wounds in rabbits to a greater extent than two antibacterial preparations, Cicatrin and Cetavlex (Orafidiya et al., 2003).

Cystitis
see **Bladder:Cystitis/Infection**

Dandruff
see **Hair:Dandruff**

Decongestant
see **Congestion**

Degenerative Disease

A degenerative disease is a disease where the affected tissues or organs are damaged due to internal mechanisms, and not due to infection. Quite a few different diseases can be categorized as degenerative diseases, including Alzheimer's disease, cancer, Parkinson's disease, atherosclerosis, diabetes, osteoporosis, rheumatoid arthritis, and many others. Support the cells and tissues through proper nutrition, reducing stress, exercising regularly, and eliminating toxins. See specific conditions in this guide for oils and other products that can support the body for each condition.

Delivery
see **Pregnancy/Motherhood:Delivery**

Dental Infection
see **Oral Conditions**

Deodorant

Oils: ⊖Cleansing Blend, ⊖melaleuca, ⊖lavender, ⊖geranium, ⊖eucalyptus, ⊖cedarwood, ⊖cypress, ⊖Joyful Blend, ⊖Calming Blend, ⊖Respiratory Blend, ⊖Women's Blend

⊖: Dilute as recommended, and apply 1–2 drops on the skin. Dilute 2–3 drops in 1 Tbs. fractionated coconut oil, and apply under the arms. Add 2–3 drops to 4 oz. unscented talcum powder and 2 oz. baking soda, and apply under the arms, on the feet, or on other areas of the body.

Deodorizing

Oils: ⊘Cleansing Blend, ⊘peppermint, ⊘cedarwood, ⊘clary sage

⊘: Diffuse into the air. Dissolve 8–10 drops in 1 tsp. perfumer's or pure grain alcohol (such as vodka), and combine with distilled water in a 1 oz. spray bottle. Spray into the air or on affected surface.

Depression

Depression is a disorder marked by excessive sadness, energy loss, feelings of worthlessness, irritableness, sudden weight loss or gain, trouble sleeping, and loss of interest in activities normally enjoyed. These symptoms can continue for weeks or months if not treated and can destroy an individual's quality of life.

Oils: ⊘⊖Olemon○, ⊘⊖frankincense○, ⊘⊘Focus Blend, ⊘⊖Olavender○, ⊘⊖bergamot○, ⊘⊘Joyful Blend, ⊘⊖Grounding Blend, ⊘⊖Invigorating Blend○, ⊘⊖melissa, ⊘⊖clary sage○, ⊘⊘rosemary○, ⊘⊘ylang ylang○, ⊘⊘grapefruit○, ⊘⊖clary sage, ⊘⊖Calming Blend, ⊘⊖Olime, ⊘⊖geranium, ⊘⊖ginger, ⊘⊖juniper berry, ⊘⊖basil, ⊘⊖sandalwood, ⊖⊘Opatchouli

—**Postpartum Depression:** *see* **Pregnancy/Motherhood:Postpartum Depression**

—**Sedatives:**

Oils: ⊘⊖lavender○, ⊘⊖ylang ylang, ⊘⊘melissa○, ⊘⊘Roman chamomile, ⊘⊖sandalwood, ⊘⊖cedarwood, ⊘⊖rose, ⊘⊖clary sage, ⊘⊖cypress, ⊘⊖juniper berry, ⊘⊖frankincense, ⊘⊖bergamot, ⊘⊖marjoram

⊘: Diffuse into the air. Inhale directly from bottle. Apply oil to hands, tissue, or cotton wick, and inhale.

⊖: Dilute as recommended, and apply 1–2 drops to temple or forehead. Add 5–10 drops to 1 Tbs. fractionated coconut oil, and use as massage oil. Add 1–3 drops to warm bathwater, and bathe.

○: Add 1–2 drops to 8 oz. distilled water or 4 oz. rice or almond milk, and drink. Add 1–2 drops to empty capsule, and swallow.

🛈: **Additional Research:**

Lemon: Lemon oil vapor was found to have strong antistress and antidepressant effects on mice subjected to several common stress tests (Komiya et al., 2006).

Lemon: Lemon oil and its component, citral, were found to decrease depressed behavior in a similar manner to antidepressant drugs in rats involved in several stress tests (Komori et al., 1995).

Lemon: In 12 patients suffering from depression, it was found that inhaling citrus aromas reduced the needed doses of antidepressants, normalized neuroendocrine hormone levels, and normalized immune function (Komori et al., 1995).

Frankincense: Incensole acetate was found to open TRPV receptors in mice brains, indicating a possible channel for emotional regulation (Moussaieff et al., 2008).

Lavender: In patients suffering from arthritis, it was found that a blend of lavender, marjoram, eucalyptus, rosemary, and peppermint blended with carrier oils was found to reduce perceived pain and depression compared to control (Kim et al., 2005).

Lavender: Female students suffering from insomnia were found to sleep better and to have a lower level of depression during weeks they used a lavender fragrance when compared to weeks they did not use a lavender fragrance (Lee et al., 2006).

Lavender: Swiss mice fed lavender oil diluted in olive oil were found to be more sedate in several common tests (Guillemain et al., 1989).

Lavender: Exposure to inhaled lavender oil and to its constituents, linalool and linalyl acetate, was found to decrease normal movement in mice as well as to return mice to normal movement rates after caffeine-induced hyperactivity (Buchbauer et al., 1991).

Lavender: Lavandula angustifolia essential oil demonstrated ability to inhibit GABA-A receptor channels of rat brain cells (Huang et al., 2008).

Lavender: Inhaling lavender oil was found to lower agitation in older adults suffering from dementia (Lin et al., 2007).

Bergamot: In 12 patients suffering from depression, it was found that inhaling citrus aromas reduced the needed doses of antidepressants, normalized neuroendocrine hormone levels, and normalized immune function (Komori et al., 1995).

Invigorating Blend: In 12 patients suffering from depression, it was found that inhaling citrus aromas reduced the needed doses of antidepressants, normalized neuroendocrine hormone levels, and normalized immune function (Komori et al., 1995).

Clary sage: Clary sage essential oil displayed antidepressant-like effects via the dopaminergic pathway in rats submitted to the forced swim test (a common stress test) (Seol et al., 2010).

Rosemary: Many fractions of *Rosmarinus officinalis*, including its essential oil, were found to have antidepressant-like effects on mice submitted to two stress tests after oral administration of the rosemary plant fractions (Machado et al., 2013).

Ylang ylang: Transdermal absorption of ylang ylang essential oil altered physiological stress responses, like blood pressure and skin temperature, and subjects reported being more calm and relaxed than the control group (Hongratanaworakit et al., 2006).

Grapefruit: In 12 patients suffering from depression, it was found that inhaling citrus aromas reduced the needed doses of antidepressants, normalized neuroendocrine hormone levels, and normalized immune function (Komori et al., 1995).

Melissa: Melissa (lemon balm) oil applied topically in a lotion was found to reduce agitation and improve quality of life factors in patients suffering severe dementia compared to those receiving a placebo lotion (Ballard et al., 2002).

Dermatitis
see **Skin:Dermatitis/Eczema**

Despair
see **Depression**

Detoxification

Detoxification is the act of clearing toxins out of the body. These toxins may be addictive drugs, alcohol, or any other harmful substance.

Oils: ⬤helichrysum, ⬤rosemary○, ⬤juniper berry, ⬤coriander○

🜂: Dilute as recommended, and apply to liver area, intestines, and reflex points on the feet.

🗋: **Additional Research:**

Rosemary: Rosemary extracts induced CYP (cytochrome 450) activity in liver cells, suggesting a possibility of increased ability to remove toxins (Debersac et al., 2001).

Coriander: Coriander extract was found to have a protective role against lead toxicity in rat brain (Velaga et al., 2014).

Diabetes

Diabetes is a disease characterized by the body's inability to properly produce or use the hormone insulin. Insulin, produced in the pancreas, helps regulate the level of sugars in the blood, as well as the conversion of starches and sugar into the energy necessary for life. Common diabetes symptoms include a frequent need to drink and urinate, blurred vision, mental fatigue, and possibly weight loss (depending on the type). Over time, diabetes can lead to additional complications, such as strokes, heart disease, kidney failure, and even the necessity of removing a limb.

Oils: O🕲cinnamon🗋, O🕲🕲rosemary🗋, 🕲🕲geranium, O🕲🕲basil🗋, 🕲🕲ylang ylang, 🕲🕲eucalyptus, 🕲🕲Protective Blend, 🕲🕲cypress, 🕲juniper berry, O🕲dill🗋, O🕲cassia🗋, 🕲🕲ginger, 🕲🕲fennel, 🕲🕲lavender

Blend 1: Combine 8 drops clove, 8 drops cinnamon, 15 drops rosemary, and 10 drops thyme with 2 oz. fractionated coconut oil. Put on feet and over pancreas.

Blend 2: Combine 5 drops cinnamon and 5 drops cypress. Rub on feet and pancreas.

Other Products: OProtective Softgels

—Pancreas Support:

Oils: 🕲cinnamon🗋, 🕲geranium

—Sores (Diabetic):

Those suffering from diabetes have to be especially careful about sores of any kind, especially those on the feet and hands. Diabetes decreases blood flow, so wounds heal much slower. Many who suffer from diabetes experience decreased sensation in their hands and feet, making it more difficult to even notice an injury right away. Even a small sore left untreated can turn into an ulcer, ultimately making amputation necessary.

Oils: 🕲lavender, 🕲Grounding Blend

O: Place 1–2 drops of oil under the tongue or place 1–2 drops in empty capsule and swallow. Take supplements as directed on packaging.

🕲: Dilute as recommended, and apply on back, chest, feet, and over pancreas.

🕲: Diffuse into the air.

🗋: **Additional Research:**

Cinnamon: Cinnamon bark extract supplementation for three months was found to significantly improve blood glucose control in Chinese patients with type 2 diabetes taking gliclazide (a prescribed antidiabetic medication) (Lu, T. et al., 2012).

Cinnamon: Cinnamaldehyde (the major constituent of cinnamon oil) produced protective action against alloxan-induced diabetic nephropathy in rats (Mishra et al., 2010).

Cinnamon: Cinnamaldehyde (found in cinnamon oil) was found to significantly reduce blood glucose levels in diabetic wistar rats (Subash et al., 2007).

Cinnamon: Oral administration of cinnamon oil was found to significantly reduce blood glucose levels in diabetic KK-Ay mice (Ping et al., 2010).

Cinnamon: Cinnamon polyphenols were found to restore pancreatic function and exert hypoglycemic and hypolipidemic effects in a diabetic mouse model (Li, R. et al., 2013).

Rosemary: Oral rosemary extract was found to decrease blood glucose levels, while increasing insulin levels in alloxan-diabetic rabbits (Bakirel et al., 2008).

Basil: Results from a clinical trial showed that basil leaf extract decreased fasting and postprandial blood glucose in diabetes mellitus patients, suggesting that basil could be used as a dietary therapy in mild to moderate cases of type 2 diabetes mellitus (Agrawal et al., 1996) .

Melissa: Oral supplementation of melissa essential oil significantly reduced plasma glucose levels compared with the control group, and increased glucose tolerance in a type 2 diabetic mouse model (Chung et al., 2010).

Dill: Dill seed extract suppressed high-fat diet-induced hyperlipidemia through hepatic PPAR-α activation in diabetic obese mice (Takahashi et al., 2013).

Helichrysum and Grapefruit: Helichrysum and grapefruit extracts were found to improve postprandial glycemic control in a dietary model of insulin resistance in rats (da la Garza et al., 2013).

Cassia: In vitro data suggest that the constituents of cassia may be appropriate for the treatment of diabetic complications (like cataract and retinopathy) because of the constituents' ability to inhibit aldose reductase and thus prevent the conversion of glucose to corbitol (Lee, 2002).

D-Limonene (found in lime, lemon, bergamot, dill, grapefruit, lavender, lemongrass, Roman chamomile, tangerine, and wild orange essential oils): In a recent study oral intake of D-limonene ameliorated insulin resistance in mice fed a high-fat diet (Jing et al., 2013).

Diaper Rash
see **Children and Infants:Diaper Rash**

Diarrhea
see **Digestive System:Diarrhea**

Digestive System

The human digestive system is the series of organs and glands that process food. The digestive system breaks down food, absorbs nutrients for the body to use as fuel, and excretes as bowel movements the part that cannot be broken down.

Oils: ○◎❷peppermint◌, ○◎❷ginger◌, ◎❷lemongrass (purifies)◌, ○◎❷Digestive Blend, ○◎❷fennel, ○◎❷wintergreen◌, ○◎❷marjoram (stimulates), ○◎❷oregano◌, ○◎❷rosemary◌, ◎❷clary sage, ○◎❷cardamom, ○◎❷grapefruit, ○◎❷basil, ○◎❷lemon◌, ◎❷cinnamon, ○◎❷clove, ◎❷juniper berry, ○◎❷orange, ○◎❷bergamot

Regimen 1: Use ○GI Cleansing Formula for 10 days to help support the digestive system in eliminating pathogenic microorganisms, followed by ○Probiotic Defense Formula for 5 days to help rebuild friendly flora to aid digestion and prevent pathogenic bacteria.

Other Products: ○Digestive Softgels to help support healthy digestion. ○Digestive Enzyme Complex for healthy digestion, enyzmatic function, and cellular metabolism. ○Cellular Vitality Complex, ○Essential Oil Omega Complex or Vegan Essential Oil Omega Complex, ○Omega-3 Fish Oil, ○Food Nutrient Complex, ○Chewable Multivitamin to provide essential nutrients, vitamins, and minerals for digestive system cellular support.

○: Take capsules as directed on package. Add 1–2 drops of oil to 16 oz. of water, and drink. Add oils as flavoring to food. Place 1–2 drops of oil in an empty capsule, and swallow.

◎: Dilute oil as recommended, and apply 1–2 drops on stomach or reflex points on feet. Dilute 1–2 drops in 1 Tbs. fractionated coconut oil, and massage over abdomen and lower back. Apply as a warm compress over affected area.

Personal Guide

🕭: Diffuse into the air. *See Negative Ions* for oils that produce negative ions when diffused to help stimulate the digestive system. Inhale oil directly or applied to hands, tissue, or cotton wick.

—Bloating:

Bloating is an abnormal swelling, increase in diameter, or feeling of fullness and tightness in the abdominal area as gas and liquid are trapped inside. Common causes of bloating can include overeating, menstruation, constipation, food allergies, and irritable bowel syndrome.

Oils: ©©Digestive Blend

Other Products: ○Digestive Softgels

🕭: Dilute as recommended, and apply to stomach and to reflex points on the feet.

🕭: Diffuse into the air.

—Constipation:

Constipation is a condition characterized by infrequent or difficult bowel movements. A person is considered constipated if he or she has fewer than three bowel movements a week or if the stools are hard and difficult to expel. Common causes of constipation include a lack of fiber, dehydration, ignoring the urge to have a bowel movement, depression, medications, large dairy intake, stress, and abuse of laxatives.

Oils: ©rosemary©, ©lemon©, ©peppermint©, ©marjoram, ©Digestive Blend, ©ginger, ©fennel, ©orange, ©rose, ©juniper berry, ©sandalwood

Other Products: ○Digestive Softgels to help support healthy digestion.

🕭: Dilute as recommended, and apply oils on abdomen. Add 1–2 drops to 1 Tbs. fractionated coconut oil, and massage onto abdomen.

○: Take capsules as directed.

—Cramps (Abdominal):

Cramps are sudden, involuntary muscle contractions that often cause severe pain. Abdominal cramps are commonly caused by stress, menstruation, mild food poisoning, and *Irritable Bowel Syndrome (below)*.

Oils: ©©Digestive Blend, ©©basil, ©clary sage

Other Products: ○Digestive Softgels to help support healthy digestion.

Recipe 1: Flavor water with 5 drops Digestive Blend, and drink for stomach pains and cramps.

○: Place 3 drops Digestive Blend and 3 drops basil in an empty capsule; swallow. Take capsules as directed.

🕭: Dilute as recommended, and massage oil onto abdomen over area of pain.

—Diarrhea:

Diarrhea is an abnormal increase in the frequency of bowel movements, marked by loose, watery stools. Diarrhea is defined as more than three bowel movements a day. Cases of Diarrhea that last more than two days can become a serious problem and cause dehydration. Rehydration with an oral rehydration solution is the most effective way to prevent dehydration. If no commercially-prepared oral rehydration solution is available, a solution made from 1 tsp. salt, 8 tsp. sugar, and 1 liter clean water (with some mashed fresh banana, if available, to add potassium) can work in an emergency. Diarrhea is usually caused by a viral, parasitic, or bacterial infection.

Oils: O©peppermint, O©ginger, ©geranium, O©Digestive Blend, ©orange, ©patchouli, ©melaleuca, ©sandalwood, ©lavender, ©Roman chamomile, ©cypress, ©eucalyptus

Other Products: ODigestive Softgels to help support healthy digestion.

–Children:

Oils: ©geranium, ©ginger, ©sandalwood

O: Place 1–2 drops in an empty capsule, and swallow. Take supplement as directed.

©: Dilute as recommended, and apply 1–2 drops on abdomen. Apply as a warm compress over affected area.

—Gas/Flatulence:

Oils: O©lavender, O©ginger, ©peppermint, O©cardamom, ©eucalyptus, ©bergamot, ©myrrh, ©juniper berry, ©rosemary

Other Products: ODigestive Softgels to help support healthy digestion.

O: Place 1–2 drops in an empty capsule, and swallow. Take supplement as directed.

©: Dilute as recommended, and apply 1–2 drops on stomach, abdomen, or reflex points on the feet

—Gastritis: *see also Inflammation*

Gastritis is inflammation of the stomach lining.

Oils: O©Digestive Blend, O©peppermint, Olemongrass☺, ©Ofennel

Other Products: ODigestive Softgels to help support healthy digestion.

O: Add 1 drop of oil to rice or almond milk; take as a supplement. Place 1–2 drops in an empty capsule; swallow capsule. Take supplement as directed.

©: Dilute as recommended, and apply 1–2 drops on stomach. Apply as a warm compress over stomach.

—Giardia:

Giardia are parasites that infect the gastrointestinal tract of humans and animals. The form of *Giardia* that affects humans causes severe diarrhea. *See Diarrhea above* for information on rehydration.

Oils: O©lavender☺

O: Place 1–2 drops in an empty capsule; swallow capsule.

©: Dilute as recommended, and apply 1–2 drops on abdomen or reflex points on the feet.

—Heartburn:

Heartburn is a painful burning sensation in the chest or throat. It occurs as a result of backed up stomach acid in the esophagus. Heartburn is often brought on by certain foods, medication, pregnancy, and alcohol.

None

Oils: ⬤lemon, ⬤peppermint, ⬤⭕Digestive Blend

Blend 1: Blend 2 drops lemon, 2 drops peppermint, and 3 drops sandalwood in 1 Tbs. fractionated coconut oil. Apply to breast bone in a clockwise motion using the palm of the hand. Apply to reflex points on the feet.

Other Products: ⭕Digestive Softgels to help support healthy digestion.

⬤: Dilute as recommended, and apply 1–2 drops to chest.

⭕: Add 1 drop of oil to rice or almond milk; take as a supplement. Place 1–2 drops in an empty capsule; swallow capsule. Take supplement as directed.

—Indigestion:

The term "indigestion" is used to describe abdominal discomfort felt after a meal. Symptoms of indigestion include belching, bloating, nausea, heartburn, a feeling of fullness, and general abdominal discomfort. Indigestion can be caused by overeating or eating too fast, alcoholic or carbonated drinks, particular foods, etc.

Oils: ⭕⬤🌀peppermint, ⭕⬤🌀ginger, ⭕⬤Digestive Blend, ⬤🌀lavender, ⬤🌀orange, ⬤⭕🌀lime, ⬤🌀thyme, ⬤🌀myrrh, ⬤🌀grapefruit

Other Products: ⭕Digestive Softgels to help support healthy digestion. ⭕Digestive Enzyme Complex for healthy digestion, enyzmatic function, and cellular metabolism.

⭕: Add 1–2 drops of oil to 8 oz. of almond or rice milk; drink. Place 1–2 drops of oil in an empty capsule; swallow capsule. Take capsules as directed on package.

⬤: Dilute oil as recommended, and apply 1–2 drops on stomach or reflex points on feet. Dilute 1–2 drops in 1 Tbs. fractionated coconut oil, and massage over abdomen and lower back. Apply as a warm compress over stomach area.

🌀: Diffuse into the air.

—Intestines:

The intestines are the largest organs in the digestive track. The intestines include the small intestine, which begins just below the stomach and is responsible for digesting and absorbing nutrients from the food, and the large intestine, which begins at the end of the small intestine and is responsible for reabsorbing water and some vitamins before the undigested food and waste is eliminated.

Oils: ⬤⭕basil, ⬤⭕marjoram, ⬤🌀ginger, ⬤⭕rose🌀, ⬤⭕rosemary

Other Products: ⭕GI Cleansing Formula to help the digestive system eliminate pathogens. ⭕Probiotic Defense Formula to provide friendly intestinal flora to aid digestion and help prevent pathogenic bacteria. ⭕Digestive Enzyme Complex for healthy digestion, enyzmatic function, and cellular metabolism.

⬤: Dilute oil as recommended, and apply 1–2 drops on stomach or reflex points on feet. Dilute 1–2 drops in 1 Tbs. fractionated coconut oil, and massage over abdomen and lower back. Apply as a warm compress over affected area.

⭕: Take capsules as directed on package. Add 1–2 drops of oil to 16 oz. of water; drink. Add oils as flavoring to food. Place 1–2 drops of oil in a capsule, and swallow.

—Intestinal Parasites: *see Parasites:Intestinal*

—Irritable Bowel Syndrome:

Irritable bowel syndrome is an intestinal disorder characterized by reoccurring diarrhea, bloating, gas, constipation, cramping, and abdominal pain. Irritable bowel syndrome is one of the most commonly diagnosed disorders by doctors.

Oils: O☺peppermint☺, O☺Digestive Blend

○: Add 2 drops of each oil to 8 oz. distilled water, and drink 1–2 times per day. Place 2 drops of each oil in an empty capsule; swallow capsule.

☜: Dilute 1–2 drops in 1 Tbs. fractionated coconut oil, and apply over the abdomen with a hot compress.

—Nausea/Upset Stomach:

Oils: ☺ODigestive Blend, O☺ginger☺, ☺☺peppermint, ☺lavender, ☺☺Women's Monthly Blend, ☺clove

Other Products: ODigestive Softgels to help support healthy digestion.

○: Place 1–2 drops in an empty capsule; swallow capsule. Place 1 drop in 8 oz. rice or almond milk, and drink. Take supplement as directed.

☜: Dilute as recommended, and apply behind ears, on stomach, or on reflex points on the feet.

�it: Diffuse into the air. Inhale directly from bottle. Apply oil to hands, tissue, or cotton wick, and inhale.

—Parasites: *see Parasites*

—Stomach:

The stomach is the organ mainly responsible for breaking food apart using strong acids. It is located below the esophagus and before the intestines.

Oils: O☺basil, O☺peppermint, Olemongrass☺, O☺ginger, O☺Digestive Blend

Other Products: ODigestive Softgels to help support healthy digestion.

○: Place 1–2 drops in an empty capsule, and swallow. Take supplement as directed.

☜: Dilute as recommended, and apply 1–2 drops on stomach, abdomen, or reflex points on the feet

—Ulcers: *see Ulcers*

⊡: **Additional Research:**

Peppermint: A combination of peppermint and caraway oil was found to reduce visceral hyperalgesia (pain hypersensitivity in the gastrointestinal tract) after induced inflammation in rats (Adam et al., 2006).

Peppermint: Peppermint oil was found to be as effective as Buscopan (an antispasmodic drug) at preventing spasms during a barium enema (a type of enema used to place barium in the colon for X-ray imaging purposes) (Asao et al., 2003).

Peppermint: The use of rosemary, lemon, and peppermint oils in massage demonstrated an ability to reduce constipation and increase bowel movements in elderly subjects, compared to massage without the oils (Kim et al., 2005).

Peppermint: Peppermint oil in enteric-coated capsules was found to relieve symptoms of irritable bowel syndrome better than a placebo in patients suffering from IBS (Rees et al., 1979).

Peppermint: Patients with IBS symptoms who took a peppermint-oil formulation in an enteric-coated capsule were found to have a significantly higher reduction of symptoms than did patients taking a placebo (Liu et al., 1997).

Peppermint: Children suffering from irritable bowel syndrome (IBS) who received peppermint oil in enteric-coated capsules (encapsulated so the capsules wouldn't open until they reached the intestines) reported a reduced severity of pain associated with IBS (Kline et al., 2001).

Peppermint: In irritable bowel syndrome patients without bacterial overgrowth, lactose intolerance, or celiac disease, peppermint oil was found over 8 weeks to reduce IBS symptoms significantly more than a placebo (Capello et al., 2007).

Peppermint: An enteric-coated capsule with peppermint and caraway oil was found to reduce pain and symptoms in patients with non-ulcer dyspepsia (indigestion), compared to a control (May et al., 1996).

Ginger: Ginger root given one hour before major gynecological surgery resulted in lower nausea and fewer incidences of vomiting compared to control (Nanthakomon et al., 2006).

Ginger: Ginger root given orally to pregnant women was found to decrease the severity of nausea and frequency of vomiting compared to control (Vutyavanich et al., 2001).

Ginger: In a trial of women receiving gynecological surgery, women receiving ginger root had less incidences of nausea than did those receiving a placebo. Ginger root has similar results to the antiemetic drug (a drug effective against vomiting and nausea) metoclopramide (Bone et al., 1990).

Lemongrass: Lemongrass and lemon verbena oil were found to be bactericidal to Helicobacter pylori (a pathogen responsible for gastroduodenal disease) at very low concentrations. Additionally, it was found that this bacteria did not develop a resistance to lemongrass oil after 10 passages, while this bacteria did develop resistance to clarithromycin (an antibiotic) under the same conditions (Ohno et al., 2003).

Wintergreen: Methyl salicylate (found in wintergreen or birch oils) was found to inhibit leukotriene C4 (a chemical messenger involved in inflammatory response), while also demonstrating gastroprotective against ethanol-induced gastric injury in rats (Trautmann et al., 1991).

Oregano: Oregano oil administered orally was found to improve gastrointestinal symptoms in 7 of 11 patients who had tested positive for the parasite Blastocystis hominis and was also found to cause disappearance of this parasite in 8 cases (Force et al., 2000).

Rosemary: The use of rosemary, lemon, and peppermint oils in massage demonstrated an ability to reduce constipation and increase bowel movements in elderly subjects, compared to massage without the oils (Kim et al., 2005).

Lemon: The use of rosemary, lemon, and peppermint oils in massage demonstrated an ability to reduce constipation and increase bowel movements in elderly subjects, compared to massage without the oils (Kim et al., 2005).

Lavender: Essential oil from Lavandula angustifolia demonstrated ability to eliminate protozoal pathogens Giardia duodenalis, Trichomonas vaginalis, and Hexamita inflata at concentrations of 1% or less (Moon et al., 2006).

Rose: Rose essential oil and its main constituents were found to inhibit rat isolated ileum (a section of the small intestine), suggesting that rose oil can be used as an antispasmodic remedy for treatment of abdominal spasm (Sadraei et al., 2013).

Disinfectant

A disinfectant is any substance that destroys microorganisms on non-living surfaces.

Oils: ⊙⊘lemon, ⊙⊘Cleansing Blend, ⊙⊘grapefruit, ⊘lemongrass⊙, ⊘geranium⊙

Other Products: Protective Hand Wash to cleanse hands and protect against harmful microorganisms.

Blend 1: Add 10 drops lavender, 20 drops thyme, 5 drops eucalyptus, and 5 drops oregano to a large bowl of water. Use to disinfect small areas.

🖐: Add 1–2 drops of oil to a wet cloth, and use to wipe down counters and other surfaces. Use hand wash as directed on packaging.

🌀: Diffuse into the air.

📖: **Additional Research:**

Lemongrass: A formulation of lemongrass and geranium oil was found to reduce airborne bacteria by 89% in an office environment after diffusion for 15 hours (Doran et al., 2009).

Geranium: A formulation of lemongrass and geranium oil was found to reduce airborne bacteria by 89% in an office environment after diffusion for 15 hours (Doran et al., 2009).

Diuretic

A diuretic is a substance that increases the rate of urination and fluid elimination from the body.

Oils: ⁰lemongrass, ⁰rosemary, ⁰cedarwood, ⁰lavender, ⁰patchouli, ⁰grapefruit, ⁰cypress, ⁰fennel, ⁰orange, ⁰lemon, ⁰oregano, ⁰juniper berry, ⁰marjoram

◎: Dilute as recommended, and apply oils to kidney area on back and to bottoms of feet.

Diverticulitis

see **Colon:Diverticulitis**

Dysentery

see also **Antibacterial, Digestive System:Diarrhea**

Dysentery is severe, frequent diarrhea, often with blood or mucus, that occurs due to infection by bacteria or amoeba. Dysentery can be fatal due to dehydration if left untreated. *See Digestive System:Diarrhea* for information on rehydrating the body.

Oils: ⁰myrrh, ⁰eucalyptus, ⁰lemon, ⁰Roman chamomile, ⁰cypress, ⁰clove (amoebic), ⁰melissa

◎: Dilute as recommended, and apply on abdomen and on bottoms of feet.

Dyspepsia

see **Digestive System:Indigestion**

Ears

Oils: ⁰⁰helichrysum, ⁰⁰Cleansing Blend, ⁰⁰eucalyptus, ⁰⁰melaleuca, ⁰juniper berry, ⁰⁰geranium, ⁰⁰Grounding Blend, ⁰⁰marjoram

—**Earache:**

Oils: ⁰basil, ⁰melaleuca, ⁰helichrysum

—**Hearing in a Tunnel:**

Oils: ⁰Cleansing Blend

—**Infection:**

Oils: ⁰melaleuca, ⁰Cleansing Blend, ⁰lavender

—**Inflammation:**

Oils: ⁰eucalyptus

—**Tinnitus:**

Tinnitus is a ringing or other audible noise in the ears caused by ear infection, wax buildup, or a block in the eustachian tube.

Oils: ⁰helichrysum, ⁰juniper berry

◎: Caution: Never put oils directly into the ear canal. Dilute as recommended, and apply 1–2 drops on surface of the ear and behind the ear on the mastoid bone. Apply 1 drop oil to small cotton ball, and place over opening to ear canal (do not press into the ear canal). Place 1 drop oil on cotton swab, and swab around the ear canal.

◎: Diffuse into the air.

Eating Disorders

—Anorexia:

Anorexia is a psychological disorder where a person becomes obsessed with body size and weight, often depriving him or herself of food to avoid gaining weight.

Oils: ⊘grapefruit, ⊘Invigorating Blend

⊘: Diffuse into the air. Inhale directly from bottle. Apply oil to hands, tissue, or cotton wick, and inhale.

—Bulimia:

Bulimia is a disorder categorized by periods of overeating, or binging, followed by periods of self-induced vomiting, fasting, or abuse of laxatives and diuretics to purge the body of the food or to compensate for the overeating.

Oils: ⊘grapefruit, ⊘Invigorating Blend

⊘: Diffuse into the air. Inhale directly from bottle. Apply oil to hands, tissue, or cotton wick, and inhale.

—Overeating:

Overeating is eating too much food for the body. It can include binging (eating so much at one time that the stomach is overly filled and uncomfortable or painful) or chronic overeating (eating more than the body needs over a long period of time). Consistently overeating can lead to obesity and other health problems.

Oils: O⊘Metabolic Blend, ⊘grapefruit⊙, ⊘lemon⊙, ⊘peppermint, ⊘ginger

Other Products: OTrim Shakes

O: Add 8 drops of Metabolic Blend to 16 oz. of water, and drink throughout the day between meals. Drink Trim or V Shake 1–2 times per day as a meal alternative.

⊘: Diffuse into the air. Inhale directly from bottle. Apply oil to hands, tissue, or cotton wick, and inhale.

○: **Additional Research:**

Grapefruit: The scent of grapefruit oil and its component, limonene, was found to affect the autonomic nerves and to reduce appetite and body weight in rats exposed to the oil for 15 minutes three times per week (Shen et al., 2005).

Lemon: The scent of grapefruit oil and its component, limonene, was found to affect the autonomic nerves and to reduce appetite and body weight in rats exposed to the oil for 15 minutes three times per week (Shen et al., 2005).

Eczema

see **Skin:Dermatitis/Eczema**

Edema

see also **Allergis, Diuretic, Inflammation**

Edema is swelling caused by the abnormal accumulation of fluids in a tissue or body cavity. This can be caused by an allergic reaction, inflammation, injury, or as a signal of problems with the heart, liver, or kidneys.

Oils: ⊙Ograpefruit, ⊙lemongrass, ⊙cypress, ⊙geranium, ⊙rosemary, ⊙cedarwood, ⊙juniper berry

---

🜄: Dilute as recommended, and apply 1–2 drops on location.

◯: Add 1–2 drops to 8 oz. of water, and drink every 3 hours.

Elbow

see **Joints:Tennis Elbow**

Emergency Oils

The following oils are recommended to have on hand in case of an emergency:

Clove: Use as an analgesic (for topical pain relief) and a drawing salve (to pull toxins/infection from the body). Good for acne, constipation, headaches, nausea, and toothaches.

Frankincense: Enhances effect of any other oil. It facilitates clarity of mind, accelerates all skin recovery issues, and reduces anxiety and mental and physical fatigue. Reduces hyperactivity, impatience, irritability, and restlessness. Helps with focus and concentration.

Lavender: Use for agitation, bruises, burns (can mix with melaleuca), leg cramps, herpes, heart irregularities, hives, insect bites, neuropathy, pain (inside and out), bee stings, sprains, sunburn (combine with frankincense), and sunstroke. Relieves insomnia, depression, and PMS and is a natural antihistamine (asthma or allergies).

Lemon: Use for arthritis, colds, constipation, coughs, cuts, sluggishness, sore throats, sunburn, and wounds. It lifts the spirits and reduces stress and fatigue. Internally it counteracts acidity, calms an upset stomach, and encourages elimination.

Lemongrass: Use for sore and cramping muscles and charley horses (with peppermint; drink lots of water). Apply to bottoms of feet in winter to warm them.

Melaleuca: Use for bug bites, colds, coughs, cuts, deodorant, eczema, fungus, infections (ear, nose, or throat), microbes (internally), psoriasis, rough hands, slivers (combine with clove to draw them out), sore throats, and wounds.

Oregano: Use as heavy-duty antibiotic (internally with olive oil or coconut oil in capsules or topically on bottoms of feet—follow up with lavender and peppermint). Also for fungal infections and for reducing pain and inflammation of arthritis, backache, bursitis, carpal tunnel syndrome, rheumatism, and sciatica. Always dilute.

Peppermint: Use as an analgesic (for topical pain relief, bumps, and bruises). Can also be used for circulation, fever, headache, indigestion, motion sickness, nausea, nerve problems, or vomiting.

Massage Blend: Use for relaxation and stress relief. It is soothing and anti-inflammatory and enhances massage.

Respiratory Blend: Use for allergies, anxiety, asthma, bronchitis, congestion, colds, coughs, flu, and respiratory distress.

Soothing Blend: Use for pain relief. Works well in cases of arthritis, bruises, carpel tunnel, headaches, inflammation, joint pain, migraines, muscle pain, sprains, and rheumatism. Follow with peppermint to enhance affects.

Digestive Blend: Use for all digestion issues such as bloating, congestion, constipation, diarrhea, food poisoning (internal), heartburn, indigestion, motion sickness, nausea, and stomachache. Also works well on diaper rash.

Protective Blend: Use to disinfect all surfaces. It eliminates mold and viruses and helps to boost the immune system (bottoms of feet or internally; use daily).

Cleansing Blend: Use for airborne pathogens, cuts, germs (on any surface), insect bites, itches (all types and varieties), and wounds. Also boosts the immune system.

Repellent Blend: Deters all flying insects and ticks from human bodies and pets.

Emotions

see also **Anxiety, Calming, Depression, Fear, Grief/Sorrow, Stress:Emotional Stress, Uplifting**

To put it simply, emotions are the way we currently feel. These feelings come in response to what we see, smell, hear, feel, taste, think, or have experienced and can affect our future thoughts and behavior. While much is still being discovered about the complex psychological and physiological processes involved in emotions, researchers have discovered that emotions involve many different systems in the body, including the brain, the sensory system, the endocrine/hormonal system, the autonomic nervous system, the immune system, and the release or inhibition of neurotransmitters (such as dopamine) in the brain. Recent research has also begun to uncover compelling evidence that various essential oils and their components have the ability to affect each one of these systems, making the use of essential oils an intriguing tool for helping to balance emotions in the human body.

Oils: ⊘⊜Massage Blend, ⊘⊜Grounding Blend, ⊘⊜Invigorating Blend, ⊘⊜Joyful Blend, ⊘⊜Calming Blend, ⊘⊜Women's Monthly Blend, ⊘⊜Women's Blend, ⊘⊜Detoxification Blend, ⊘⊜cypress, ⊘⊜geranium, ⊘⊜lavender, ⊘⊜rose, ⊘⊜orange, ⊘⊜peppermint

—Acceptance:

Oils: ⊘⊜Joyful Blend

—Alertness: *see also* **Alertness**

Oils: ⊘⊜peppermint◐, ⊘ylang ylang◐, ⊘black pepper, ⊘⊜juniper berry, ⊘cinnamon

—Anger:

Oils: ⊘⊜Calming Blend, ⊘⊜lavender◐, ⊜⊘Focus Blend, ⊘⊘ylang ylang◐, ⊘⊜melissa◐, ⊘⊜Joyful Blend, ⊘⊜Grounding Blend, ⊘⊜helichrysum

—Anxious: *see also* **Anxiety**

Oils: ⊘⊜lavender◐, ⊘orange◐, ⊘lemon◐, ⊘⊘Focus Blend, ⊘⊜Calming Blend, ⊜Massage Blend, ⊘Joyful Blend, ⊜Grounding Blend (on back of neck), ⊜Respiratory Blend (on chest)

—Balance:

Oils: ⊘⊜Grounding Blend, ⊘⊜Massage Blend, ⊘⊜Invigorating Blend, ⊘⊜geranium, ⊘⊜juniper berry, ⊘⊜lavender, ⊘⊜orange, ⊘⊜sandalwood, ⊘⊜vetiver

—Blocks:

Oils: ⊘⊜cypress, ⊘⊜frankincense, ⊘⊜helichrysum, ⊘⊜sandalwood, ⊘⊜Grounding Blend

—Clearing:
  Oils: ◎◎Joyful Blend, ◎◎juniper berry, ◎◎Grounding Blend
—Coldness:
  Oils: ◎◎myrrh, ◎◎ylang ylang
—Concentration: *see also Concentration*
  Oils: ◎◎Focus Blend, ◎lavender◎, ◎lemon, ◎peppermint
—Confidence:
  Oils: ◎◎Joyful Blend, ◎◎Women's Blend, ◎◎cedarwood, ◎◎orange
—Creativity:
  Oils: ◎◎frankincense, ◎◎sandalwood, ◎◎Joyful Blend, ◎◎cypress, ◎◎lemon
—Defeated:
  Oils: ◎◎cypress, ◎◎white fir, ◎◎Joyful Blend, ◎◎juniper berry, ◎◎Grounding Blend
—Depression: *see also Depression*
  Oils: ◎◎◎lemon◎, ◎◎frankincense◎, ◎◎Focus Blend, ◎◎◎lavender◎, ◎◎berga-
  mot◎, ◎◎Joyful Blend, ◎◎Grounding Blend, ◎◎Invigorating Blend ◎
—Emotional Trauma:
  Oils: ◎◎sandalwood
—Expression (self-expression):
  Oils: ◎◎Grounding Blend, ◎◎Joyful Blend
—Fear: *see also Fear*
  Oils: ◎◎Grounding Blend, ◎◎ylang ylang◎, ◎orange◎, ◎◎sandalwood, ◎◎Calming
  Blend, ◎◎Joyful Blend
—Focus: *see Concentration*
—Grief/Sorrow: *see also Grief/Sorrow*
  Oils: ◎◎lemon◎, ◎◎Joyful Blend, ◎Grounding Blend, ◎◎lavender, ◎◎bergamot,
  ◎◎orange, ◎◎Invigorating Blend, ◎◎grapefruit, ◎◎wintergreen
—Guilt:
  Oils: ◎◎Joyful Blend, ◎◎Soothing Blend (on outer earlobes)
—Happiness/Joy:
  Oils: ◎◎Joyful Blend, ◎◎Invigorating Blend, ◎◎lemon, ◎◎orange, ◎◎spearmint,
  ◎◎sandalwood, ◎◎bergamot
—Loss:
  Oils: ◎◎Joyful Blend, ◎◎tangerine, ◎◎orange
—Mind (open):
  Oils: ◎◎frankincense, ◎◎sandalwood, ◎◎Grounding Blend

—Negative Emotions:

    Oils: ⊘⊜Joyful Blend, ⊘⊜Invigorating Blend, ⊘⊜orange, ⊘⊜grapefruit, ⊘⊜Grounding Blend, ⊘⊜white fir, ⊘⊜wintergreen, ⊘⊜lavender

—Overburdened/Overwhelmed:

    Oils: ⊘⊜Grounding Blend, ⊘⊜Invigorating Blend, ⊘⊜orange

—Peace:

    Oils: ⊘⊜Calming Blend, ⊘⊜lavender◌, ⊜⊘Focus Blend, ⊘⊘ylang ylang◌, ⊘⊘melissa◌

—Pity (self-pity):

    Oils: ⊘⊜Joyful Blend, ⊘⊜Invigorating Blend, ⊘⊜orange

—Positive (feeling):

    Oils: ⊘⊜Joyful Blend, ⊘⊜basil, ⊘⊜peppermint, ⊘⊜frankincense, ⊘⊜cedarwood, ⊘⊜juniper berry

—Rejection:

    Oils: ⊘⊜Grounding Blend, ⊘⊜lavender, ⊘⊜geranium

—Release:

    Oils: ⊘⊜Roman chamomile

—Stress: *see also Stress:Emotional Stress*

    Oils: ⊘⊜Joyful Blend, ⊘⊜clary sage, ⊘⊜bergamot, ⊘⊜Calming Blend

—Suicidal:

    Oils: ⊘⊜Joyful Blend, ⊜⊘Massage Blend, ⊘⊜Invigorating Blend, ⊘⊜Calming Blend

—Uplifting: *see also* **Uplifting**

    Oils: ⊘lemon◌, ⊘orange, ⊘Joyful Blend, ⊘⊜Invigorating Blend

—Worried:

    Oils: ⊘bergamot, ⊘⊜Calming Blend, ⊘⊜Joyful Blend, ⊘⊜Grounding Blend, ⊜⊘Massage Blend

⊘: Inhale directly from bottle. Diffuse into the air. Apply oil to hands, tissue, or cotton wick, and inhale.

⊜: Massage oils on back, chest, and/or legs. Gently massage 1–2 drops of oil into the outer lobes of the ear (avoid the ear canal). Add 1–2 drops of oil to a bath or shower gel or to bath salts, and use during a bath or shower.

○: Add 1–2 drops to 8 oz. distilled water or to 4 oz. rice or almond milk before drinking. Add 1–2 drops to an empty capsule, and swallow.

▢: **Additional Research:**

    Peppermint: In human trials, the aroma of peppermint was found to enhance memory and increase alertness (Moss et al., 2008).

    Ylang ylang: Inhaled ylang ylang oil was found to decrease blood pressure and pulse rate and to enhance attentiveness and alertness in volunteers compared to an odorless control (Hongratanaworakit et al., 2004).

    Ylang ylang: In human trials, the aroma of peppermint was found to enhance memory and to increase alertness, while ylang ylang aroma was found to increase calmness (Moss et al., 2008).

Ylang ylang: Subjects who had ylang ylang oil applied to their skin had decreased blood pressure, increased skin temperature, and reported feeling more calm and relaxed, as compared to subjects in a control group (Hongratanaworakit et al., 2006).

Lavender: Lavandula angustifolia essential oil demonstrated ability to inhibit GABA-A receptor channels of rat brain cells (Huang et al., 2008).

Lavender: Inhaling lavender oil was found to be effective at alleviating agitated behaviors in older Chinese patients suffering from dementia (Lin et al., 2007).

Lavender: Female patients waiting for dental treatment were found to be less anxious, more positive, and more calm when exposed to orange oil odor than were patients who were not exposed to the orange oil odor (Lehrner et al., 2000).

Lavender: Exposure to lavender odor was found to decrease anxiety in gerbils in the elevated plus maze, with a further decrease in anxiety in females after prolonged (2 week) exposure (Bradley et al., 2007).

Lavender: Subjects receiving a lozenge containing lavender oil, hops extract, lemon balm, and oat were found to have increases in alpha 1, alpha 2, and beta 1 electrical output (Dimpfel et al., 2004).

Lavender: In patients admitted to an intensive care unit, those receiving lavender aromatherapy reported a greater improvement in mood and perceived levels of anxiety compared to those receiving massage or a period of rest (Dunn et al., 1995).

Lavender: Female patients being treated for chronic hemodialysis demonstrated less anxiety when exposed to lavender aroma compared to control (Itai et al., 2000).

Lavender: Lavender oil was found to demonstrate anti-conflict effects in mice similar to the anxiolytic (antianxiety) drug diazepam (Umezu, 2000).

Lavender: Subjects who smelled a cleansing gel with lavender aroma were more relaxed and able to complete math computations faster (Field et al., 2005).

Lavender: Subjects exposed to 3 minutes of lavender aroma were more relaxed and able to perform math computations faster and more accurately. Subjects exposed to rosemary aroma were more alert and completed math computations faster (but not more accurately) (Diego et al., 1998).

Lavender: In patients suffering from arthritis, it was found that a blend of lavender, marjoram, eucalyptus, rosemary, and peppermint blended with carrier oils was found to reduce perceived pain and depression compared to control (Kim et al., 2005).

Lavender: Female students suffering from insomnia were found to sleep better and to have a lower level of depression during weeks they used a lavender fragrance when compared to weeks they did not use a lavender fragrance (Lee et al., 2006).

Lavender: Swiss mice fed lavender oil diluted in olive oil were found to be more sedate in several common tests (Guillemain et al., 1989).

Melissa: Melissa (lemon balm) oil applied topically in a lotion was found to reduce agitation and to improve quality of life factors in patients suffering from severe dementia, as compared to those receiving a placebo lotion (Ballard et al., 2002).

Orange: Bitter orange peel oil taken orally by mice was found to reduce anxiety, increase sleeping time, and increase the time before a chemically-induced seizure started (Carvalho-Freitas et al., 2002).

Orange: Female patients waiting for dental treatment were found to be less anxious, more positive, and more calm when exposed to orange oil odor than patients who were not exposed to the orange oil odor (Lehrner et al., 2000).

Lemon: Rats exposed long-term to lemon essential oil were found to demonstrate different anxiety and pain threshold levels than untreated rats. It was also found that exposure to lemon oil induced chemical changes in the neuronal circuits involved in anxiety and pain (Ceccarelli et al., 2004).

Lemon: Lemon oil was found to have an antistress effect on mice involved in several behavioral tasks (Komiya et al., 2006).

Lemon: Lemon oil vapor was found to have strong antistress and antidepressant effects on mice subjected to several common stress tests (Komiya et al., 2006).

Lemon: Lemon oil and its component, citral, were found to decrease depressed behavior in a similar manner to antidepressant drugs in rats involved in several stress tests (Komori et al., 1995).

Lemon: In 12 patients suffering from depression, it was found that inhaling citrus aromas reduced the needed doses of antidepressants, normalized neuroendocrine hormone levels, and normalized immune function (Komori et al., 1995).

Lemon: Lemon odor was found to enhance the positive mood of volunteers exposed to a stressor (Kiecolt-Glaser et al., 2008).

Frankincense: Incensole acetate was found to open TRPV receptors in mice brains, indicating a possible channel for emotional regulation (Moussaieff et al., 2008).

Melissa: Melissa (lemon balm) oil applied topically in a lotion was found to reduce agitation and to improve quality of life factors in patients suffering severe dementia, as compared to those receiving a placebo lotion (Ballard et al., 2002).

Emphysema

Emphysema is a chronic pulmonary disease where airflow is restricted through the lungs due to destruction (typically caused by airborne toxins such as those in cigarette smoke) of the wall of the alveoli (small air sacs in the lungs where oxygen and carbon dioxide is exchanged with the blood). This destruction of the alveolar wall causes the alveoli to collapse when air is expelled from the lungs, trapping air inside.

Oils: ⊘⊜eucalyptus, ⊘⊜Respiratory Blend

⊘: Diffuse into the air.

⊜: Dilute as recommended, and apply 1–2 drops to chest and back. Apply as a warm compress on chest.

Endocrine System

see also **Adrenal Glands, Ovaries, Pancreas, Pineal Gland, Pituitary Gland, Testes, Thymus, Thyroid**

The endocrine system is the series of hormone-producing glands and organs that help regulate metabolism, reproduction, blood pressure, appetite, and many other body functions. The endocrine system is mainly controlled by the hypothalamus region of the brain that either produces hormones that stimulate the other endocrine glands directly, or that stimulates the pituitary gland located just below it to release the hormones needed to stimulate the other endocrine glands. These hormones are released into the blood stream where they travel to other areas of the body to either stimulate other endocrine glands or to stimulate tissues and organs of the body directly. Some essential oils may act as hormones or stimulate the endocrine system to produce hormones that have a regulating effect on the body.

Oils: ⭘⊜Detoxification Blend, ⊘⊜rosemary, ⊘⊜cinnamon

Other Products: ⭘Detoxification Complex to help support healthy endocrine cleansing and filtering.

—Hormonal Balance:

Oils: ⊜⊘clary sage, ⊘clove, ⊘⊜ylang ylang

Other Products: ⭘Phytoestrogen Complex

–Female:

Oils: ⊜⊘Women's Monthly Blend, ⊜⊘Women's Blend

–Sexual Energy:

Oils: ⊘⊜ylang ylang

⭘: Take capsules as directed on package. Place 1–2 drops of oil under the tongue, or add 3–5 drops of essential oil to an empty capsule; swallow capsule.

⊘: Diffuse into the air. Inhale directly from bottle. Apply oil to hands, tissue, or cotton wick, and inhale.

⊜: Dilute as recommended, and apply 1–2 drops to the reflex points on the feet, lower back, thyroid, liver, kidneys, gland areas, the center of the body, or both sides of the spine and clavicle area. Add 1–2 drops to 1 Tbs. fractionated coconut oil, and use as massage oil.

Endometriosis

Endometriosis is a chronic disorder in women where endometrium cells (cells from the lining of the uterus) grow outside of the uterus—typically around the ovaries, the ligaments that support the uterus, or the peritoneal (abdominal) cavity. These cells are often still responsive to the monthly hormone cycle that effects the changes in the uterus and can cause abnormal abdominal pain and irregularities in the menstrual cycle.

Oils: ⊙geranium, ⊙cypress, ⊙clary sage, ⊙Protective Blend, ⊙eucalyptus, ⊙Women's Blend

⊙: Dilute as recommended, and apply 1–2 drops on lower abdomen or on feet. Apply as a warm compress. Place 1–2 drops in warm bathwater, and bathe.

Endurance

Oils: ⊘Opeppermint⊙

Other Products: OEnergy & Stamina Complex, OCellular Vitality Complex, OChewable Multivitamin, OEssential Oil Omega Complex or Vegan Essential Oil Omega Complex, OOmega-3 Fish Oil, OFood Nutrient Complex to provide nutrients and antioxidants that help support healthy cellular function and energy levels.

⊘: Diffuse into the air. Inhale directly from bottle. Apply oil to hands, tissue, or cotton wick, and inhale.

O: Take capsules as directed on package.

⊡: **Additional Research:**

Peppermint: A quasi experiment comparing exercise performance before and after consumption of mineral water containing peppermint essential oil for 10 days found that exercise performance improved after consumption of peppermint oil (including increases in respiratory efficiency, energy expenditure, time to exhaustion, and distance during exercise and decreases in resting and exercise heart rates) (Meamarbashi et al., 2013).

Energy

Oils: ⊘O⊙peppermint⊙, ⊘⊙white fir, ⊘⊙Joyful Blend, ⊘⊙Grounding Blend, ⊘⊙lemon, ⊘⊙basil, ⊘⊙thyme, ⊘⊙rosemary, ⊘⊙orange, ⊘⊙lemongrass, ⊘⊙eucalyptus

Other Products: OEnergy & Stamina Complex, OCellular Vitality Complex, OChewable Multivitamin, OEssential Oil Omega Complex or Vegan Essential Oil Omega Complex, OOmega-3 Fish Oil, OFood Nutrient Complex to provide nutrients and antioxidants that help support healthy cellular function and energy levels.

—Exhaustion:

Oils: First, work with one or more of the following nervous system oils to help calm and relax: ⊙lavender, ⊙ylang ylang, ⊙Roman chamomile, ⊙frankincense, ⊙clary sage. Secondly, use an energizing oil such as ⊙lemon, ⊙sandalwood, ⊙rosemary, ⊘⊙lime, ⊙basil, ⊙grapefruit.

—Fatigue:

Oils: ⊙⊘rosemary (nervous fatigue), ⊘⊘thyme (general fatigue)

−Mental Fatigue:

Oils: ⊘⊙Calming Blend, ⊘⊙lemongrass, ⊘⊙basil

Blend 1: Blend equal parts basil and lemongrass together. Apply to temples, back of neck, and feet. Diffuse into the air.

–Physical Fatigue:

Oils: ©@Calming Blend

—Physical:

Oils: @lemon, @cinnamon, @bergamot

—Sexual:

Oils: @ylang ylang

@: Diffuse into the air. Inhale directly from bottle. Apply oil to hands, tissue, or cotton wick, and inhale.

©: Dilute 1–2 drops in 1 Tbs. fractionated coconut oil, and massage into muscles. Place 1–2 drops in warm bathwater, and bathe. Dilute as recommended, and apply 1–2 drops on temples, back of neck, liver area, or feet.

○: Take capsules as directed on package.

▥: **Additional Research:**

Peppermint: A quasi experiment comparing exercise performance before and after consumption of mineral water containing peppermint essential oil for 10 days found that exercise performance improved after consumption of peppermint oil (including increases in respiratory efficiency, energy expenditure, time to exhaustion, and distance during exercise and decreases in resting and exercise heart rates) (Meamarbashi et al., 2013).

Epilepsy
see **Seizure:Epilepsy**

Epstein-Barr
see **Mono;** *see also* **Antiviral:Epstein-Barr Virus**

Estrogen
Estrogens are hormones produced by the ovaries that regulate the development of female characteristics and the menstrual cycle in females.

Oils: ©@Women's Monthly Blend, ©@clary sage

Other Products: ○Phytoestrogen Complex

©: Apply on the lower abdomen. Dilute 1–2 drops in 1 Tbs. fractionated coconut oil, and use as massage oil.

○: Take capsules as directed on package.

@: Diffuse into the air. Inhale directly from bottle. Apply oil to hands, tissue, or cotton wick, and inhale.

Exhaustion
see **Energy:Exhaustion**

Expectorant
see **Congestion:Expectorant**

Eyes

Eyes are the organs of the body responsible for detecting and adjusting to light and focusing images of the surrounding environment onto the optical nerve for transfer to the brain for processing.

Oils: ©lemongrass, ©sandalwood, ©cypress, ©lemon, ©fennel, ©eucalyptus, ©lavender, ©Protective Blend

Other Products: OFood Nutrient Complex for nutrients that help support healthy eye cell function.

Recipe 1: Eye Drop Recipe: Combine 5 parts distilled water, 2 parts honey, and 1 part apple cider vinegar (do not use white vinegar). Mix together, and store in a bottle. Does not need to be refrigerated. This special eye drop formula is found in Stanley Burroughs' book, *Healing for the Age of Enlightenment* and has proven over the years to be superior to most commercial eye drops. These drops have been used for glaucoma, cataracts, spots, film, and growths of various kinds. Apply drops one at a time to each eye several times a day until condition has cleared.

—Blocked Tear Ducts:

Tears from the eye normally drain through small tubes called tear ducts. The tear ducts carry tears from the surface of the eye into the nose where they are reabsorbed or evaporate. When these tear ducts are blocked, the eyes become watery and irritated. Blocked tear ducts are most common in babies and in older adults.

Oils: ©lavender

—Cataracts:

A cataract is a clouding of the normally transparent lens of the eye. This clouding results in blurry vision, seemingly faded colors, double vision, glare, and difficulty seeing at night. Over time, the clouding can increase and lead to severe vision problems.

Oils: ©clove, ©lavender

Blend 1: Combine 8 drops lemongrass, 6 drops cypress, and 3 drops eucalyptus. Apply around the eye area two times a day. Do not get oil in the eyes.

—Dry/Itchy Eyes:

Oils: ⊘melaleuca (in humidifier)

—Eye Lid Drop/Drooping Eyelid:

A drooping eyelid is characterized by an excessive sagging of the upper eyelid. Drooping can be present at birth as a result of underdeveloped eyelid muscles, or it can occur with aging. Drooping eyelids can cause visual impairment if they droop enough to partially cover the eye.

Blend 2: Combine equal parts helichrysum and peppermint, and apply 1–2 drops on the eyelid. Do not get oil in the eyes.

—Improve Vision:

Oils: ©frankincense, ©lemongrass, ©juniper berry, ©Protective Blend, ©sandalwood, ©lavender

Blend 3: Combine 10 drops lemongrass, 5 drops cypress, and 3 drops eucalyptus with 2 Tbs. fractionated coconut oil. Apply around the eyes morning and night, or apply on reflex points on the feet or on the ears.

—Iris Inflammation:

The iris is the colored part of the eye that regulates the amount of light entering the eye through the pupil. When the iris becomes inflamed, it results in a condition called iritis. Iritis is normally related to a disease or infection in another part of the body, but it can also be caused by injury to the eye. Symptoms of iritis include blurred vision, pain, tearing, light sensitivity, red eye, and a small pupil size.

Oils: ◔eucalyptus

—Macular Degeneration:

Macular degeneration is an eye disease common in individuals 65 and older. It is marked by degeneration of a small, oval-shaped part of the retina called the macula. Because the macula is responsible for capturing the light from the central part of images coming into the eye, macular degeneration causes blurring or a blind spot in the central vision, making it difficult to drive, recognize faces, read, or do any kind of detail work.

Oils: ◔clove

—Pink Eye:

Pink eye, also know as conjunctivitis, is an inflammation or infection of the membranes covering the whites of the eyes (conjunctiva) and the inner part of the eyelids. Swelling, redness, itching, discharge, and burning of the eyes are common symptoms of pink eye. Frequent causes include allergies, bacterial or viral infection, contact lenses, and eye drops.

Oils: ◔◔melaleuca, ◔◔lavender

—Retina (strengthen):

The retina is a layer of nerves lining the back of the eye. The retina is responsible for sensing light and then sending impulses (via the optic nerve) back to the brain so that visual images can be formed.

Oils: ◔cypress, ◔lemongrass, ◔helichrysum, ◔juniper berry, ◔peppermint, ◔lavender, ◔sandalwood

—Swollen Eyes:

Oils: ◔cypress, ◔helichrysum, ◔peppermint (allergies), ◔lavender

◔: Caution: Never put essential oils directly in the eyes! Be careful when applying oils near the eyes. Be sure to have some fractionated coconut oil handy for additional dilution if irritation occurs. Never use water to wash off an oil that irritates. Dilute as recommended, and apply 1–2 drops around eyes or to feet, thumbs, ankles, pelvis, base of neck, or reflex points on the feet.

◔: Diffuse into the air.

◔: Take capsules as directed on package.

Facial Oils
see **Skin**

Fainting
see also **Shock**

Fainting is a temporary loss of consciousness caused by a momentary disruption of blood flow to the brain. Fainting can result from standing in one place too long, coughing very hard, fear, emotional trauma, heavy bleeding, or severe dehydration. Fainting can sometimes be a symptom of a more serious condition.

Oils: ⊘peppermint, ⊘rosemary, ⊘basil, ⊘lavender

⊘: Inhale directly from bottle.

Fatigue
see **Energy:Fatigue**

Fear
see also **Anxiety, Calming**

Fear causes the blood vessels to tighten, restricting the amount of oxygen and nutrients that can reach the cells.

Oils: ⊘⊘Grounding Blend, ⊘⊘ylang ylang⊙, ⊘orange⊙, ⊘⊘sandalwood, ⊘⊘clary sage, ⊘⊘geranium, ⊘⊘juniper berry, ⊘⊘myrrh, ⊘⊘bergamot, ⊘⊘white fir, ⊘⊘cypress, ⊘⊘marjoram

⊘: Diffuse into the air. Inhale directly from bottle. Apply oil to hands, tissue, or cotton wick, and inhale.

⊜: Dilute as recommended, and apply 1–2 drops to temples, back of neck, or bottoms of feet.

▭: **Additional Research:**

> **Ylang ylang:** Subjects who had ylang ylang oil applied to their skin had decreased blood pressure, increased skin temperature, and reported feeling more calm and relaxed compared to subjects in a control group (Hongratanaworakit et al., 2006).
>
> **Orange:** Female patients waiting for dental treatment were found to be less anxious, more positive, and more calm when exposed to orange oil odor than were patients who were not exposed to the orange oil odor (Lehrner et al., 2000).

Feet
see **Foot**

Female Specific Conditions
see also **Endometriosis, Pregnancy/Motherhood**

—**Hemorrhaging**: *see* **Blood:Hemorrhaging**

—**Hot Flashes**:

> A hot flash is a sudden, intense feeling of heat in the face and upper body, often accompanied by an increased heart rate, sweating, dizziness, headache, weakness, or anxiety. Hot flashes are generally associated with the symptoms of menopause and premenopause.
>
> Oils: ⊙⊘Women's Monthly Blend, ⊙Grounding Blend, ⊙peppermint, ⊙clary sage

Other Products: ᴏPhytoestrogen Complex, ᴏDaily Supplements Pack (contains Cellular Vitality Complex, Essential Oil Omega Complex or Vegan Essential Oil Omega Complex, ᴏᴏOmega-3 Fish Oil, and Food Nutrient Complex)

Recipe 1: Both morning and evening, apply 1–2 drops each of Grounding Blend and peppermint to back of neck; then apply 1–2 drops clary sage to forearms in the morning and to ankles in the evening. The Daily Supplements Pack may also be taken to help regulate the hormonal system.

—**Hormones (balancing):**

Oils: ☺☻Women's Monthly Blend, ☺☻ylang ylang, ☺☻clary sage

Other Products: ᴏPhytoestrogen Complex

—**Infertility:**

Infertility is clinically defined as the inability to get pregnant after a year of trying. This could be due to any of several underlying causes.

Oils: ☺clary sage, ☺geranium, ☺melissa, ☺cypress, ☺thyme, ☺fennel, ☺Roman chamomile, ☺ylang ylang

—**Menopause:**

Menopause is the permanent ending of a female's menstruation and fertility. For most American women, Menopause occurs around age 51 and is often recognized by hot flashes, irregular periods, vaginal dryness, mood swings, difficulty sleeping, thinning hair, abdominal weight gain, and decreased fertility.

Oils: ☺☻Women's Monthly Blend, ☺cypress, ☺lavender☉, ☺Roman chamomile, ☺orange, ☺clary sage, ☺ᴏfennel☉, ☺basil, ☺geranium, ☺rosemary, ☺thyme

Other Products: ᴏPhytoestrogen Complex, ᴏBone Nutrient Complex

—**Premenopause:**

Oils: ☺☻Women's Monthly Blend, ☺clary sage, ☺lavender

Other Products: ᴏPhytoestrogen Complex, ᴏBone Nutrient Complex

—**Menstruation:**

Menstruation, also known as a woman's "period," is the regular shedding of the uterus lining and vaginal discharge of blood when a woman is not pregnant. A woman's period lasts between two and seven days and reoccurs on an average of every 28 days.

—**Amenorrhea:**

Amenorrhea is the absence of menstruation. The following oils may help induce menstrual flow (emmenagogic) and may need to be avoided during pregnancy for this reason. See Pregnancy/Motherhood for further safety data.

Oils: ☺☻Women's Monthly Blend, ☺basil, ☺clary sage, ☺peppermint, ☺rosemary, ☺juniper berry, ☺marjoram, ☺lavender, ☺Roman chamomile

Other Products: ᴏPhytoestrogen Complex

—Dysmenorrhea:

Dysmenorrhea is painful menstruation. Apply one or more of these oils to the abdomen. It may also help to use a hot compress.

Oils: ◐⊘Women's Monthly Blend, , ◐clary sage◔, ◐geranium ◐lavender◔, ◐rose◔, ◐cypress, ◐peppermint, ◐marjoram, ◐Roman chamomile, ◐basil, ◐rosemary, ◐fennel

Other Products: ○Phytoestrogen Complex

—Irregular:

Oils: ◐⊘Women's Monthly Blend, ◐peppermint, ◐rosemary, ◐Roman chamomile, ◐clary sage, ◐fennel, ◐lavender, ◐rose

Other Products: ○Phytoestrogen Complex

—Menorrhagia:

Menorrhagia is abnormally heavy or extended menstrual flow. It may also refer to irregular bleeding at any time. This situation may be a sign of a more serious condition, so please see your doctor.

Oils: ◐⊘Women's Monthly Blend, ◐cypress, ◐geranium, ◐Roman chamomile, ◐rose

Other Products: ○Phytoestrogen Complex

—Scanty:

Oils: ◐⊘Women's Monthly Blend, ◐peppermint, ◐lavender, ◐melissa

Other Products: ○Phytoestrogen Complex

—Ovaries:

Ovaries are the female reproductive organs in which eggs are produced and stored.

Oils: ◐⊘Women's Monthly Blend, ◐rosemary, ◐geranium, ◐Digestive Blend

Other Products: ○Phytoestrogen Complex

—Ovarian Cyst:

Oils: ◐basil

—PMS:

Premenstrual syndrome (PMS) is a group of symptoms such as irritability, anxiety, moodiness, bloating, breast tenderness, headaches, and cramping that occurs in the days or hours before menstruation begins and then disappear once menstruation begins. PMS is thought to be caused by the fluctuation in hormones during this time or by the way progesterone is broken down by the body. Caffeine intake from beverages or chocolate is also thought to enhance PMS symptoms.

Oils: ◐⊘Women's Monthly Blend, ◐⊘clary sage, ◐⊘geranium, ◐⊘fennel, ◐lavender, ◐⊘bergamot, ◐⊘grapefruit

Other Products: ○Phytoestrogen Complex, ○Bone Nutrient Complex or ○Food Nutrient Complex contain calcium, which has been found to help lessen PMS symptoms.

–Apathetic-Tired-Listless:

Oils: ☉⊘Women's Monthly Blend, ☉⊘grapefruit, ☉⊘geranium, ☉⊘bergamot, ☉⊘fennel

Other Products: ⓞPhytoestrogen Complex

–Irritable:

Oils: ☉⊘Women's Monthly Blend, ☉⊘clary sage, ☉⊘bergamot, ☉⊘Roman chamomile

Other Products: ⓞPhytoestrogen Complex

–Violent Aggressive:

Oils: ☉⊘Women's Monthly Blend, ☉⊘geranium, ☉⊘bergamot

Other Products: ⓞPhytoestrogen Complex

–Weeping-Depression:

Oils: ☉⊘Women's Monthly Blend, ☉⊘clary sage, ☉⊘bergamot, ☉⊘geranium

Other Products: ⓞPhytoestrogen Complex

–Postpartum Depression: *see **Pregnancy/Motherhood:Postpartum Depression***

☉: Dilute as recommended, and apply to the abdomen, lower back, shoulders, or reflex points on the feet. Add 1–2 drops to 1 Tbs. fractionated coconut oil, and massage into abdomen, lower back, and shoulders. Apply as a warm compress to the abdomen. Add 1–2 drops to 2 tsp. olive oil, insert into vagina, and retain overnight with a tampon.

⊘: Place in hands and inhale. Diffuse into the air.

ⓞ: Take capsules as directed on package.

▭: **Additional Research:**

Lavender: Inhalation of linalool or *Lavandula burnatii* super-derived essential oil (composed from the five main lavender oils and containing a high levels of linalool) was found to aid in the recovery of ether-inhalation induced decrease in adrenaline, noradrenaline, and dopamine levels in female menopausal model rats. The researchers stated that these results suggest that lavender or linalool may contribute to relieving tension and may be applicable to the treatment of menopausal disorders (Yamada et al., 2005).

Fennel: Using a mouse model of postmenopausal bone loss researchers found that oral administration of fennel oil for six weeks had an intermediate effect on the prevention of femoral bone mineral density and bone mineral content when compared to controls. These findings suggest that fennel oil has potential in preventing bone loss in postmenopausal osteoporosis (Kim et al., 2012).

Clary Sage: In an experiment with 67 female college students, an aromatherapy massage with lavender, clary sage, and rose essential oils proved to be more effective at treating dysmenorrhea than a placebo treatment of almond oil or the control (Han et al., 2006).

Clary sage, lavender, and marjoram: Compared to a synthetic fragrance, dysmenorrhea pain decreased and shortened in duration when subjects massaged a blend of lavender, marjoram, and clary sage essential oils (in a ratio of 2:1:1) daily on the abdomen between menstruations (Ou et al., 2012).

Rose: A study with 92 university age female students with primary dysmenorrhea found that ingestion of a capsule containing 200 mg of Rosa damascena extract every 6 hours at the first 3 days of menstruation was as effective as administration of Mefenamic acid (a drug with possible adverse reactions and side effects) (Bani et al., 2014).

Thyme: A study comparing administration of thyme essential oil, ibuprofen, and placebo treatment revealed that thyme essential oil alleviates dysmenorrhea pain as well as ibuprofen and works significantly better than the placebo treatment (Salmalian et al., 2014).

Fertility

see **Female Specific Conditions:Infertility, Male Specific Conditions:Infertility**

Fever

see also **Cooling Oils**

Fever is an increase of the body's core temperature, typically in response to an infection or injury. A fever is the body's natural response to help enhance the immune system's ability to fight the infection.

Oils: O☯❀peppermint, O☯lemon, O☯❀lime, ☯eucalyptus, Oclove, O☯❀patchouli, ☯melaleuca, ☯ginger, ☯lavender, ☯basil, ☯white fir, ☯bergamot

—**To Cool the System:**

> **Oils:** Oclove, O☯❀peppermint, ☯eucalyptus, ☯bergamot

—**To Induce Sweating:**

> **Oils:** ☯basil, ☯fennel, ☯melaleuca, ☯peppermint, ☯rosemary, ☯lavender, ☯cypress

O: Place 1–2 drops of oil under the tongue or place 1–2 drops of essential oil into capsule; then swallow capsule. Place 1–2 drops in 8 oz. of rice milk or water, and sip slowly.

➲: Dilute as recommended, and apply to back or to bottoms of the feet.

∂: Diffuse into the air.

Fibrillation

see **Cardiovascular System**

Fibroids

Fibroids are noncancerous growths of muscle and connective tissue in the uterus. Fibroids can be painful and may affect fertility and pregnancy.

Oils: ☯frankincense, ☯helichrysum, ☯oregano, ☯Grounding Blend, ☯lavender

➲: Place 3 drops of oil in douche. Dilute as recommended, and apply to reflex points on the feet.

Fibromyalgia

Fibromyalgia is long-term localized or generalized aches, pain, or tenderness in the muscles, ligaments, or other soft tissue that can interfere with normal movement, sleep, or other activities. There is no known cause of fibromyalgia, and many different factors may contribute to the development of this condition. Some have suggested eliminating refined sugar from the diet. Others have recommended reducing stress, stretching exercises, massage, or better sleep.

Oils: ☯Soothing Blend, ☯wintergreen, ☯helichrysum, ☯lavender, ☯rosemary, ☯thyme

Other Products: OEnergy & Stamina Complex, OCellular Vitality Complex, OChewable Multivitamin, OEssential Oil Omega Complex or Vegan Essential Oil Omega Complex, OOmega-3 Fish Oil, OFood Nutrient Complex for nutrients needed for healthy muscle and nerve cell function.

➲: Add 1–2 drops of oil to 1 Tbs. fractionated coconut oil, and massage on location. Apply as a warm compress over affected area.

○: Take capsules as directed on package.

Finger (mashed)

Recipe 1: Apply 1 drop geranium (for bruising), 1 drop helichrysum (to stop the bleeding), 1 drop lavender, 1 drop lemongrass (for tissue repair), and 1 drop Soothing Blend (for pain).

Flatulence

see Digestive System:Gas/Flatulence

Flu

see Influenza

Fluids

see Edema, Diuretic

Food Poisoning

see also Antibacterial, Antifungal, Antiviral, Digestive System, Parasites

Food poisoning refers to the effects on the digestive tract by pathogenic organisms—or the toxins they produce—that are ingested into the body in food. Symptoms of food poisoning can include stomach pain, cramps, diarrhea, nausea, and vomiting.

Oils: ○Digestive Blend☺, ○Protective Blend, ○rosemary

Other Products: ○Digestive Softgels ○Protective Softgels

○: Add 6 drops to 8 oz. of water. Swish around in the mouth, and swallow. Place 1–2 drops in an empty capsule, and swallow.

▢: **Additional Research:**

> **Digestive Blend:** Peppermint and spearmint oils inhibited resistant strains of Staphylococcus, E. coli, Salmonella, and Helicobacter pylori (Imai et al., 2001).

Foot

Oils: ◎lemon, ◎lavender, ◎Roman chamomile

—Athlete's Foot: *see* Antifungal:Athlete's Foot

—Blisters:

> **Oils:** ◎lavender, ◎geranium, ◎melaleuca, ◎Cleansing Blend

—Bunion: *see also* Bursitis

> A bunion is bursitis located at the base of the big toe. It is often caused by constrictive shoes that force the big toe to point inward and the base of the big toe to jut outward. This misplacement can irritate the bursa located at the base of the toe and cause it to become inflamed, which causes further irritation.
>
> **Oils:** ◎cypress

—Calluses:

> A callus is a flat, thick growth of skin that develops on areas of the skin where there is constant friction or rubbing. Calluses typically form on the bottoms of the feet, but they can also form on the hands or other areas of the body exposed to constant friction.

Oils: ⊘oregano

—Club Foot:

Oils: ⊘ginger, ⊘rosemary, ⊘lavender, ⊘Roman chamomile

—Corns:

Corns are painful growths that develop on the small toes due to repetitive friction in that area (often from ill-fitting footwear). If untreated, corns can cause increased pressure on underlying tissue, causing tissue damage or ulcerations.

Oils: ⊘clove, ⊘peppermint, ⊘grapefruit, ⊘Invigorating Blend

⊘: Dilute as recommended, and apply to area. Combine 1–2 drops with fractionated coconut oil, and massage on location.

Forgetfulness
see **Memory**

Free Radicals
see **Antioxidant**

Frigidity
see **Sexual Issues:Female Frigidity**

Fungus
see **Antifungal**

Gallbladder

The gallbladder is a small sac that stores extra bile from the liver until it is needed to help with digestion in the small intestine. The gallbladder is located just below the liver.

Oils: ⊘geranium, ⊘rosemary, ⊘lavender,

⊘juniper berry

—Infection:

Oils: ⊘helichrysum

—Stones:

Gallstones are formed by cholesterol that has crystallized from the bile stored in the gallbladder. These stones can sometimes block the duct that comes from the gallbladder or the small opening from the common hepatic duct that allows bile to flow into the small intestine. Gallstones blocking these ducts can be painful and can lead to more serious complications, such as infections or jaundice.

Oils: ⊘grapefruit, ⊘geranium, ⊘rosemary, ⊘juniper berry, ⊘wintergreen, ⊘lime

⊘: Dilute as recommended, and apply 1–2 drops over gallbladder area. Apply as a warm compress over the gallbladder area.

Gallstones
see **Gallbladder:Stones**

Gangrene

Gangrene is the localized decay of body tissue caused by a loss of blood to that area. Gas gangrene is caused by bacteria invading a deep wound that has lessened the blood supply or cut it off entirely. The bacteria create gases and pus in the infected area, causing severe pain and accelerating decay of the tissue.

Oils: ◐lavender, ◐Protective Blend, ◐thyme

◐: Dilute as recommended, and apply 1–3 drops on location.

Gas

see **Digestive System: Gas/Flatulence**

Gastritis

see **Digestive System:Gastritis**

Genitals

see **Female Specific Conditions, Male Specific Conditions/Issues**

Germs

see **Antibacterial, Antifungal, Antiviral**

Gingivitis

see **Oral Conditions:Gum Disease**

Goiter

see **Thyroid:Hyperthyroidism**

Gout

Gout is a painful inflammation of a joint caused by a buildup of uric acid crystals deposited in the joint. Uric acid is formed during the natural breakdown of dead tissues in the body. An excess of uric acid in the bloodstream can lead to the formation of crystals in the joints or kidneys (kidney stones). Some good ways to prevent the formation of uric acid crystals include maintaining a healthy body weight (which leaves less body tissue to be broken down), exercising, and drinking plenty of water.

Oils: ◐◐lemon, ◐geranium, ◐Soothing Blend, ◐wintergreen, ◐thyme

◯: Place 1–2 drops in 8 oz. of water, and drink. Place 1–2 drops of oil under the tongue or place 1–2 drops in an empty capsule, and swallow.

◐: Dilute as recommended, and apply on location. Add 1–2 drops to 1 Tbs. fractionated coconut oil, and massage on location.

Grave's Disease

see **Thyroid:Hyperthyroidism**

Grave's disease is an autoimmune disease caused by an abnormally-shaped protein stimulating the thyroid to make and secrete more hormones. This can cause an enlargement of the thyroid (goiter), bulging eyes, increased heart rate, high blood pressure, and anxiety.

Oils: ◐◐lemongrass, ◐◐myrrh

Personal Guide

F

G

Other Products: ○Food Nutrient Complex for nutrients and minerals to help support thyroid function.

🔧: Dilute as recommended, and apply on thyroid area or on reflex points on the feet.

🗲: Diffuse into the air.

○: Take capsules as directed on package.

Grief/Sorrow

Oils: ⊘○lemon○, ⊘○Joyful Blend, ○Grounding Blend, ⊘○lavender, ⊘○bergamot○, ⊘○clary sage, ⊘○juniper berry, ⊘○eucalyptus, ⊘○helichrysum

🗲: Diffuse into the air. Inhale directly from bottle. Apply oil to hands, tissue, or cotton wick, and inhale. Wear 1–2 drops as perfume or cologne.

🔧: Dilute as recommended, and apply 1–2 drops to the forehead, shoulders, or feet. Add 1–2 drops to 1 Tbs. fractionated coconut oil, and massage over whole body.

📖: **Additional Research:**

Lemon: Lemon odor was found to enhance the positive mood of volunteers exposed to a stressor (Kiecolt-Glaser et al., 2008).

Lemon: Lemon oil vapor was found to have strong antistress and antidepressant effects on mice subjected to several common stress tests (Komiya et al., 2006).

Lemon: Lemon oil and its component, citral, were found to decrease depressed behavior in a similar manner to antidepressant drugs in rats involved in several stress tests (Komori et al., 1995).

Lemon: In 12 patients suffering from depression, it was found that inhaling citrus aromas reduced the needed doses of antidepressants, normalized neuroendocrine hormone levels, and normalized immune function (Komori et al., 1995).

Bergamot: Lemon oil and its component, citral, were found to decrease depressed behavior in a similar manner to antidepressant drugs in rats involved in several stress tests (Komori et al., 1995).

Gum Disease
see Oral Conditions:Gum Disease

Gums
see Oral Conditions:Gums

Habits
see Addictions

Hair

Other Products: ○Smoothing Conditioner, ○Protecting Shampoo, ○Hair Serum, ○Hair Glaze.

—**Beard:**

　Oils: ○rosemary, ○lemon, ○lavender, ○thyme, ○cypress

—**Children:**

　Oils: ○lavender

—**Damaged:**

　Other Products: ○Smoothing Conditioner, ○Protecting Shampoo, ○Hair Serum

—Dandruff: *see also* **Antifungal**

Dandruff is a scalp condition characterized by the excessive shedding of dead skin cells. A small amount of flaking on the scalp is normal as old skin cells die off and fall away, but dandruff results when the amount of dead skin cells becomes excessive and visible. Dandruff can be caused by many possible factors: hormonal imbalance, poor hygiene, allergies, excessive use of hair sprays and gels, excessive use of curling irons, cold weather, infrequent shampooing, etc. Many specialists believe that dandruff is caused by a tiny fungus called *Pityrosporum ovale.*

Oils: ◎lavender, ◎wintergreen, ◎cypress, ◎rosemary, ◎cedarwood, ◎thyme

—Dry:

Oils: ◎geranium, ◎sandalwood, ◎lavender, ◎rosemary, ◎wintergreen

Other Products: ◎Smoothing Conditioner, ◎Protecting Shampoo, ◎Hair Serum

—Estrogen Balance:

Estrogen is a steroid hormone that causes the development of female characteristics such as breasts and larger hips, helps with calcium uptake and balance, and plays many other important roles. Estrogen also helps hair to grow faster and to stay on the head longer. If estrogen levels fall, hair loss can quickly result.

Oils: ◎clary sage

—Fragile Hair:

Oils: ◎clary sage, ◎lavender, ◎thyme, ◎sandalwood, ◎wintergreen, ◎Roman chamomile

Other Products: ◎Smoothing Conditioner, ◎Protecting Shampoo, ◎Hair Serum

—Greasy/Oily Hair:

Oils: ◎basil, ◎cypress, ◎thyme, ◎lemon, ◎rosemary

Other Products: ◎Smoothing Conditioner, ◎Protecting Shampoo

—Growth (stimulate):

Oils: ◎thyme◎, ◎lavender◎, ◎rosemary◎, ◎ylang ylang, ◎cedarwood, ◎clary sage, ◎geranium, ◎ginger, ◎lemon, ◎grapefruit

—Itching:

Oils: ◎peppermint, ◎lavender

—Loss:

One common form of hair loss, especially in males, is androgenic alopecia (also known as male-pattern baldness in males). This condition is thought to be caused by a genetically-predisposed sensitivity within the hair follicles to androgen hormones that causes them to shrink when exposed to this hormone. This shrinking of the hair follicles inhibits their ability to produce hair, leading to a receding hairline and partial baldness on the top and sides of the head in males and thinning hair in females. Another common form of baldness, especially in females, is alopecia areata, which is a condition in which hair loss occurs on all or part of the body. The most common form of alopecia areata involves the loss of round patches of hair on the scalp, leading this condition to be commonly referred to as "spot baldness."

Oils: ⊘rosemary◷, ⊘lavender, ⊘thyme, ⊘ylang ylang, ⊘cedarwood, ⊘wintergreen, ⊘lemon, ⊘clary sage, ⊘cypress, ⊘Roman chamomile

⊖: Apply 1–2 drops of oil to hands, and massage into hair and scalp before bath or shower; then shampoo and rinse hair as normal. Add 1–2 drops of oil to 2 Tbs. of an unscented shampoo or shower gel, and use to shampoo hair. Use shampoo and conditioner as directed on bottles.

▭: **Additional Research:**

Thyme: Patients with alopecia areata (hair loss) that massaged carrier oils containing a blend of thyme, rosemary, lavender, and cedarwood oils into their scalps were more likely to show improvement when compared to a control group that massaged carrier oils alone into their scalps (Hay et al., 1998)

Lavender: Patients with alopecia areata (hair loss) that massaged carrier oils containing a blend of thyme, rosemary, lavender, and cedarwood oils into their scalps were more likely to show improvement when compared to a control group that massaged carrier oils alone into their scalps (Hay et al., 1998)

Rosemary: Patients with alopecia areata (hair loss) that massaged carrier oils containing a blend of thyme, rosemary, lavender, and cedarwood oils into their scalps were more likely to show improvement when compared to a control group that massaged carrier oils alone into their scalps (Hay et al., 1998)

Halitosis
see **Oral Conditions:Halitosis**

Hands
Oils: ⊘geranium, ⊘lemon, ⊘lemongrass, ⊘sandalwood, ⊘rosemary, ⊘eucalyptus

—Dry:
Oils: ⊘geranium, ⊘sandalwood

—Neglected:
Oils: ⊘geranium, ⊘lemon

—Tingling In:
Oils: ⊘lemongrass

⊖: Dilute as recommended, and apply 1–2 drops to hands. Dilute 1–2 drops in 1 Tbs. almond or olive oil, and use as massage oil to massage into hands.

Hangovers
A hangover is a set of unpleasant physical effects that comes after heavy alcohol consumption. Common symptoms of a hangover include nausea, headache, lack of energy, diarrhea, and increased sensitivity to light and noise.

Oils: ⊘⊘lemon, ⊘⊘grapefruit, ⊘⊘lavender, ⊘⊘rosemary, ⊘⊘sandalwood

⊖: Add 3–4 drops to warm bathwater, and bathe. Dilute as recommended, and apply 1–2 drops to back of neck or over liver. Add 1–2 drops to 1 Tbs. fractionated coconut oil, and massage onto back and neck.

⊘: Inhale directly from bottle. Apply oil to hands, tissue, or cotton wick, and inhale. Drop 1–2 drops in bowl of hot water, and inhale vapors. Diffuse into the air.

Hashimoto's Disease
see also **Thyroid:Hypothyroidism.**

Hashimoto's disease is an autoimmune disorder where the immune system attacks the thyroid, causing it to swell up and become irritated. Hashimoto's disease does not have a unique set of symptoms, but possible symptoms include abnormal fatigue, weight gain, muscle pain and stiffness, a hoarse voice, prolonged menstrual bleeding, constipation, a feeling of tightness in the throat, sensitivity to cold, dry skin, and depression.

Oils: ⊖❷lemongrass, ⊖❷myrrh

Other Products: ⭘Food Nutrient Complex , ⭘Cellular Vitality Complex, ⭘Chewable Multivitamin to help provide nutrients essential for thyroid cell health.

⊖: Dilute as recommended, and apply 1–2 drops over thyroid area or on reflex points on the feet.

❷: Diffuse into the air. Inhale oil applied to hands.

⭘: Take capsules as directed on package.

Hay Fever
see Allergies:Hay Fever

Head Lice
see Insects/Bugs:Lice

Headaches

Oils: ⊖❷Tension Blend, ⊖❷peppermint⁰, ⊖❷rosemary, ⊖❷Soothing Blend, ⊖❷cardamom, ⊖❷eucalyptus, ⊖❷frankincense, ⊖❷patchouli, ⊖❷basil, ⊖❷marjoram, ⊖❷lavender⁰, ⊖❷clove

Recipe 1: Apply 1–2 drops each of peppermint, lavender, and frankincense to back of neck, temples, and forehead.

—Migraine Headache:

A migraine is a severe and painful type of headache. Symptoms of migraines include throbbing pain accompanied by nausea, vomiting, and heightened sensitivity to light. Women are much more likely than men to suffer from migraines. Migraines can be triggered by stress, anxiety, sleep or food deprivation, bright lights, loud noises, and hormonal changes.

Oils: ⊖❷Tension Blend, ⊖❷peppermint, ⊖❷basil, ⊖❷Soothing Blend, ⊖❷wintergreen, ⊖❷ylang ylang

—Tension Headache:

Tension headaches (also called "stress headaches") are the most common type of headache. Tension headaches are characterized by dull, constant pressure or pain (usually on both sides of the head). Tension headaches can last from thirty minutes to several days and tend to come back when a person is under stress.

Oils: ⊖❷Tension Blend, ⊖❷peppermint, ⊖❷Soothing Blend

—Sugar Headache (caused by low blood sugar):

Oils: ⊖❷Protective Blend

⊖: Dilute as recommended, and apply 1–2 drops to temples, back of neck, and forehead.

⊘: Diffuse into the air. Inhale directly from bottle. Apply oil to hands, tissue, or cotton wick, and inhale.

📖: **Additional Research:**

Peppermint: A combination of peppermint oil and ethanol was found to have a significant analgesic effect with a reduction in sensitivity to headache, while a combination of peppermint, eucalyptus, and ethanol was found to relax muscles and to increase cognitive performance in humans (Göbel et al., 1994).

Lavender: Inhalation of lavender essential oil was found to be more effective than inhalation of a placebo for reducing the severity of headaches in subjects diagnosed with migraine headaches (Sasannejad et al., 2012).

Hearing
see **Ears**

Heart
see **Cardiovascular System:Heart**

Heartburn
see **Digestive System:Heartburn**

Heatstroke

Heatstroke is when the body's temperature rises dangerously high due to the body's inability to dissipate heat, typically because of high environmental temperatures and high levels of exertion. If not corrected, the body can overheat too much, causing organs and body systems to become damaged and possibly shut down—possibly leading to death. Symptoms of heatstroke include perspiration, dizziness, confusion, headaches, and nausea.

Oils: ⌀peppermint, ⌀lavender

⊜: Dilute as recommended, and apply 3–5 drops on neck and forehead. Cool the body as soon as possible in a cool bathtub, lake, river, or soaked linens.

Hematoma
see also **Blood:Hemorrhaging.**

A hematoma is a collection of blood outside of the blood vessels. The most common form of a hematoma is a bruise. Hematomas can also form into hard, blood-filled sacs that look like welts and can move to different locations. These often dissolve on their own. Hematomas can also form in other organs as the result of injury or hemorrhaging.

Oils: ⌀helichrysum

⊜: Dilute as recommended, and apply 1–2 drops on location.

Hemorrhaging
see **Blood:Hemorrhaging**

Hemorrhoids

Hemorrhoids are swollen, twisted veins that occur in the rectum or anus. They are caused by increased pressure within the veins, often due to pregnancy, frequent lifting, or constipation.

Oils: ⌀cypress, ⌀geranium, ⌀clary sage, ⌀helichrysum, ⌀patchouli, ⌀peppermint, ⌀sandalwood, ⌀juniper berry, ⌀frankincense, ⌀myrrh

Blend 1: Mix 1 drop cypress with 1 drop of either helichrysum or geranium, and apply on location.

🜚: Dilute as recommended, and apply 1–2 drops on location. Mix 1–2 drops with 1 tsp. fractionated coconut oil, and apply on location using a rectal syringe.

Hepatitis
see **Liver:Hepatitis**

Hernia
see also **Back:Herniated Discs**

A hernia is the protrudence of a tissue or organ through tissue or muscle outside of the body cavity in which it is normally contained. There are several different types of hernias, and the symptoms vary with each type.

—Hiatal:

A hiatal (hiatus) hernia is when a portion of the stomach protrudes through the diaphragm into the chest cavity above. This can cause pain, acid reflux, and heartburn. It can be caused by a birth defect or may be brought on by heavy lifting, stress, or being overweight.

Oils: 🜚basil, 🜚peppermint, 🜚cypress, 🜚ginger, 🜚geranium, 🜚lavender, 🜚fennel, 🜚rosemary

—Incisional:

An incisional hernia is caused by a protrusion through scar tissue from an abdominal wound or incision that hasn't healed correctly.

Oils: 🜚basil, 🜚helichrysum, 🜚lemongrass, 🜚geranium, 🜚lavender, 🜚ginger, 🜚lemon, 🜚melaleuca

—Inguinal:

An inguinal hernia is when the intestines protrude into the inguinal canal (a small opening that leads from the abdominal cavity into the groin area). This can sometimes be seen as a bulge in the groin area and is usually painless, but it may become painful if the blood supply to the herniated portion of the intestine is restricted (strangulated).

Oils: 🜚lemongrass, 🜚lavender

🜚: Dilute as recommended, and apply on location, lower back, and reflex points on the feet.

Herpes Simplex
see also **Antiviral**

Herpes simplex type 1 and type 2 viruses are the two viruses that cause genital and oral herpes infections. These viruses cause painful outbreaks of blisters and sores to occur in the affected area when the virus is active in the skin or mucus membranes, followed by periods of latency when the virus resides in the nerve cells around the infected area.

Oils: 🜚peppermint○, 🜚melaleuca○, 🜚helichrysum○, 🜚clove○, 🜚lavender, 🜚eucalyptus○, 🜚lemon, 🜚cypress, 🜚rose, 🜚bergamot

🜚: Dilute as recommended, and apply oil directly on the lesions at the first sign of outbreak.

📖: **Additional Research:**

⊘=Aromatic, 🜚=Topical, ○=Internal (See page 33 for further details.)   169

Peppermint: Peppermint oil demonstrated a direct virucidal activity against herpes type 1 and type 2 viruses (Schuhmacher et al., 2003).

Melaleuca: Tea tree and eucalyptus oil demonstrated ability to inhibit Herpes simplex virus (Schnitzler et al., 2001).

Helichrysum: Helichrysum was found to have significant antiviral activity against the herpes virus at non-cytotoxic concentrations (Nostro et al., 2003).

Clove: Eugenol was found to be virucidal to Herpes simplex and to delay the development of herpes-induced keratitis (inflammation of the cornea) in mice (Benencia et al., 2000).

Eucalyptus: Tea tree and eucalyptus oil demonstrated ability to inhibit Herpes simplex virus (Schnitzler et al., 2001).

Hiccups/Hiccoughs

Hiccups, or hiccoughs, are the uncontrollable spasms of the diaphragm that cause a sudden intake of breath and the closure of the glottis (the opening that stops substances from entering the trachea while swallowing). Hiccups are thought to be caused either by a lack of carbon dioxide in the blood or by something irritating the diaphragm.

Oils: ❂❂sandalwood

🕭: Diffuse into the air. Inhale directly from bottle. Apply oil to hands, tissue, or cotton wick, and inhale.

🜄: Dilute as recommended, and apply 1–2 drops to the diaphragm area or reflex points on the feet.

High Blood Pressure
See Blood:Blood Pressure:High

Hives
see also Allergies, Antiviral

Hives are itchy patches of inflamed spots on the skin surrounded by redness, typically caused by an allergic reaction or a viral infection.

Oils: ❂melaleuca❂, ❂peppermint, ❂lavender❂

🜄: Dilute as recommended, and apply 1–2 drops on location. Add 1–2 drops to 1 Tbs. fractionated coconut oil, and massage on location.

🗀: **Additional Research:**

Melaleuca: Tea tree oil applied to histamine-induced weal and flare in human volunteers was found to decrease the mean weal volume when compared to a control (Koh et al., 2002).

Melaleuca: Tea tree oil applied to histamine-induced edema (swelling) in mice ears was found to significantly reduce swelling (Brand et al., 2002).

Lavender: Lavender oil was found to inhibit immediate-type allergic reactions in mice and rats by inhibiting mast cell degranulation (Kim et al., 1999).

Hodgkin's Disease
see also Cancer

Hodgkin's disease (or Hodgkin's lymphoma) is a type of cancer that affects lymphocytes (white blood cells). It can cause enlarged lymph nodes, fever, sweating, fatigue, and weight loss.

Oils: ❂clove

🜄: Dilute as recommended, and apply 1–2 drops to the liver, kidney, and reflex points on the feet.

Hormonal System/Imbalance
see **Endocrine System**

Hot Flashes
see **Female Specific Conditions**

Housecleaning

—Bathrooms/Kitchens:

Oils: ⊘lemon, ⊘white fir (for cleaning and disinfecting)

Other Products: ⊘Protective Cleaner to help eliminate microorganisms from household surfaces.

⊘: Place a few drops on your cleaning rag or dust cloth; or place 10 drops in a small spray bottle with distilled water, and mist on surfaces before cleaning.

—Carpets:

Oils: ⊘lemon, ⊘Cleansing Blend

⊘: Apply on carpet stains to help remove. To freshen carpet, add 50–70 drops of these (or another favorite oil) to 1/2 cup baking soda. Sprinkle over carpets, wait 15 minutes, and then vacuum.

—Dishes:

Oils: ⊘lemon

Other Products: ⊘Protective Cleaner to help purify dishes.

⊘: Add a couple of drops to dishwater for sparkling dishes and a great smelling kitchen. Can add to dishwasher as well.

—Furniture Polish:

Oils: ⊘lemon, ⊘white fir, ⊘Invigorating Blend, ⊘Cleansing Blend

⊘: Place a few drops on a clean rag, and use to polish furniture.

—Gum/Grease:

Oils: ⊘lemon, ⊘lime

⊘: Place 1–2 drops on gum or grease to help dissolve.

—Laundry:

Oils: ⊘lemon, ⊘Cleansing Blend

Other Products: ⊘Protective Laundry Detergent to help naturally fight stains and brighten clothes.

⊘: Add a few drops of oil to the water in the washer. Add a few drops on a washcloth with clothes in the dryer. Add a few drops to a small spray bottle of water, and mist on laundry in the dryer before drying. Any of these methods can increase the antibacterial benefits and help clothes to smell fresh and clean.

—Mold/Fungus: *see also* **Antifungal:Mold**

Oils: ⊘⊘Protective Blend, ⊘Cleansing Blend

②: Diffuse into the air.

◉: Place a few drops on a cleaning rag, and wipe down the affected area.

—Stains:

Oils: *◉*lemon (has been used to remove black shoe polish from carpets)

◉: Apply on location.

Hyperactivity
see **Calming:Hyperactivity**

Hyperpnea
see **Respiratory System:Hyperpnea**

Hypertension
see **Blood:Blood Pressure:High**

Hypoglycemia

Hypoglycemia is a condition of low levels of sugar in the blood. It is most common in people with diabetes but can be caused by drugs or by a tumor in the pancreas that causes the pancreas to create too much insulin. Symptoms of hypoglycemia can include hunger, sweating, weakness, palpitations, shaking, dizziness, and confusion.

Oils: *◉*eucalyptus, *◉*Protective Blend, *◉*cinnamon, *◉*clove, *◉*thyme

Other Products: *O*Probiotic Defense Formula to help maintain a healthy digestive system.

◉: Dilute as recommended and apply 1–2 drops over pancreas and on reflex points on the feet.

○: Take capsules as directed on package.

Hysteria
see **Calming**

Immune System
see also **Allergies, Antibacterial, Antifungal, Antiviral, Cancer, Lymphatic System, Parasites**

The immune system is the body's defense against disease. The immune system protects the body by identifying and killing bacteria, viruses, parasites, other microorganisms, and tumor cells that would harm the body. The immune system is comprised of several different types of white blood cells (lymphocytes) that recognize, process, or destroy foreign objects, the bone marrow that creates several types of white blood cells, the thymus that creates white blood cells and teaches them to recognize foreign objects and distinguish them from the body's cells, lymphatic vessels that help transport lymph and white blood cells, and several other organs, such as the lymph nodes, tonsils, spleen, and appendix, that filter out foreign objects and serve as a place for white blood cells to gather, interact, and share information about infections.

Oils: *◉②O*Protective Blend, *◉②O*oregano*◉*, *◉②*melaleuca, *◉②*rosemary, *◉②*clove, *◉②*frankincense, *◉②*geranium, *◉②*lemon, *◉②*thyme, *◉②*lavender, *◉②*lime

Other Products: *O*Protective Softgels, *O*Energy & Stamina Complex, *O*Cellular Vitality Complex, *O*Chewable Multivitamin, *O*Essential Oil Omega Complex or Vegan Essential Oil

Omega Complex, OOmega-3 Fish Oil, OFood Nutrient Complex to provide nutrients essential for healthy immune system function.

—Stimulates:

Oils: ⊜⊜Ooregano⊜, ⊜cinnamon, ⊜⊜frankincense, ⊜⊜melaleuca, ⊜Protective Blend, ⊜⊜lavender

⊜: Dilute as recommended, and apply 1–2 drops to bottoms of feet, along spine, or under arms (around lymph nodes). Add 1–2 drops to 1 Tbs. fractionated coconut oil, and massage onto back, arms, and feet.

O: Take capsules as recommended. Place 1–2 drops of oil under the tongue or place 2–3 drops in an empty capsule, and swallow.

⊘: Diffuse into the air.

⊡: **Additional Research:**

Oregano: Growth-retarded pigs receiving a supplementation of oregano leaves and flowers enriched with cold-pressed oregano oil were found to have increased growth, decreased mortality, and higher numbers of immune-system cells and compounds when compared to control pigs who did not receive supplementation (Walter et al., 2004).

Impetigo
see **Skin:Impetigo**

Impotence
see **Male Specific Conditions:Impotence**

Incontinence
see **Bladder:Bed Wetting and Incontinence**

Indigestion
see **Digestive System:Indigestion**

Infection
see also **Antibacterial, Antifungal, Antiviral**

Oils: ⊜⊜cinnamon, ⊜⊜clary sage, ⊜⊜Protective Blend, ⊜⊜bergamot, ⊜⊜myrrh (with oregano), ⊜⊜basil, ⊜⊜cypress, ⊜⊜rosemary (with myrrh for oral infection), ⊜⊜thyme (for urinary infection), ⊜⊜lemongrass, ⊜⊜lime, ⊜⊜patchouli, ⊜⊜lavender, ⊜⊜oregano, ⊜⊜juniper berry, ⊜⊜fennel, ⊜⊜peppermint

Other Products: OProtective Softgels. OFood Nutrient Complex for nutrients that help provide immune support.

—Infected Wounds:

Oils: ⊜⊜frankincense, ⊜⊜melaleuca

Blend 1: Apply 1 drop thyme on location with hot compress daily. After infection and pus have been expelled, mix 3 drops lavender, 2 drops melaleuca, and 2 drops thyme combined with 1 tsp. fractionated coconut oil, and apply a little of this mixture on location twice daily.

⊜: Dilute as recommended, and apply 1–2 drops on location. Mix 1–2 drops with 1 Tbs. fractionated coconut oil, and massage on location or on neck, arms, chest, or feet.

⮐: Diffuse into the air. Add 1–2 drops to a bowl of hot water, and inhale the vapors.

◯: Take capsules as directed on package.

Infertility

see Female Specific Conditions: Infertility, Male Specific Conditions:Infertility

Inflammation

see also Antioxidant

Inflammation is the body's reaction to infection and injury. It is characterized by redness, swelling, warmth, and pain. Inflammation is an immune system response that allows the body to contain and fight infection or repair damaged tissue by dilating the blood vessels and allowing vascular permeability to increase blood supply to an injured or infected tissue. While a certain amount of inflammation can be beneficial in fighting disease and healing injuries, too much inflammation or chronic inflammation can actually be debilitating.

Oils: ⬤⬤◯frankincense▢, ⬤⬤melaleuca▢, ⬤⬤eucalyptus▢, ⬤oregano, ⬤Soothing Blend, ⬤lavender▢, cardamom▢, ⬤◯⬤patchouli, ⬤Roman chamomile▢, ⬤myrrh▢, ⬤rosemary▢, ⬤◯⬤peppermint▢, ⬤◯wintergreen▢, ◯⬤clove▢, ⬤thyme▢, ⬤geranium▢, ⬤helichrysum▢, ⬤Anti-Aging Blend, ⬤juniper berry, ⬤cedarwood▢, ⬤⬤Calming Blend, ⬤⬤lemongrass, ⬤⬤cypress

Other products: ◯Cellular Vitality Complex and ◯Food Nutrient Complex or ◯Chewable Multivitamin for polyphenols and other antioxidants to help relieve oxidative stress associated with inflammation. ◯Essential Oil Omega Complex or Vegan Essential Oil Omega Complex or ◯◯Omega-3 Fish Oil for omega-3 fatty acids that help balance the inflammatory response.

🖐: Dilute as recommended, and apply 1–2 drops on location and on the back of neck by the base of the skull. Add 3–4 drops to 1 Tbs. fractionated coconut oil, and massage on location.

◯: Place 1–2 drops of oil under the tongue, or place 2–3 drops of in an empty capsule, and swallow. Place 1–2 drops in 8 oz. of rice or almond milk, and drink. Take supplements as directed on package.

⮐: Diffuse into the air. Add 1–2 drops to a bowl of hot water or humidifier, and inhale the vapors to help relieve inflammation within the respiratory system.

📖: **Additional Research:**

Frankincense: Alpha-pinene was found to block proinflammatory responses in THP-1 cells (Zhou et al., 2004).

Frankincense: Boswellia frereana extracts were found to inhibit proinflammatory molecules involved in joint cartilage degredation (Blain et al., 2009).

Frankincense: Compounds from Boswellia serrata were found to carry out anti-inflammatory activity by switching off the pro-inflammatory cytokines and mediators that initiate the inflammatory process (Gayathri et al., 2007).

Frankincense: An acetone extract of frankincense was found to decrease arthritic scores, reduce paw edema (swelling), and suppress pro-inflammatory cytokines (cellular messengers) (Fan et al., 2005).

Frankincense: Incensole acetate, isolated from frankincense resin, was found to demonstrate an anti-inflammatory and neuroprotective effect in mice with closed head injuries (Moussaieff et al., 2008).

Melaleuca: Melaleuca alternifolia oil was found to mediate the reactive oxygen species (ROS) production of leukocytes (white blood cells), indicating possible anti-inflammatory activity (Caldefie-Chézet et al., 2004).

Melaleuca: Tea tree oil applied to histamine-induced edema (swelling) in mice ears was found to significantly reduce swelling (Brand et al., 2002).

Melaleuca: Tea tree oil applied to histamine-induced edema (swelling) in mice ears was found to significantly reduce swelling (Brand et al., 2002).

Melaleuca: Tea tree oil was found to reduce swelling during a contact hypersensitivity response in the skin of mice sensitized to the chemical hapten (Brand et al., 2002).

Melaleuca: Several water-soluble components of tea tree oil were found to suppress the production of superoxide by monocytes (a type of white blood cell involved in the immune system) (Brand et al., 2001).

Melaleuca: The water soluble terpinen-4-ol component of tea tree was found to suppress the production of pro-inflammatory mediators in human monocytes (a type of white blood cell that is part of the human immune system (Hart et al., 2000).

Melaleuca: Inhaled tea tree oil was found to have anti-inflammatory influences on male rats with induced peritoneal inflammation (Golab et al., 2007).

Melaleuca: Tea tree oil applied to histamine-induced weal and flare in human volunteers was found to decrease the mean weal volume when compared to a control (Koh et al., 2002).

Melaleuca: Tea tree oil was found to reduce inflammation in nickel-sensitive human skin exposed to nickel (Pearce et al., 2005).

Eucalyptus: Eucalyptus oil was shown to ameliorate inflammatory processes by interacting with oxygen radicals and interfering with leukocyte activation (Grassmann et al., 2000).

Eucalyptus: 1,8 cineole (eucalyptol) was found to display an anti-inflammatory effect on rats in several tests and was found to exhibit antinociceptive (pain-reducing) effects in mice, possibly by depressing the central nervous system (Santos et al., 2000).

Eucalyptus: Eucalyptus oil was found to have an anti-inflammatory and mucin-inhibitory effect in rats with lipopolysaccharide-induced bronchitis (Lu et al., 2004).

Eucalyptus: Oils of three eucalyptus species (citriodora, tereticornis, and globulus) were found to have analgesic (pain-relieving) and anti-inflammatory properties in rats (Silva et al., 2003).

Eucalyptus: Extracts from eucalyptus and thyme were found to have high nitrous oxide (NO) scavenging abilities and to inhibit NO production in macrophage cells. This could possibly explain their role in aiding respiratory inflammatory diseases (Vigo et al., 2004).

Lavender: Oil from Lavandula angustifolia was found to reduce writhing in induced writhing in rats and to reduce edema (swelling) in carrageenan-induced paw edema, indicating an anti-inflammatory effect (Hajhashemi et al., 2003).

Lavender: Linalool and linalyl acetate (from lavender and other essential oils) were found to exhibit anti-inflammatory activity in rats subjected to carrageenin-induced edema (inflammation) (Peana et al., 2002).

Cardamom: Cardamom essential oil reduced rat paw edema by 76% of the control value, illustrating significant anti-inflammatory activity (al-Zuhair et al., 1996).

Roman Chamomile: Chamazulene, a chemical in chamomile oil, was found to block formation of leukotriene (a signaling chemical involved in the inflammation process) in neutrophilic (immune system) granulocytes (white blood cells containing granules). It also demonstrated an antioxidant effect (Safayhi et al., 1994).

Myrrh: At subtoxic levels, myrrh oil was found to reduce interleukin (chemical signals believed to play a role in the inflammation response) by fibroblast cells in the gums (Tipton et al., 2003).

Myrrh: Subtoxic levels of myrrh oil were found to inhibit interleukin (chemical messenger involved in inflammation), in part by inhibiting PGE(2) (Prostaglandin E, a lipid compound that has several messenger functions in the body, including in the inflammatory response) (Tipton et al., 2006).

Rosemary: An ethanol extract of rosemary was found to have an antiproliferative effect on human leukemia and breast carcinoma cells as well as an antioxidant effect (Cheung et al., 2007).

Rosemary: An ethanol extract of rosemary was found to demonstrate antinociceptive (pain blocking) and anti-inflammatory activity in mice and rats (González-Trujano et al., 2007).

Rosemary: Rosemary oil was found to have anti-inflammatory and peripheral-antinociceptive (pain sensitivity blocking) properties in mice (Takaki et al., 2008).

Peppermint: A combination of peppermint and caraway oil was found to reduce visceral hyperalgesia (pain hypersensitivity in the gastrointestinal tract) after induced inflammation in rats (Adam et al., 2006).

Peppermint: L-menthol was found to inhibit production of inflammation mediators in human monocytes (a type of white blood cell involved in the immune response) (Juergens et al., 1998).

Wintergreen: Methyl salicylate (found in wintergreen or birch oils) was found to inhibit leukotriene C4 (a chemical messenger involved in inflammatory response), while also demonstrating a gastroprotective effect against ethanol-induced gastric injury in rats (Trautmann et al., 1991).

Clove: Eugenol (found in clove EO) was found to increase the anti-inflammatory activity of cod liver oil (lowered inflammation by 30%) (Reddy et al., 1994).

Clove: Clove oil was found to increase humoral immunity and decrease cell-mediated immunity in rats, illustrating that clove oil can modulate the immune response and overall acts as an anti-inflammatory agent (Halder et al., 2011).

Thyme: Extracts from eucalyptus and thyme were found to have high nitrous oxide (NO) scavenging abilities and to inhibit NO production in macrophage cells. This could possibly explain their role in aiding respiratory inflammatory diseases (Vigo et al., 2004).

Geranium: Topical application of geranium oil was found to reduce the inflammatory response of neutrophil (white blood cell) accumulation in mice (Maruyama et al., 2005).

Helichrysum: Arzanol, extracted from helichrysum, inhibited HIV-1 replication in T cells and also inhibited the release of pro-inflammatory cytokines (chemical messengers) in monocytes (Appendino et al., 2007).

Cedarwood: *Juniperus virginiana* oil was found to have anti-inflammatory activity in mice (Tumen et al., 2013).

Dill: Oil-based dill extract displayed greater anti-inflammatory activity when topically applied to inflamed rat paws than the anti-inflammatory drug diclofenac (Naseri et al., 2012).

Influenza

see also **Antiviral**

Influenza, commonly referred to as "the flu," is a highly contagious viral infection of the respiratory system. Influenza is marked by a sudden onset of high fever, dry cough, sore throat, muscle aches and pains, headache, fatigue, loss of appetite, nausea, and nasal congestion.

Oils: ⊘⊙Respiratory Blend, ⊘⊙melaleuca⊙, ⊘⊙Opeppermint, ⊘⊙rosemary, ⊘⊙eucalyptus, ⊙⊘Protective Blend, ⊘⊙white fir (aches/pains), ⊘⊙lavender, ⊘⊙oregano, ⊘⊙thyme, ⊘orange, ⊘⊙clove, O⊙ginger

Other Products: OProtective Softgels. ⊙Protective Hand Wash to help prevent the spread of influenza viruses. OFood Nutrient Complex for nutrients to help support immune function.

⊘: Diffuse into the air.

⊜: Dilute as recommended, an apply to thymus area, chest, back, sinuses, or reflex points on the feet. Add 1–2 drops to hot bathwater, and bathe. Dilute 1–2 drops in 1 Tbs. fractionated coconut oil, and massage on chest, back, and feet.

O: Place 1–2 drops of ginger or peppermint oil in an empty capsule, and swallow to help reduce feelings of nausea. Take supplements as directed on package.

⊡: **Additional Research:**

Melaleuca: In vitro research has found that *Melaleuca alternifolia* concentrate can disturb the normal viral membrane fusion of the influenza virus and inhibit entry of influenza virus into the host cell (Li et al., 2013).

Injuries

see **Bones, Bruises, Cuts, Inflammation, Joints, Muscles/Connective Tissue, Pain, Skin:Scarring, Tissue:Scarring, Wounds**

Insects/Bugs

see also **Bites/Stings**

—Bees, Wasps, and Hornet Stings:

Oils: ⊙Roman chamomile, ⊙basil, ⊙Cleansing Blend, ⊙lavender, ⊙lemongrass, ⊙lemon, ⊙peppermint, ⊙thyme.

Recipe 1: Remove the stinger, and apply a cold compress of Roman chamomile to the area for several hours or as long as possible.

⊖: Dilute as recommended, and apply 1–2 drops on location after making certain that the stinger is removed.

—Gnats and Midges:

Oils: ⊖lavender, ⊖⊘Repellent Blend

Recipe 2: Mix 3 drops thyme in 1 tsp. cider vinegar or lemon juice. Apply to bites to stop irritation.

⊖: Dilute as recommended, and apply 1–2 drops to bite area.

⊘: Diffuse into the air. Place 1–2 drops on small ribbons, strings, or cloth, and hang around area to help repel mosquitoes.

—Itching:

Oils: ⊖lavender

⊖: Dilute as recommended, and apply 1–2 drops to affected area.

—Lice:

Oils: ⊖eucalyptus◌, ⊖⊘Repellent Blend, ⊖rosemary, ⊖melaleuca◌, ⊖geranium, ⊖lemon, ⊖lavender

⊖: Dilute as recommended, and rub 1–2 drops into the scalp three times a day, and apply to feet.

—Mosquitoes:

Oils: ⊖⊘Repellent Blend, ⊖⊘patchouli◌, ⊖lavender, ⊖helichrysum

⊖: Dilute as recommended, and apply 1–2 drops to feet and exposed skin. Add 3–5 drops to 1 Tbs. fractionated coconut oil, and apply to exposed skin. Add 2–3 drops to 1–2 oz. distilled water in a small spray bottle; shake well, and mist onto the skin or into small openings where bugs may come through.

⊘: Diffuse into the air. Place 1–2 drops on small ribbons, strings, or cloth, and hang around area to help repel mosquitoes.

—Repellent:

Oils: ⊖⊘Repellent Blend, ⊖⊘patchouli, ⊖⊘basil, ⊖⊘lavender◌, ⊖⊘lemongrass, ⊖⊘cedarwood◌, ⊖⊘eucalyptus, ⊖⊘arborvitae, ⊖⊘thyme, ⊖⊘Cleansing Blend

Blend 1: Combine 5 drops lavender, 5 drops lemongrass, 3 drops peppermint, and 1 drop thyme. Place neat on feet. Add to 1 cup (8 oz.) of water, and spray on using a fine-mist spray bottle. Or place drops of this blend on ribbons or strings and tie near windows or around picnic or camping area.

Blend 2: Combine equal parts clove, lemon, and orange, and apply 2–3 drops on skin.

Blend 3: Place 5 drops lemon and 5 drops Cleansing Blend in a small spray bottle with distilled water. Shake well, and mist on your skin to help protect against insects, flies, and mosquitoes.

⊖: Dilute as recommended, and apply 1–2 drops to feet and exposed skin. Add 3–5 drops to 1 Tbs. fractionated coconut oil, and apply to exposed skin. Add 2–3 drops

---

to 1–2 oz. distilled water in a small spray bottle; shake well, and mist onto the skin or into small openings where bugs may come through.

⊘: Diffuse into the air. Place 1–2 drops on small ribbons, strings, or cloth, and hang around area to help repel insects.

—Spiders:

Oils: ◎basil, ◎Cleansing Blend (with melaleuca), ◎lavender, ◎lemongrass, ◎lemon, ◎peppermint, ◎thyme

◎: Dilute as recommended, and apply 1–2 drops to affected area. Apply oil as a cold compress.

—Termites:

Oils: ◎⊘patchouli◌, ◎⊘vetiver◌ (repels), ⊘⊘clove◌ (kills)

◎: Apply oils around foundation and to soil around wood structures to help repel termites.

⊘: Diffuse into the air.

—Ticks:

Oils: ◎⊘Repellent Blend, ◎lavender ◌

Removing Ticks:

Do not apply mineral oil, Vaseline, or anything else to remove the tick as this may cause it to inject the spirochetes into the wound.

Be sure to remove the entire tick. Get as close to the mouth as possible, and firmly tug on the tick until it releases its grip. Don't twist. If available, use a magnifying glass to make sure that you have removed the entire tick.

Save the tick in a jar, and label it with the date, where you were bitten on your body, and the location or address where you were bitten for proper identification by your doctor, especially if you develop any symptoms.

Do not handle the tick.

Wash hands immediately.

Check the site of the bite occasionally to see if any rash develops. If it does, seek medical advice promptly.

◎: After getting the tick out, apply 1 drop lavender every 5 minutes for 30 minutes.

▣: **Additional Research:**

Melaleuca: Tea tree oil was found to be effective against both lice and dust mites in a mite chamber assay (Williamson et al., 2007).

Melaleuca: Tea tree oil was found to prevent some blood feeding by lice on treated skin; and while not highly effective at the studied dosages, tea tree oil was found to be more effective than DEET at repelling head lice (Canyon et al., 2007).

Patchouli: Clove, citronella, and patchouli oils were found to effectively repel 3 species of mosquitoes (Trongtokit et al., 2005).

Lavender: An infestation of the red bud borer pest was reduced by more than 95% in the grafted buds of apple trees by application of the essential oil of Lavandula angustifolia (van Tol et al., 2007).

Lavender: Lavender oil was found to be comparable to DEET in its ability to repel ticks (Hyalomma marginatum) (Mkolo et al., 2007).

Eucalyptus: Researchers found that an 8% eucalyptus oil spray was the most effective treatment (when compared against other concentrations of eucalyptus and clove oil sprays) against lice and insecticide-resistant head lice (Choi et al., 2010).

Patchouli: Both patchouli oil and its constituent, patchouli alcohol (patchoulol), were found to be repellent and insecticidal to Formosan termites when applied topically (Zhu et al., 2003).

Vetiver: Vetiver oil was found to repel termites and to prevent tunneling (with long-lasting effects), while clove oil was found to be highly termiticidal (Zhu et al., 2001).

Clove: Vetiver oil was found to repel termites and to prevent tunneling (with long-lasting effects), while clove oil was found to be highly termiticidal (Zhu et al., 2001).

Lavender: Lavender oil was found to be comparable to DEET in its ability to repel ticks (Hyalomma marginatum) (Mkolo et al., 2007).

Cedarwood: Cedarwood was found to possess highly insecticidal activity against adult mosquitos and other household insects (Singh et al., 1984).

Cassia: Cassia oil and its components were found to repel adult female mosquitoes for about 50 minutes post-application when applied to human subjects (Chang et al., 2006).

Geranium: A sesquiterpene alcohol from geranium essential oil proved to be an effective repellant of the lone star tick (*Amblyomma americanum*) and at concentrations greater than 0.052 mg the oil was comparable to the repellant capability of DEET (Tabanca et al., 2013).

Grapefruit: Nootkatone, found in grapefruit essential oil, was found to be toxic to four tick species (Flor-Weiler et al., 2011).

Insomnia

Insomnia is difficulty falling or staying asleep. It can be triggered by stress, medications, drug or alcohol use, anxiety, or depression.

Oils: lavender, orange, Calming Blend, Roman chamomile, cypress, ylang ylang, Invigorating Blend, marjoram, lemon, rosemary, sandalwood, clary sage, bergamot

Blend 1: Combine 6 drops Invigorating Blend with 6 drops lavender. Apply blend to big toes, bottoms of the feet, 2 drops around the navel, and 3 drops on the back of the neck.

Recipe 1: Combine 2 drops Roman chamomile, 6 drops geranium, 3 drops lemon, and 4 drops sandalwood. Add 6 drops of this blend to your bath at bedtime, and combine 5 drops with 2 tsp. fractionated coconut oil for a massage after the bath.

—For Children:

–1–5 years:

Oils: lavender, Roman chamomile

–5+ years:

Oils: clary sage, geranium, ylang ylang

: Diffuse into the air. Dissolve 3 drops essential oil in 1 tsp. pure grain alcohol (such as vodka) or perfumers alcohol, and combine with distilled water in a 2 oz. spray bottle; shake well, and spray into the air before sleep. Place 1–2 drops on bottom of pillow or stuffed animal.

: Dilute as recommended, and apply 1–2 drops on feet and back of neck. Combine 1–2 drops essential oil with 1 Tbs. fractionated coconut oil, and massage onto back, legs, feet, and arms.

: **Additional Research:**

Lavender: Female students suffering from insomnia were found to sleep better and to have a lower level of depression during weeks they used a lavender fragrance when compared to weeks they did not use a lavender fragrance (Lee et al., 2006).

Lavender: Twenty-four sessions of lavender essential oil aromatherapy was found to improve sleep quality in midlife women with insomnia up to one week after the end of the intervention when compared to the control group (Chien et al., 2012).

Orange: Bitter orange peel oil taken orally by mice was found to reduce anxiety, increase sleeping time, and increase the time before a chemically-induced seizure started (Carvalho-Freitas et al., 2002).

Intestinal Problems
see Digestive System

Invigorating

Oils: ⚬⊘wintergreen, ⚬⊘eucalyptus, ⚬⊘peppermint

⚬: Dilute as recommended, and apply 1–2 drops to back of neck or temples.

⊘: Diffuse into the air. Inhale directly from bottle. Apply oil to hands, tissue, or cotton wick, and inhale.

Irritability
see Calming

Irritable Bowel Syndrome
see Digestive System

Itching

Itching is a tingling or irritation of the skin that produces a desire to scratch. Itching can be brought on by many factors including stress, bug bites, sunburns, allergic reactions, infections, and dry skin.

Oils: ⚬lavender, ⚬Calming Blend, ⚬peppermint

⚬: Dilute as recommended, and apply 1–2 drops on location and on ears. Add 2–3 drops to 1 Tbs. fractionated coconut oil, and apply a small amount on location.

Jaundice

Jaundice is a condition characterized by a yellow appearance of the skin and the whites of the eyes. Jaundice is a result of excessive levels in the blood of a chemical called bilirubin. Bilirubin is a pigment that is made when hemoglobin from old or dead red blood cells is broken down. Jaundice occurs when the liver is unable to pass bilirubin from the body as fast as it is being produced. Jaundice is often a symptom of other diseases or conditions.

Oils: ⚬⊘geranium, ⊘⚬lemon, ⚬⊘rosemary

⚬: Dilute as recommended, and apply 1–2 drops to liver area, abdomen, and reflex points on the feet.

⊘: Diffuse into the air.

Jet Lag
see also Insomnia

Jet lag is the disruption of normal sleep patterns experienced while the body's internal clock adjusts to rapid changes in daylight and nighttime hours when flying to different areas of the world. Jet lag can cause tiredness, fatigue, and insomnia during normal sleeping hours. It is recommended to drink lots of fluids and to avoid alcohol or caffeine while flying to help prevent jet lag. Avoiding naps and forcing yourself to stay awake until your normal bedtime the first day can also help the body recover more quickly.

Oils: ⚬Grounding Blend, ⚬peppermint, ⚬eucalyptus, ⚬geranium, ⚬lavender, ⚬grapefruit, ⚬lemongrass

⊘: Use invigorating oils such as peppermint and eucalyptus in the morning and calming oils such as lavender and geranium at night. Dilute as recommended, and apply 1–2 drops to temples, thymus, lower back, and bottoms of feet. Add 2–3 drops to 1 Tbs. fractionated coconut oil, and massage onto back, legs, shoulders, and feet. Add 1–2 drops to warm bathwater, and bathe.

Joints

see also **Arthritis, Bones, Inflammation, Muscles/Connective Tissue**

A joint is an area where two bones come together. Joints can offer limited or no movement between the bones (such as in the skull) or can offer a wide range of motion (such as in the shoulders, hands, and knees).

Oils: ⊘Soothing Blend, ⊘wintergreen, ⊘Roman chamomile (inflammation)

Other Products: ⊘Soothing Blend Rub to help comfort joint stiffness and soreness.

—Rotator Cuff (sore):

The rotator cuff is the group of muscles and tendons that connect and hold the upper arm in the shoulder joint. The rotator cuff can become sore due to repetitive stressful shoulder motions or injury.

Oils: ⊘wintergreen, ⊘Soothing Blend, ⊘lemongrass, ⊘peppermint, ⊘white fir

Other Products: ⊘Soothing Rub to help comfort joint stiffness and soreness.

—Shoulder (frozen): *see also* **Inflammation**

A frozen shoulder refers to a condition where the range of motion of the shoulder is severely limited and painful. This can be caused by inflammation, stiffness, abnormal tissue growth within the joint capsule (connective tissue that helps cushion, lubricate, and protect the joint) around the shoulder, arthritis, or inflammation of the bursa (small fluid-filled sacs that cushions muscle, ligament, and tendon tissue from the bones as they move across them). These conditions can be extremely painful and can take a long time to heal.

Oils: ⊘Soothing Blend, ⊘white fir, ⊘lemongrass, ⊘basil, ⊘wintergreen, ⊘oregano, ⊘peppermint

Other Products: ⊘Soothing Rub to help comfort joint stiffness and soreness.

Regimen 1: Begin by applying 1–2 drops of white fir to the shoulder reflex point on the foot on the same side as the frozen shoulder to help with any inflammation. Check for any improvement in pain and/or range of motion. Repeat these steps using lemongrass (for torn or pulled ligaments), basil (for muscle spasms), and wintergreen (for bone problems). After determining which of these oils gets the best results for improving pain and/or range of motion, apply 1–2 drops of the oil (or oils) to the shoulder. Then apply 1–2 drops of peppermint (to help soothe the nerves) and 1–2 drops oregano (to help enhance muscle flexibility). Finally, apply white fir to the opposite shoulder to create balance as it compensates for the sore one. Drink lots of water.

—Tennis Elbow:

Tennis elbow (epicondylitis) is an injury to the tendons that connect the humerus bone near the elbow to the muscles that pull the hand backwards (lateral) and forward (medial) at the wrist. This type of injury is often associated with the repetitive forehand and backhand motions of playing tennis but can be caused by other activities that stress these tendons as well.

Oils: ⬯Soothing Blend, ⬯eucalyptus, ⬯peppermint, ⬯helichrysum, ⬯wintergreen, ⬯rosemary, ⬯lemongrass

Other Products: ⬯Soothing Rub to help comfort joint stiffness and soreness.

Blend 1: Combine 10 drops eucalyptus, 10 drops peppermint, 10 drops rosemary, and 1 Tbs. fractionated coconut oil. Apply on location; then apply an ice pack. Can also try alternating cold and hot packs.

Blend 2: Combine 1 drop each of lemongrass, helichrysum, marjoram, and peppermint. Apply on location; then apply an ice pack.

⬮: Dilute as recommended, and apply 1–2 drops on location or on reflex points on the feet. Combine 5–10 drops with 1 Tbs. fractionated coconut oil, and massage on location.

Kidneys

The kidneys are paired organs located just below the rib cage on either side of the spine that function to filter waste and extra water from the blood. The kidneys convert the waste and extra water into urine that is then excreted through urination. The kidneys also play an important role in hormone production.

Oils: ⬯lemongrass, Othyme⬯, ODetoxification Blend, Obergamot⬯, ⬯juniper berry, ⬯grapefruit, ⬯geranium, ⬯clary sage

Other Products: OEssential Oil Omega Complex or Vegan Essential Oil Omega Complex or OOmega-3 Fish Oil to provide omega-3 fatty acids that help support kidney function. ODetoxification Complex to help support healthy kidney functioning.

⬮: Dilute as recommended, and apply to kidneys and reflex points on the feet. Apply as a hot compress.

◔: Take capsules as directed on package. Add 1–2 drops of essential oil to an empty capsule; swallow capsule.

—Diuretic: *see Diuretic*

—Infection:

Kidney infections occur when bacteria enters the urinary tract. They are marked by fever, abdominal pain, chills, painful urination, dull kidney pain, nausea, vomiting, and a general feeling of discomfort.

Oils: ⬯rosemary

⬮: Dilute as recommended, and apply to kidneys and reflex points on the feet.

◔: Drink 1 gallon of distilled water and 2 quarts cranberry juice in one day.

—Inflammation (nephritis):

◯: Drink 1 gallon of distilled water and 2 quarts cranberry juice in one day.

—Kidney Stones:

A kidney stone is a solid piece of material that forms as chemicals in the urine crystal-lize and adhere together in the kidney. Small stones may pass through urination without causing pain. Larger stones with sharp edges and corners, however, can cause an extreme amount of pain as they are passed out of the body through the urinary tract.

Oils: ◯lemon, ◒eucalyptus, ◒juniper berry

◒: Apply as a hot compress over kidneys. Dilute as recommended, and apply 1–2 drops on location.

◯: Add 1–2 drops oil to 8 oz. of water, and drink. To help pass a stone, drink 4 oz. dis-tilled water with juice from 1/2 lemon every 30 minutes for 6 hours; then take 2 Tbs. extra-light virgin olive oil with the juice from 1 full lemon, and repeat daily until stone passes. Drinking plenty of water can help prevent the formation of kidney stones.

◻: **Additional Research:**

Thyme: Older rats whose diets were supplemented with thyme oil were found to have a higher level of the antioxidant enzymes superoxide dismutase and glutathione peroxidase in the heart, liver, and kidneys than did older rats without this supplementation (Youdim et al., 1999).

Bergamot: The antioxidant activity of bergamot juice was found to have protective action against renal (kidney) injury of diet-induced hypercholesterolemia in rats (Trovato et al., 2010).

Knee Cartilage Injury
see **Muscles/Connective Tissue:Cartilage Injury**

Labor
see **Pregnancy/Motherhood:Labor**

Lactation
see **Pregnancy/Motherhood:Lactation**

Lactose Intolerance
Lactose intolerance is the inability of the body to fully digest lactose, a sugar found in milk and in other dairy products. Symptoms of lactose intolerance include abdominal pain and bloating, diarrhea, nausea, and gas.

Oils: ◯◒lemongrass

◯: Add 1–2 drops to 1 tsp. honey, and swallow; or add 1–2 drops to 4 oz. rice or almond milk, and drink. Place 1–2 drops in an empty capsule, and swallow.

◒: Dilute as recommended, and apply 1–2 drops on abdomen or reflex points on the feet.

Laryngitis
see also **Allergies, Antiviral**

Laryngitis is an inflammation and swelling of the voice box (called the larynx) that causes the voice to sound hoarse or raspy. Laryngitis is most commonly caused by viruses, allergies, or overuse of the voice and will generally go away by itself within two weeks.

Oils: ◉◎sandalwood, ◎frankincense, ◎thyme, ◎lavender

◔: Diffuse into the air.

◔: Dilute as recommended, and apply to neck and reflex points on the feet.

Laundry
see **Housecleaning:Laundry**

Leukemia
see **Cancer:Leukemia**

Libido
see **Sexual Issues:Libido**

Lice
see **Insects/Bugs:Lice**

Ligaments
see **Muscles/Connective Tissue:Ligaments**

Lipoma
see **Tumor:Lipoma**

Lips

Oils: ◎lavender, ◎melaleuca, ◎lemon

—Dry lips:

   Blend 1: Combine 2–5 drops geranium with 2–5 drops lavender. Apply 1–2 drops on lips.

◔: Dilute as recommended, and apply 1 drop on lips. Combine 1–2 drops essential oil with 1 Tbs. fractionated coconut oil, and apply a small amount to lips.

Liver

The liver is the largest internal organ of the body. It is located in the upper abdomen and helps with digestion, produces cholesterol used to make several hormones and cellular membranes, removes waste products and old cells from the blood, and metabolizes harmful substances and toxins into harmless chemicals. The liver also has amazing regenerative abilities. Left with as little as 25% of its original mass, the liver can regrow what was lost and return to normal size.

Oils: ◎◎geranium, ◎helichrysum, ◎◉Digestive Blend, ◉cilantro◔, ◉rosemary◔, ◉ginger◔, ◎cypress◔, ◎◎◉grapefruit, ◉Detoxification Blend, ◎◉myrrh, ◎◎Calming Blend, ◎◎Roman chamomile

Other Products: ◉Essential Oil Omega Complex or Vegan Essential Oil Omega Complex, ◉Omega-3 Fish Oil, ◉Cellular Vitality Complex, ◉Food Nutrient Complex, ◉Chewable Multivitamin for omega-3 fatty acids and other nutrients that help support healthy liver cell functions. ◉Detoxification Complex to help support healthy liver functioning.

—Cirrhosis:

Cirrhosis is scarring of the liver that occurs as the liver tries to repair damage done to itself. When extensive liver damage occurs, the massive scar tissue buildup makes it impossible for the liver to function. The most common causes of cirrhosis are fatty liver (resulting from obesity or diabetes) and alcohol abuse; but any damage done to the liver can cause cirrhosis.

Oils: ©©frankincense, ©©myrrh, ©©geranium, ©©rosemary©, ©©juniper berry, ©©rose, ©©Roman chamomile

—Cleansing:

Oils: ©©clove, ©©geranium, ©©helichrysum, ©©myrrh

—Hepatitis: *see also* **Antiviral.**

Hepatitis is any swelling or inflammation of the liver. This can interfere with normal liver functioning and can possibly lead to cirrhosis or cancer over time. The most common cause of hepatitis is from one of the five different forms of hepatitis viruses, but it can also be caused by alcohol consumption, other viruses, or medications. Possible symptoms of hepatitis include diarrhea, jaundice, stomach pain, loss of appetite, dark-colored urine, pale bowel movements, nausea, and vomiting.

Oils: ©©myrrh, ©©melaleuca, ©©frankincense©, ©cypress©, ©©rosemary, ©©oregano, ©©thyme, ©©basil, ©©cinnamon, ©©eucalyptus, ©©peppermint

–Viral:

Oils: O©myrrh, ©©rosemary, ©©basil

Other Products: OProbiotic Defense Formula to help maintain friendly intestinal flora that help prevent toxins from pathogenic bacteria and viruses.

—Jaundice: *see* **Jaundice**

—Stimulant:

Oils: ©©helichrysum

©: Dilute as recommended, and apply 1–2 drops over liver area and on reflex points on the feet. Apply 1–2 drops on spine and liver area for viral infections. Apply as a warm compress over the liver area.

©: Diffuse into the air. Inhale directly from bottle. Apply oil to hands, tissue, or cotton wick, and inhale.

O: Take capsules as directed on package. Add 1–2 drops essential oil to an empty capsule; swallow capsule.

©: **Additional Research:**

Frankincense: A methanol extract of Boswellia carterii was found to have a high inhibition rate of hepatitis C virus protease (Hussein et al., 2000).

Cypress: Oral administration of cypress methanolic extract displayed preventive action against CCl4-induced hepatotoxicity in rats. These results suggest that the antioxidant activity of the flavonoid content of cypress could have potential use as a treatment for liver diseases (Ali et al., 2010).

Cilantro: Ethanolic extract of the cilantro leaf was found to protect against carbon tetrachloride induced liver injury in rats, validating its use as a liver protective agent (Pandey et al., 2011).

Cilantro: In rat livers, the antioxidant activity of cilantro leaves improved the adverse effect of the repeated administration of a potent liver toxin (Moustafa et al., 2012).

Rosemary: Daily administration of rosemary essential oil displayed a protective effect against chemical-induced liver injury in rats (Ra Kovi et al., 2014).

Ginger: Daily oral administration of ginger (*Z. officinale R.*) essential oil and isolated citral (the main constituent of ginger essential oil) displayed preventative effects on the formation alcohol fatty liver disease in mice administered an alcoholic liquid diet for four weeks (Liu et al., 2013).

Loss of Smell

see **Nose:Olfactory Loss**

Lou Gehrig's Disease

Lou Gehrig's disease (also known as amyotrophic lateral sclerosis) is a progressive and fatal neurological disease that affects nerve cells in the brain and spinal cord. As the disease progresses, motor neurons die and the brain loses its ability to control muscle movement. Later stages of the disease can lead to complete paralysis. Eventually, control is lost of the muscles needed to breathe, to speak, and to eat.

Oils: ☁cypress, ☁Grounding Blend, ☁☯frankincense, ☁☯sandalwood, ☁Calming Blend, ☁☯geranium, ☁☯rosemary, ☁☯thyme

Other Products: ○Essential Oil Omega Complex or Vegan Essential Oil Omega Complex or ○Omega-3 Fish Oil for omega fatty acids essential for nerve cell function.

☁: Dilute as recommended, and apply 1–2 drops on brain stem, neck, spine, and reflex points on the feet. Add 1–2 drops to 1 Tbs. fractionated coconut oil, and apply on back, neck, and feet.

☯: Diffuse into the air. Inhale directly from bottle. Apply oil to hands, tissue, or cotton wick, and inhale.

○: Take capsules as directed on package.

Lumbago

see **Back:Lumbago/Lower Back Pain**

Lungs

see **Respiratory System:Lungs**

Lupus

Lupus is an autoimmune disease that occurs when the immune system begins attacking its own tissues and organs. Lupus can cause pain, damage, and inflammation in the joints, blood vessels, skin, and organs. Common symptoms include joint pain or swelling, fever, muscle pain, and red rashes (often on the face). Lupus is more common in women than in men.

Oils: ☁clove, ☁☯Joyful Blend, ☁Protective Blend, ☁Grounding Blend, ☯☯melissa

☁: Dilute as recommended, and apply 1–2 drops on adrenal glands, under the arms, on neck, or on bottoms of the feet.

☯: Diffuse into the air. Inhale directly from bottle. Apply oil to hands, tissue, or cotton wick, and inhale.

Lymphatic System

see also **Immune System**

The lymphatic system is made up of the tissues and organs (bone marrow, thymus, spleen, lymph nodes, etc.) that produce and store the cells used to fight infection and disease. The lymphatic system transports immune cells through a fluid called lymph.

Oils: ✪cypress, ✪✪sandalwood, ✪✪Digestive Blend

Blend 1: Combine 5 drops Roman chamomile, 5 drops lavender, and 5 drops orange with 2 Tbs. fractionated coconut oil, and massage onto the skin over lymph nodes.

Other Products: ○Cellular Vitality Complex, ○Chewable Multivitamin, ○Essential Oil Omega Complex or Vegan Essential Oil Omega Complex or ○Omega-3 Fish Oil, and ○Food Nutrient Complex for nutrients that help support healthy immune function.

—Cleansing:

Oils: ✪✪lemon, ✪✪lime

—Decongestant For:

Oils: ✪✪cypress, ✪✪grapefruit, ✪✪Invigorating Blend, ✪✪lemongrass, ✪helichrysum, ✪✪orange, ✪✪rosemary, ✪✪thyme

—Drainage Of:

Oils: ✪helichrysum, ✪✪lemongrass

—Eliminates Waste Through:

Oils: ✪✪lavender

—Increase Function of:

Oils: ✪✪lemon

✪: Diffuse into the air. Inhale directly from bottle. Apply oil to hands, tissue, or cotton wick, and inhale.

✪: Dilute as recommended, and apply 1–2 drops on neck, arms, thyroid area, and reflex points on the feet. Add 1–2 drops to warm bathwater, and bathe.

○: Take capsules as directed on package.

Malaria

Malaria is a disease caused by single-celled *Plasmodium* parasites. These parasites are spread by mosquitoes from one infected person to another. Symptoms of malaria include light-headedness, shortness of breath, fever, chills, nausea, and, in some cases, coma and death. The best way to prevent malaria is to avoid being bit by using mosquito repellent and mosquito nets, especially between dusk and dawn, in areas of the world where malaria is common.

Oils: ✪✪Repellent Blend, ✪✪eucalyptus, ✪✪lemongrass, ✪✪lavender, ○lemon

✪: Dilute as recommended, and apply 1–2 drops to feet and exposed skin. Add 3–5 drops to 1 Tbs. fractionated coconut oil, and apply to exposed skin. Add 2–3 drops to 1–2 oz. distilled water in a small spray bottle; shake well, and mist onto the skin or into small openings where bugs may come through.

🕸: Diffuse into the air. Place 1–2 drops on small ribbons, strings, or cloth, and hang around area to help repel mosquitoes.

○: Mix 1–2 drops lemon with 1 tsp. honey and 8 oz. distilled water, and drink.

⬜: **Additional Research:**

Eucalyptus: A eucalyptus-based repellent containing p-menthane-3,8-diol as the active ingredient was found to be as effective as DEET in repelling the mosquito commonly known to carry a deadly malaria disease (complete protection for 6–7.75 hours) (Trigg, 1996).

Male Specific Conditions/Issues

—Genital Area

    −Infection:

        Oils: 🔹melaleuca, 🔹oregano, 🔹eucalyptus, 🔹lavender

    −Inflammation:

        Oils: 🔹lavender, 🔹Roman chamomile

    −Swelling:

        Oils: 🔹cypress, 🔹lavender, 🔹rosemary, 🔹eucalyptus

—Impotence:

Impotence, also known as erectile dysfunction, is the frequent inability to have or sustain an erection. This may be caused by circulation problems, nerve problems, low levels of testosterone, medications, or psychological stresses.

Oils: 🔹○clary sage, 🔹○cassia⬜, 🔹○clove, 🔹○ginger, 🔹○dill⬜, 🔹○sandalwood

—Infertility:

Infertility is clinically defined as the inability to achieve pregnancy after a year of trying.

Oils: 🔹🕸basil, 🔹🕸clary sage, 🔹thyme, 🔹○geranium⬜, 🔹○cinnamon⬜

—Jock Itch: *see also* **Antifungal:Ringworm**

Jock itch is a type of fungal infection that infects the skin of the genital area, causing itching or painful red patches of skin. It occurs more often during warm weather.

Oils: 🔹melaleuca, 🔹lavender, 🔹cypress

Recipe 1: Place 2 drops of any of the above oils in 1 tsp. fractionated coconut oil, and apply to area morning and night. Alternately, place 2 drops oil in a small bowl of water, and wash the area with the water and then dry well each morning and night.

🔄: Dilute as recommended, and apply 1–2 drops on location or on reflex points on the feet. Dilute 1–2 drops in 1 Tbs. fractionated coconut oil, and massage on location. Add 1–2 drops essential oil to warm water, and bathe.

○: Place 1–2 drops in an empty capsule, and swallow.

🕸: Diffuse into the air. Inhale directly from bottle. Apply oil to hands, tissue, or cotton wick, and inhale.

⬜ **Additional Research:**

Cassia: Methanol extract of cassia was found to effectively manage sexual dysfunction in aged rats (Goswami et al., 2013).

Dill: Male mice internally administered low doses of dill extracts displayed a short-term increase in mounting frequency and an enhanced protein phosphorylation level in testicular lysate, suggesting that low doses of dill enhances aphrodisiac activity in males and may be beneficial in treating male sexual dysfunction (Iamsaard et al., 2013). (It should be noted that high doses of dill extract have been shown to decrease fertility in male rats, but no significant difference in sperm count, sperm motility, or testosterone concentrations occur (Monsefi et al., 2011).)

Geranium: Male mice exposed to a harmful insecticide, known to cause sperm damage, were successfully treated with geranium essential oil through its antioxidant effects. Compared to the control group, the oral administration of geranium oil prevented testicular oxidative damage, reduced lipid peroxidation, and improved total sperm motility, viability, and morphology in mice spermatozoa (Slima et al., 2013).

Cinnamon: Cinnamon bark essential oil was found to have a protective effect against damages in male rat reproductive organs and cells induced by carbon tetrachloride (a common toxic substance) (Yüce et al., 2014).

Cassia: Methanol extract of Cinnamonum cassia was found to increase the sexual function of young male rats (Goswami et al., 2014).

Massage

For oils that can be used of an aromatic massage for a specific purpose, see also **Anxiety, Arthritis, Asthma, Back, Bones, Calming, Cardiovascular System, Cooling Oils, Edema, Energy, Fever, Foot, Hair, Hands, Headaches, Inflammation, Invigorating, Joints, Lymphatic System, Muscles/ Connective Tissue, Nervous System, Pain, Pregnancy/Motherhood, Respiratory System, Skin, Sleep, Stress, Tissue, Uplifting, Warming Oils**

Massage is the manipulation of the soft tissues in the body through holding, moving, compressing, or stroking. Massage can be done to help aid circulation, relax muscles, relieve pain, reduce swelling, speed healing after strains and sprains, restore function to the body, and release tension and stress.

Oils: ⊘Massage Blend—a blend specifically created to aid in therapeutic massage to relax and soothe muscles, to increase circulation, and to stimulate tissues. See other conditions for specific oils that can be used to create a massage oil for that condition.

Other Products: ⊘Soothing Rub to help soothe tired, achy, and sore muscles and improve circulation within the tissue.

Blend 1: Combine 5 drops Roman chamomile, 5 drops lavender, and 5 drops orange with 2 Tbs. fractionated coconut oil, and use as massage oil for a relaxing massage.

⊘: Add 1–10 drops of essential oil to 1 Tbs. fractionated coconut oil or another carrier oil such as almond, olive, jojoba, sesame seed, or flaxseed to create a massage oil. *See also the section on the Aroma Massage Technique in the Science and Application of Essential Oils section of this book.*

Measles

see **Childhood Diseases:Measles**

Melanoma

see **Cancer:Skin/Melanoma**

Memory

see also **Alzheimer's Disease**

Memory is the mental capacity to retain and recall facts, events, past experiences, and impressions. Memory retention can be enhanced by memory exercises, adequate sleep, and associations with previous knowledge. Aroma also plays a role in memory. At least one study has indicated that individuals exposed to an aroma while learning had an easier time remembering what they had learned when exposed to the same aroma, while those who were exposed to a differing aroma had a more difficult time remembering what they had learned⊕.

Oils: ⊘◉rosemary⊕, ⊘◉peppermint⊕, ⊘◉frankincense, ⊘◉basil⊕, ⊘◉Invigorating Blend, ⊘◉clove⊕, ⊘◉lemon, ⊘◉juniper berry, ⊘◉cedarwood, ⊘◉ginger, ⊘◉grapefruit, ◉⊘lime, ⊘◉bergamot, ⊘◉◉rose⊕, ⊘◉dill⊕, ⊘◉lavender, ⊘◉lemongrass

Other Products: ◯Essential Oil Omega Complex or Vegan Essential Oil Omega Complex, ◯Omega-3 Fish Oil, ◯Food Nutrient Complex for omega-3 fatty acids and other nutrients essential to brain cell health.

—Improve:

    Oils: ⊘◉clove, ⊘clary sage

—Stimulate:

    Oils: ⊘rosemary

⊘ Diffuse into the air. Inhale directly from bottle. Apply oil to hands, tissue, or cotton wick, and inhale. Wear as a perfume or cologne.

◉ Dilute as recommended, and apply 1–2 drops on temples or back of neck.

◯ Take capsules as directed on package.

▥ **Additional Research:**

Subjects who had learned a list of 24 words when exposed to an odor had an easier time relearning the list when exposed to the same odor compared to those who were exposed to an alternate odor (Smith et al., 1992).

Rosemary: Volunteers completing a battery of tests were found to be more content when exposed to lavender and rosemary aromas. Rosemary aroma also was found to enhance quality of memory compared to control (Moss et al., 2003).

Peppermint: In human trials, the aroma of peppermint was found to enhance memory and to increase alertness (Moss et al., 2008).

Basil: A study evaluating memory retention and retrieval of mice revealed that the hydroalcoholic extract of Ocimum basilicum significantly increased memory retention and retrieval. The memory enhancing effects were attributed to the antioxidant activity of flavonoids, tannins and terpenoids in the basil extract (Sarahroodi et al., 2012).

Clove: Administration of clove essential oil for three weeks before treatment with scopolamine (a known agent causing memory impairment) was shown to significantly reverse the scopolamine-induced memory deficit, when compared to pretreatment with saline only (Halder et al., 2011).

Rose: Oral administration of Rosa damascena extract for one month was found to enhance adult neurogenesis, hippocampal volume, and synaptic plasticity, as well as reverse the amyloid-β-associated memory abnormalities in a rat model of amyloid-β-induced Alzheimer's disease. These results indicate that rose extract may have memory-enhancing ability (Esfandiary et al., 2014).

Dill: A combined extract of *Cissampelos pareira* and *Anethum graveolens* was found to produce cognitive-enhancing and neuroprotective effects on spatial memory in memory deficit induced rats (Thukham-Mee et al., 2012).

Menopause
see **Female Specific Conditions:Menopause**

Menstruation
see **Female Specific Conditions:Menstruation**

Mental
see **Alertness, Brain, Energy, Memory, Stress**

Metabolism

Metabolism refers to the processes involved in converting ingested nutrients into substances that can be used within the cells of the body for energy or to create needed cellular structures. This process is carried out by various chemical reactions facilitated by enzymes within the body.

—Balance:

    Oils: ⌀clove, ⌀⌀Grounding Blend, ⌀⌀oregano

    ⌀ Diffuse into the air. Inhale oil applied to tissue or cotton wick.

    ⌀ Dilute as recommended, and apply 1–2 drops on neck or on bottoms of the feet.

Metals

see **Detoxification**

Mice (Repel)

Oils: ⌀⌀Cleansing Blend

    ⌀ Apply 1–2 drops in small openings or crevices where mice are likely to appear. Add 1–5 drops to small cotton balls, and place in openings where mice may come in.

    ⌀ Diffuse into the air.

Migraines

see **Headaches:Migraine Headache**

Mildew

see also **Antifungal**

Mildew is a whitish fungus that forms a flat growth on plants and organic material. Mildew attacks clothing, leather, paper, ceilings, walls, floors, shower walls, windowsills, and other places with high moisture levels. Mildew can produce a strong musty odor, especially in places with poor air circulation.

Oils: ⌀Cleansing Blend

    ⌀: Place a few drops in a small spray bottle with distilled water, and spray into air or on surface to help neutralize mildew.

Mind

see **Alertness, Brain, Energy:Fatigue:Mental Fatigue, Memory**

Minerals (Deficiency)

Minerals are naturally-occurring, inorganic substances with a chemical composition and structure. Some minerals are essential to the human body. A person is considered to have a mineral deficiency when the concentration level of any mineral needed to maintain optimal health is abnormally low in the body.

Other Products: ⭕Food Nutrient Complex contains a balanced blend of minerals essential for optimal cellular health, including calcium, magnesium, zinc, selenium, copper, manganese, chromium, and molybdenum; ⭕Fruit & Veggie Drink Mix for a whole food source of essential nutrients.

⚪: Take capsules as directed on package.

Miscarriage
see **Pregnancy/Motherhood:Miscarriage**

Moles
see **Skin:Moles**

Mono (Mononucleosis)
see also **Antiviral**

Mononucleosis is a viral disease caused by the Epstein-Barr virus that usually spread through contact with infected saliva, tears, and mucous. Most adults have been exposed to this virus sometime in their lives, but many display no symptoms or only very mild flu-like symptoms. Mononucleosis symptoms are most often seen in adolescents and young adults. Symptoms of this disease include fatigue, weakness, severe sore throat, fever, swollen lymph nodes, swollen tonsils, headache, loss of appetite, and a soft or swollen spleen. Once individuals are exposed to the Epstein-Barr virus, they carry the virus for the rest of their lives. The virus sporadically becomes active, but the symptoms do not appear again. Whenever the virus is active, however, it can be spread to others—even if the person carrying it shows no symptoms.

Oils: ©@Respiratory Blend, ©@Protective Blend

Other Products: ⭕Protective Softgels

Blend 1: Combine 3 drops oregano, 3 drops Protective Blend, and 3 drops thyme. Rub the blend on the feet.

🔹: Dilute as recommended, and apply 1–3 drops on throat and feet.

🌀: Diffuse into the air. Inhale oil directly from bottle, or inhale oil that is applied to the hands.

Mood Swings

A mood swing is a rapid change of mood caused by fatigue or by a sudden shift in the body's hormonal balance.

Oils: ⊘clary sage, ⊘Calming Blend, ⊘lavender, ⊘Grounding Blend, ⊘rosemary, ⊘Joyful Blend, ⊘geranium, ⊘rose, ⊘ylang ylang, ⊘sandalwood, ⊘lemon, ⊘peppermint, ⊘bergamot, ⊘fennel

🌀: Diffuse into the air. Inhale oil directly or applied to the hands.

Morning Sickness
see **Pregnancy/Motherhood:Morning Sickness**

Mosquitoes
see **Insects/Bugs:Mosquitoes**

Motion Sickness
see **Nausea:Motion Sickness**

MRSA
see **Antibacterial**

Mucus

see **Congestion**

Multiple Sclerosis

see also **Brain:Myelin Sheath**

Multiple sclerosis (MS) is an autoimmune disease in which the immune system attacks and gradually destroys the myelin sheath (which covers and insulates the nerves) and the underlying nerve fibers of the central nervous system. This destruction of the myelin sheath interferes with communication between the brain and the rest of the body. Symptoms of MS include partial or complete loss of vision, tingling, burning, pain in parts of the body, tremors, loss of coordination, unsteady gait, dizziness, and memory problems.

Oils: ⊘❷frankincense, ❷sandalwood, ❷peppermint, ❷cypress, ❷juniper berry, ❷❷Calming Blend, ❷oregano, ❷thyme, ❷birch, ❷rosemary, ❷wintergreen

Other Products: ❍Essential Oil Omega Complex or Vegan Essential Oil Omega Complex or ❍❍Omega-3 Fish Oil for omega-3 fatty acids that help support nerve and brain function.

❂: Dilute as recommended, and apply 1–2 drops to spine, back of neck, and feet. Dilute 1–3 drops in 1 Tbs. fractionated coconut oil, and massage on back and neck.

❍: Take capsules as directed on package.

❷: Diffuse into the air. Inhale directly from bottle. Apply oil to hands, tissue, or cotton wick, and inhale.

Mumps

see **Childhood Diseases: Mumps**

Muscles/Connective Tissue

see also **Cardiovascular System:Heart Tissue**

Muscle is the tissue in the body that has the ability to contract, making movement possible. The three main types of muscle in the body are smooth muscle (such as that in the stomach, intestines, and blood vessels), cardiac muscle (found in the heart), and skeletal muscle (attached to the bones). Skeletal muscles are connected to the bones with tough fibrous tissue called tendons and allow for coordinated, controlled movement of the body, such as walking, pointing, or eye movement. Smooth muscles and cardiac muscles move automatically without conscious control to perform their functions.

Oils: ❷marjoram, ❷Soothing Blend, ❷peppermint⊙, ❷Massage Blend, ❷birch, ❷cypress, ❷wintergreen, ❷lemongrass, ❷lavender

Other Products: ❷Soothing Rub to help relieve sore muscles, ❍Energy & Stamina Complex, ❍Cellular Vitality Complex, ❍Chewable Multivitamin, ❍Essential Oil Omega Complex or Vegan Essential Oil Omega Complex, ❍❍Omega-3 Fish Oil, ❍Food Nutrient Complex for coenzyme Q10 and other nutrients to support muscle cell energy and function.

—**Aches and Pains:** *see also* **Pain**

Muscle pain usually results from overuse, tension, stress, strain, or injury. However, muscle pain can also be caused by a disease or infection affecting the whole body, such as the flu, fibromyalgia, or a connective tissue disorder.

Oils: ♻marjoram, ♻Soothing Blend, ♻birch, ♻clove, ♻Massage Blend, ♻oregano, ♻peppermint, ♻wintergreen, ♻white fir (with inflammation), ♻vetiver, ♻Roman chamomile, ♻helichrysum, ♻ginger, ♻lavender, ♻rosemary, ♻thyme

Other Products: ♻Soothing Rub to help relieve sore muscles.

—Bruised: *see Bruises*

—Cardiac Muscle: *see also Cardiovascular System:Heart*

Cardiac muscle is the type of muscle found in the walls of the heart.

Oils: ♻⊘marjoram, ♻⊘lavender, ♻⊘peppermint, ♻⊘rosemary, ♻cinnamon

—Cartilage Injury:

Cartilage is a type of connective tissue in the body. It is firmer than other tissues and is used to provide structure and support without being as hard or as rigid as bone. Types of cartilage include hyaline cartilage, elastic cartilage, and fibrocartilage. Hyaline cartilage lines the bones and joints, helping them move smoothly. Elastic cartilage is found in the ear and larynx and is used to keep other tubular structures, such as the nose and trachea, open. Fibrocartilage is the strongest and most rigid cartilage. It is found in the intervertebral discs and other high-stress areas and serves to connect tendons and ligaments to bones. The hyaline cartilage surrounding bones and joints can become torn or injured if the joint is bent or twisted in a traumatic way. This can cause pain, swelling, tenderness, popping, or clicking within the joint and can limit movement.

Oils: ♻birch, ♻wintergreen, ♻marjoram, ♻lemongrass, ♻white fir, ♻peppermint

—Cramps/Charley Horses:

A muscle cramp or charley horse is the sudden, involuntary contraction of a muscle. Muscle cramps can occur in any muscle in the body, but they usually occur in the thigh, calf, or arch of the foot. Cramps can be caused by excessive strain to the muscle, injury, overuse, dehydration, or lack of blood flow to the muscle. Muscle cramps can happen during or after a physical activity and while lying in bed.

Oils: ♻lemongrass with ♻peppermint, ♻marjoram, ♻Soothing Blend, ♻rosemary, ♻basil, ♻thyme, ♻vetiver, ♻Roman chamomile, ♻cypress, ♻grapefruit, ♻clary sage, ⊘lavender

—Development:

When muscles are stretched or used during exercise, they produce a substance that activates stem cells already present in the tissue. Once these cells are activated, they begin to divide—creating new muscle fiber and thereby increasing the size and strength of the muscles.

Oils: ♻birch, ♻wintergreen, ♻Soothing Blend

—Fatigue:

Muscle fatigue is the muscle's temporary reduction in strength, power, and endurance. This happens when there is an increase in lactic acid and blood flow to the muscle, a depletion of glycogen, or a deprivation of oxygen to the tissue.

Oils: ♻marjoram, ♻white fir, ♻cypress, ♻peppermint, ♻eucalyptus, ♻grapefruit, ♻rosemary, ♻thyme

Other Products: ♻Soothing Blend Rub

—Inflammation: *see Inflammation*

—Ligaments:

A ligament is a sheet or band of tough connective tissue and fibers that connects bones together or helps bind and support a joint.

Oils: ⌒lemongrass

—Over Exercised:

When a person overexercises, his or her muscles do not get sufficient rest or time to heal. This continued muscle strain can cause muscle sprains, strain, and even tears to soft tissue. It may also cause stiffness and soreness to the neck, upper or lower back, shoulder, arm, or joint.

Oils: ⌒white fir, ⌒eucalyptus, ⌒lavender, ⌒thyme, ⌒ginger

Other Products: ⌒Soothing Rub to help provide comfort to tired and sore muscles.

Recipe 1: Add 3 drops marjoram and 2 drops lemon to warm bathwater, and soak.

Blend 1: Combine 2 drops eucalyptus, 2 drops peppermint, and 2 drops ginger with 1 Tbs. fractionated coconut oil, and massage into muscles.

—Rheumatism (Muscular): *see Fibromyalgia*

—Smooth Muscle:

Oils: ⌒marjoram, ⌒rosemary⌒, ⌒Opeppermint, ⌒fennel, ⌒cypress, ⌒juniper berry, ⌒clary sage, ⌒melissa, ⌒lavender, ⌒sandalwood, ⌒bergamot

—Spasms:

A muscle spasm is a sudden, involuntary contraction or twitching of a muscle. This may or may not cause pain.

Oils: ⌒basil, ⌒marjoram, ⌒Soothing Blend, ⌒Roman chamomile, ⌒peppermint, ⌒cypress, ⌒clary sage, ⌒lavender

—Sprains:

A sprain is an injury to a ligament caused by excessive stretching. The ligament can have little tears in it or it can be completely torn apart to be considered a sprain. The most common areas to receive a sprain are the ankle, knee, and wrist. After a person receives a sprain, the area will swell rapidly and be quite painful. If the ligament is torn apart, surgery may be required.

Oils: ⌒marjoram, ⌒lemongrass, ⌒white fir, ⌒helichrysum, ⌒rosemary, ⌒thyme, ⌒vetiver, ⌒eucalyptus, ⌒clove, ⌒ginger, ⌒lavender

—Strain:

A strain is a tear of the muscle tissue due to excessive strain or overstretching. Strains can cause inflammation, pain, and discoloration of the skin around the injured area.

Oils: ⌒lemongrass, ⌒Soothing Blend, ⌒ginger (circulation), ⌒helichrysum (pain)

—Stiffness:

Oils: ⌒Soothing Blend

Other Products: ⬥Soothing Rub

—Tendinitis:

> Tendinitis is the inflammation of a tendon due to injury, repetitive exercise or strain, or diseases such as arthritis, gout, and gonorrhea. This can cause swelling and pain in the effected tendon.

> **Oils:** ⬥marjoram, ⬥lavender

—Tension (especially in shoulders and neck):

> Muscle tension is a condition in which the muscle remains in a semi-contracted state for an extended period of time. This is usually due to physical or emotional stress.

> **Oils:** ⬥marjoram, ⬥Soothing Blend, ⬥peppermint⬤, ⬥helichrysum, ⬥juniper berry, ⬥lavender, ⬥Roman chamomile

> **Other Products:** ⬥Soothing Rub

—Tone:

> Apply these oils before exercise to help tone muscles.

> **Oils:** ⬥birch, ⬥cypress, ⬥wintergreen, ⬥marjoram, ⬥basil, ⬥peppermint, ⬥orange, ⬥thyme, ⬥rosemary, ⬥juniper berry, ⬥grapefruit, ⬥lavender

⬥: Dilute as recommended, and apply 1–2 drops on location. Add 2–4 drops to 1 Tbs. fractionated coconut oil, and massage into desired muscles or joints. Add 1–2 drops to warm bathwater, and bathe. Apply as hot or cold (for strains or sprains) compress.

⬤: Take capsules as directed on package. Place 1–2 drops of oil under the tongue or add 1–2 drops essential oil to empty capsule, and swallow.

⬥: Diffuse into the air.

⬥: **Additional Research:**

> **Peppermint:** A combination of peppermint oil and ethanol was found to have a significant analgesic effect with a reduction in sensitivity to headache; while a combination of peppermint, eucalyptus, and ethanol were found to relax muscles, and increase cognitive performance in humans (Göbel et al., 1994).

> **Rosemary:** Rosemary oil demonstrated a relaxant effect on smooth muscle from the trachea of rabbits and guinea pigs (Aqel, 1991).

Muscular Dystrophy

Muscular dystrophy is any of several genetic diseases that cause gradual weakening of the skeletal muscles. The most common forms, Duchenne and Becker muscular dystrophies, are caused by a gene defect that inhibits or alters the production of dystrophin, a protein necessary for proper muscle cell structure.

Oils: ⬥marjoram, ⬥lemongrass, ⬥basil, ⬥rosemary, ⬥Massage Blend, ⬥Soothing Blend, ⬥geranium, ⬥lavender, ⬥lemon, ⬥orange, ⬥ginger

Other Products: ⬥Soothing Rub to help relieve and relax tense and aching muscles.

⬥: Dilute as recommended, and apply 1–2 drops on location. Add 2–4 drops to 1 Tbs. fractionated coconut oil, and massage into desired muscles. Add 1–2 drops to warm bathwater and bathe. Apply as cold compress.

Myelin Sheath

see **Brain:Myelin Sheath**

Nails

Oils: ⬡lemon, ⬡frankincense, ⬡myrrh, ⬡Invigorating Blend, ⬡melaleuca (infection⬡), ⬡eucalyptus, ⬡lavender, ⬡grapefruit, ⬡rosemary, ⬡cypress, ⬡oregano, ⬡thyme

Blend 1: Combine 2 drops frankincense, 2 drops lemon, and 2 drops myrrh with 2 drops wheat germ oil. Apply 2–3 times per week.

Other Products: ⬡Food Nutrient Complex for nutrients essential to healthy nail growth.

⬡: Dilute as recommended, and apply 1–2 drops to nails. Add 1–2 drops to 1 tsp. fractionated coconut oil, and apply to nails.

⬡: Take capsules as directed on package.

⬡: **Additional Research:**

Melaleuca: Topical application of 100% tea tree oil was found to have results similar to topical application of 1% clotrimazole (antifungal drug) solution on onychomycosis (also known as tinea, or fungal nail infection) (Buck et al., 1994).

Nasal

see **Nose**

Nausea

Nausea is a sick feeling in the stomach producing an urge to vomit.

Oils: ⬡⬡⬡ginger⬡, ⬡peppermint⬡, ⬡⬡lavender, ⬡⬡⬡cardamom, ⬡⬡Digestive Blend, ⬡⬡patchouli, ⬡⬡juniper berry, ⬡⬡clove

Other Products: ⬡Digestive Softgels

—**Morning Sickness:** *see* **Pregnancy/Motherhood:Morning Sickness**

—**Motion Sickness:**

Motion sickness is a feeling of illness that occurs as a result of repeated movement, such as that experienced in a car, on a boat, or on a plane. These motions interfere with the body's sense of balance and equilibrium. The most common symptoms of motion sickness include dizziness, fatigue, and nausea.

Oils: ⬡peppermint, ⬡Digestive Blend, ⬡ginger

—**Vomiting:**

Oils: ⬡⬡ginger⬡, ⬡peppermint, ⬡⬡patchouli, ⬡⬡fennel, ⬡rose, ⬡Roman chamomile

⬡: Place 1–2 drops essential oil in an empty capsule, and swallow. Take supplements as directed.

⬡: Diffuse into the air. Inhale directly from bottle. Apply oil to hands, tissue, or cotton wick, and inhale.

⬡: Dilute as recommended, and apply 1–2 drops to the feet, temples and wrists. Dilute 1–2 drops essential oil in 1 Tbs. fractionated coconut oil, and massage on stomach. Apply oil as a warm compress.

⊕: **Additional Research:**

Ginger: Ginger root given orally to pregnant women was found to decrease the severity of nausea and frequency of vomiting compared to control (Vutyavanich et al., 2001).

Ginger: Ginger root given one hour before major gynecological surgery resulted in lower nausea and fewer incidences of vomiting compared to control (Nanthakomon et al., 2006).

Ginger: In a trial of women receiving gynecological surgery, women receiving ginger root had less incidences of nausea compared to a placebo. Ginger root has similar results to the antiemetic drug (a drug effective against vomiting and nausea) metoclopramide (Bone et al., 1990).

Peppermint: Oral administration of capsules containing two drops of either spearmint or peppermint oil to cancer patients during chemotherapy cycles was found to reduce the intensity of nausea when compared to the control (Tayarani-Najaran et al., 2013).

Neck

Oils: ⚬lemon, ⚬geranium, ⚬clary sage, ⚬orange, ⚬basil, ⚬helichrysum

🝆: Dilute 1–5 drops oil in 1 Tbs. fractionated coconut oil, and massage on neck.

Nervous System

see also **Back, Brain**

The nervous system is a network of nerve cells that regulates the body's reaction to external and internal stimuli. The nervous system sends nerve impulses to organs and muscles throughout the body. The body relies on these impulses to function. The nervous system is comprised of the central nervous system (the brain and spinal cord) and the peripheral nervous system (all other nerves). The peripheral nervous system is comprised of the somatic nervous system (nerves that connect to the skeletal muscles and sensory nerve receptors in the skin) and the autonomic nervous system (nerves that connect to the cardiac and smooth muscles and other organs, tissues, and systems that don't require conscious effort to control). The autonomic system is divided further into two main parts: the sympathetic and parasympathetic nervous systems. The sympathetic nervous system functions to accelerate heart rate, increase blood pressure, slow digestion, and constrict blood vessels. It activates the "fight or flight" response in order to deal with threatening or stressful situations. The parasympathetic nervous system functions to slow heart rate, store energy, stimulate digestive activity, and relax specific muscles. It allows the body to return to a normal and calm state after experiencing pain or stress.

Oils: ⚬⚭peppermint⚓ (soothes and strengthens damaged nerves), ⚬⚭basil (stimulates), ⚬⚭lavender⚓, ⚬⚭lemon⚓, ⚬⚭grapefruit⚓, ⚬⚭frankincense⚓, ⚬⚭bergamot, ⚬⚭cedarwood (nervous tension), ⚬⚭lemongrass (for nerve damage), ⚬⚭marjoram (soothing), ⚬⚭geranium (regenerates), ⚭⚭Calming Blend, ⚬⚭Roman chamomile, ⚬⚭juniper berry, ⚬⚭vetiver, ⚬⚭cinnamon, ⚬⚭ginger, ⚬⚭orange, ⚬⚭sandalwood

Other Products: OEnergy & Stamina Complex to help support healthy nerve function. OEssential Oil Omega Complex or Vegan Essential Oil Omega Complex or OOmega-3 Fish Oil for essential omega fatty acids that help support nerve cell health. OFood Nutrient Complex, OChewable Multivitamin for nutrients and minerals necessary for proper nerve cell function. OCellular Vitality Complex for nutrients that help support nerve cell health and energy.

—Bell's Palsy:

Bell's palsy is a weakness or paralysis of muscles on one side of the face. Bell's palsy tends to set in quickly, normally in a single day. Symptoms include numbness of one side of the face, loss of ability to taste, drooling, pain in or behind the ear, facial droop, headache, and change in the amount of saliva or tears produced. In most cases Bell's palsy symptoms will begin to improve within a few weeks. But in some few cases the symptoms continue for life.

Oils: ⊙⊘peppermint, ⊙⊘rosemary, ⊙⊘thyme

—Carpal Tunnel Syndrome: *see Carpal Tunnel Syndrome*

—Huntington's Disease:

Huntington's disease (HD) is a progressive neurodegenerative disorder passed genetically from one generation to the next. As the disease develops, it causes nerve cells in the brain to waste away, resulting in a loss of control over body movement, emotions, and mental reasoning. Early symptoms include unsteady walking and decreased coordination. Later symptoms include sudden involuntary jerking body movements, slurred speech, decreased mental capacity, and psychological and emotional problems. Those carrying the HD gene have a 50 percent chance of passing it on to each of their children.

Oils: ⊙⊘peppermint, ⊙⊘basil

Other Products: Oils: ⊙Energy & Stamina Complex to help support healthy nerve function. ⊙Essential Oil Omega Complex or Vegan Essential Oil Omega Complex

—Lou Gehrig's Disease (ALS): *see Lou Gehrig's Disease*

—Multiple Sclerosis (MS): *see Multiple Sclerosis*

—Neuralgia:

Neuralgia is intense pain felt along the path of a nerve. Neuralgia results from damage or irritation to a nerve. Causes can include certain drugs, diabetes, infections, inflammation, trauma, and chemical irritation.

Oils: ⊙marjoram, ⊙eucalyptus⊙, ⊙Roman chamomile, ⊙lavender, ⊙juniper berry, ⊙helichrysum, ⊙cedarwood

—Neuritis:

Neuritis is the inflammation of a nerve or of a group of nerves. Neuritis causes pain, poor reflexes, and muscle atrophy.

Oils: ⊙eucalyptus⊙, ⊙Roman chamomile ⊙lavender, ⊙juniper berry, ⊙clove, ⊙cedarwood

—Neurotonic:

Oils: ⊙melaleuca, ⊙thyme

—Paralysis:

Paralysis is the loss of one's ability to move and control one or more specific sets of muscles. Paralysis generally occurs as a result of damage to the nervous system, especially damage to the spinal cord. Primary causes include injury, stroke, multiple sclerosis, amyotrophic lateral sclerosis (Lou Gehrig's disease), botulism, spina bifida, and Guillain-Barré syndrome.

Oils: ⊘⊙peppermint, ⊘⊙lemongrass, ⊘⊙geranium, ⊘⊙Grounding Blend, ⊘⊙Cleansing Blend, ⊘⊙cypress, ⊘⊙juniper berry, ⊘⊙ginger, ⊘⊙helichrysum

—**Parasympathetic Nervous System**: *see also Ions:Negative Ions.*

The parasympathetic nervous system functions to slow heart rate, store energy, stimulate digestive activity, and relax specific muscles. It allows the body to return to a normal and calm state after experiencing pain or stress.

Oils: ⊘⊙lavender⊙ (stimulates), ⊘⊙lemongrass (regulates), ⊘⊙marjoram (tones), ⊘⊙Calming Blend, ⊘⊙Grounding Blend

—**Parkinson's Disease**: *see Parkinson's Disease*

—**Sympathetic Nervous System**: *see also Ions:Positive Ions.*

The sympathetic nervous system functions to accelerate heart rate, increase blood pressure, slow digestion, and constrict blood vessels in most tissues and organs, while dilating arterioles in the skeletal muscles where increased blood flow is needed. It activates the "fight or flight" response in order to deal with threatening or stressful situations.

Oils: ⊘⊙grapefruit⊙ (stimulates), ⊘⊙eucalyptus, ⊘⊙peppermint, ⊘⊙ginger

—**Virus of Nerves**: *see also Antiviral*

Oils: ⊙frankincense, ⊙clove

⊜: Dilute as recommended, and apply 1–3 drops on location, spine, back of neck, and reflex points on the feet. Add 2–4 drops to 1 Tbs. fractionated coconut oil, and massage on location. Add 1–2 drops to warm bathwater, and bathe.

⊘: Diffuse into the air. Inhale directly from bottle. Apply oil to hands, tissue, or cotton wick, and inhale.

⊙: Take capsules as directed on package.

⊡: **Additional Research:**

Peppermint: Pretreatment of human and rat astrocyte cells (cells found in the nerve and brain that support the blood-brain barrier and help repair the brain and spinal cord following injuries) with peppermint oil was found to inhibit heat-shock induced apoptosis of these cells (Koo et al., 2001).

Lavender: Lavender oil scent was found to lower sympathetic nerve activity and blood pressure, while elevating parasympathetic nerve activity in rats. It was further found that applying an anosmia-inducing agent (something that causes a loss of smell) eliminated the effects of the lavender oil scent (Tanida et al., 2006).

Lavender: Lavender oil was found to inhibit sympathetic nerve activity, while exciting parasympathetic nerve activity in rats. Linalool, a component of lavender, was shown to have similar effects (Shen et al., 2005).

Lemon: Inhaling the aroma of lemon essential oil was found to decrease pain response in rats and was also found to modulate the neuronal response to formalin-induced pain (Aloisi et al., 2002).

Lemon: Several constituents of lemon oil and their metabolites (chemicals made by these chemicals in the body) were found to increase the release of monoamines (various chemicals responsible for neurotransmission and neuromodulation) in rat brain tissue, indicating a possible effect on brain nerve cell behavior (Fukumoto et al., 2006).

Lemon: Pretreatment of human and rat astrocyte cells (cells found in the nerve and brain that support the blood-brain barrier and help repair the brain and spinal cord following injuries) with lemon oil was found to inhibit heat-shock induced apoptosis of these cells (Koo et al., 2002).

Grapefruit: The scent of grapefruit oil and its component, limonene, was found to affect the autonomic nerves and reduce appetite and body weight in rats exposed to the oil for 15 minutes three times per week (Shen et al., 2005).

Grapefruit: Inhalation of essential oils such as pepper, estragon, fennel, and grapefruit was found to have a stimulating effect on sympathetic activity; while inhalation of essential oils of rose or patchouli caused a decrease in sympathetic activity in healthy adults (Haze et al., 2002).

Frankincense: Incensole acetate, isolated from frankincense resin, was found to demonstrate an anti-inflammatory and neuro-protective effect in mice with a closed head injury (Moussaieff et al., 2008).

Eucalyptus: 1,8 cineole (eucalyptol) was found to display an anti-inflammatory effect on rats in several tests and was found to exhibit antinociceptive (pain-reducing) effects in mice, possibly by depressing the central nervous system (Santos et al., 2000).

Nervousness

Nervousness is a state of high anxiety, distress, agitation, or psychological uneasiness.

Oils: ⊘⊜orange

⊘: Diffuse into the air. Inhale directly from bottle. Apply oil to hands, tissue, or cotton wick, and inhale.

⊜: Dilute as recommended, and apply 1–2 drops to temples.

Nose

Oils: ⊜⊘melaleuca, ⊜⊘rosemary

—Bleeding:

A nosebleed (medically called *epistaxis*) is the loss of blood through the nose. Nosebleeds are fairly common and can be caused by many factors. The most common causes of nosebleed are dry air that causes the nasal membrane to dry out and crack, allergies, nose trauma/injury, and colds and other viruses.

Oils: ⊜helichrysum, ⊜cypress, ⊜lemon, ⊜frankincense, ⊜lavender

Blend 1: Combine 2 drops cypress, 1 drop helichrysum, and 2 drops lemon in 8 oz. (1 cup) ice water. Soak a cloth in the water, and apply the cloth to nose and back of neck.

—Nasal Nasopharynx:

The nasopharynx is the upper part of the throat (pharynx) situated behind the nose. The nasopharynx is responsible for carrying air from the nasal chamber into the trachea.

Oils: ⊘⊜eucalyptus

—Nasal Polyp:

A nasal polyp is an abnormal tissue growth inside the nose. Since nasal polyps are not cancerous, very small polyps generally do not cause any problems. But larger polyps can obstruct the nasal passage and make it difficult to breath or smell and can cause frequent sinus infections. Possible symptoms of polyps include runny nose, decreased sense of smell, decreased sense of taste, snoring, facial pain or headache, itching around the eyes, and persistent congestion.

Oils: ⊜⊘frankincense, ⊜⊘oregano, ⊜⊘Respiratory Blend, ⊜⊘peppermint, ⊜⊘Cleansing Blend, ⊜⊘basil

—Olfactory Loss:

Olfactory loss (or anosmia) is the loss of one's ability to smell. The most common causes for olfactory loss are sinonasal disease, head injury, and infection of the upper respiratory tract.

Oils: ⊘⊜peppermint, ⊘⊜basil

⊘=Aromatic, ⊜=Topical, ○=Internal *(See page 33 for further details.)*

—**Rhinitis**: *see also Allergies, Antiviral, Colds*

Rhinitis is an inflammation of the nasal mucus membrane (the moist lining inside the nasal cavity where mucus is produced that acts as an air filtration system by trapping incoming dirt particles and moving them away for disposal). Rhinitis can cause runny nose, nasal congestion, sneezing, ear problems, and phlegm in the throat. Rhinitis is commonly caused by viral infections and allergies and can be acute (short-term) or chronic (long-term).

Oils: ⌀⊙eucalyptus, ⌀⊙peppermint, ⌀⊙lemon⊙, ⌀⊙lavender, ⌀⊙basil

Other Products: ⊙Seasonal Blend Softgels

🜄: Dilute as recommended, and apply 1–2 drops on nose (use extreme caution to avoid getting oil in the eye). Dilute as recommended, and apply 1 drop to a cotton swab, and swab the inside of the nose.

🜃: Diffuse into the air, and inhale the vapors through the nose. Inhale directly from bottle. Apply oil to hands, tissue, or cotton wick, and inhale.

🜂: **Additional Research:**

Lemon: A study including 100 patients (ages 3 to 79) suffering from vasomotor allergic rhinopathy, showed that topical application of a citrus lemon based spray resulted in a total reduction of eosinophils granulocytes and mast cells. These results suggest that the lemon-based nasal spray is a good alternative to conventional medicine for the treatment of perennial and seasonal allergic and vasomotor rhinopathy (Ferrara et al., 2012).

Nursing
see **Pregnancy/Motherhood:Lactation**

Obesity
see **Weight:Obesity**

Odors
see **Deodorant, Deodorizing**

Oral Conditions
see also **Antibacterial, Antifungal:Thrush.**

—**Abscess**:

A tooth abscess is a collection of pus at the root of an infected tooth. The main symptom of a tooth abscess is a painful, persistent, throbbing toothache. The infected tooth may be sensitive to heat, cold, and pressure caused by chewing. Later symptoms may include swelling in the face, swollen lymph nodes in the neck or jaw, and a fever. Abscesses may eventually rupture, leaving a foul-tasting fluid in the mouth. If left untreated, an abscess can spread to other areas of the head and neck.

Oils: ⊙clove, ⊙Protective Blend, ⊙Cleansing Blend, ⊙helichrysum, ⊙melaleuca, ⊙frankincense, ⊙Roman chamomile, ⊙wintergreen

Other Products: ⊙Protective Toothpaste

Blend 1: Blend 1 drop each of clove, wintergreen, myrrh, and helichrysum to help with infection.

—Cavities:

A cavity is a decayed area or hole in a tooth caused by bacteria in the mouth. A cavity that is allowed to progress without treatment can result in pain, infection, and loss of the tooth. Good oral hygiene and eating less sugar can help to reduce the risk of cavities.

Oils: ⊜Protective Blend, ⊜melaleuca⊙, ⊜peppermint⊙, ⊜eucalyptus⊙, ⊜cinnamon⊙

Other Products: ⊜Protective Toothpaste

—Gums:

The gums (also called "gingiva") are the soft pink tissue surrounding the teeth. The gums form a seal around the teeth and are snugly attached to the bone underneath to withstand the friction of food passing over them in chewing.

Oils: ⊜myrrh, ⊜lavender, ⊜melaleuca, ⊜helichrysum, ⊜Roman chamomile

Other Products: ⊜Protective Toothpaste

—Gum Disease:

Gum disease is an infection of the tissue and bones surrounding the teeth and is caused by a buildup of plaque. Gum disease consists of two parts: first gingivitis and then periodontal disease. Gingivitis is an inflammation of the gums because of bacteria associated with plaque buildup. When infected with gingivitis, the gums become red and swollen and often bleed during teeth brushing. Periodontal disease occurs when gingivitis is left untreated and becomes progressively worse. The inflamed gums begin pulling away from the teeth and leave empty pockets where food particles can easily collect and become infected. As the disease progresses, the gums pull farther away from the teeth and the bacteria eats away at the tissue and bone. As this occurs, the teeth lose their anchoring and can fall out.

Oils: ⊜melaleuca⊙, ⊜Protective Blend, ⊜myrrh, ⊜helichrysum, ⊜rose

Other Products: ⊜Protective Toothpaste

—Halitosis (Bad Breath):

Halitosis is the technical term for "bad breath." Common causes of halitosis include smoking, drinking, poor oral hygiene, gum disease, dry mouth, tooth decay, and certain foods.

Oils: ⊜peppermint⊙, ⊜Protective Blend, ⊜patchouli, ⊜lavender

Other Products: ⊜Protective Toothpaste

—Mouth Ulcers:

Mouth ulcers are open, often painful, sores that occur in the mouth. Common mouth ulcers include canker sores and cold sores. Stress, anxiety, fatigue, injury, illness, hormonal changes, and food allergies can often trigger mouth ulcers.

Oils: ⊜basil, ⊜myrrh, ⊜orange

Other Products: ⊜Protective Toothpaste

—Teeth Grinding:

Teeth grinding (also called bruxism) is the habit of clenching the teeth and rubbing them against one another. Teeth grinding often occurs unconsciously while a person is asleep. If teeth grinding is frequent, it can lead to tooth damage, jaw pain, and headaches.

⊘=Aromatic, ⊜=Topical, ⊙=Internal *(See page 33 for further details.)*   203

Oils: ⊘☉Calming Blend

—Teething Pain:

Around ages 4–7 months, a baby will get his or her first teeth. Some infants teethe without discomfort; but for other infants, teething can be a painful process. Common symptoms of teething include irritability or fussiness, drooling, chin rash, biting, difficulty sleeping, and low-grade fever.

Oils: ☉lavender

—Toothache:

A toothache is a pain around a tooth. Toothaches can result from many factors, including infection, injury, decay, jaw problems, cavities, damaged fillings, and gum disease. Common symptoms of a toothache include sharp or throbbing pain, swelling around the tooth, fever, headache, and foul-tasting drainage from the infected tooth.

Oils: ☉clove, ☉melaleuca, ☉Cleansing Blend, ☉Roman chamomile

Other Products: ☉Protective Toothpaste

—Toothpaste:

Oils: ☉Protective Blend

Other Products: ☉Protective Toothpaste

Recipe 1: Mix 1–2 drops Protective Blend blend with 1/2 tsp. baking soda to form a paste, and use as toothpaste to brush onto the teeth.

☉: Dilute as recommended, and apply 1–2 drops on location or along jawbone. Apply the oils with a hot compress on the face. Use Protective Blend toothpaste as directed. Dilute as recommended, and apply 1–2 drops to a small cotton ball or cotton swab; swab on location. Mix 1–2 drops with 4 oz. of water, and use as mouth-rinse. Add 1–2 drops to toothpaste. Place 5–6 drops with 1 oz. distilled water in a small spray bottle, and mist into the mouth.

⊘: Diffuse into the air.

⊕: **Additional Research:**

Melaleuca: Among several oils tested, tea tree (melaleuca), manuka, and eucalyptus demonstrated strong antibacterial activity against detrimental oral bacteria (Takarada et al., 2004).

Melaleuca: Tea tree, peppermint, and sage oils were found to inhibit oral bacteria, with thymol and eugenol being the most active components of these oils (Shapiro et al., 1994).

Melaleuca: Cinnamon oil exhibited a strong antimicrobial activity against two detrimental oral bacteria. Manuka, tea tree, and the component thymol also exhibited antimicrobial potency (Filoche et al., 2005).

Melaleuca: In 34 patients with fixed orthodontic appliances, a dental gel containing 5% melaleuca essential oil performed better than Colgate Total gel when comparing microbial biofilm and quantification of *Streptococcus mutans* in the patients' saliva (Santamaria et al., 2014).

Peppermint: Peppermint oil blended with toothpaste was found to be more effective at lower concentrations in inhibiting the formation of dental plaque than chlorhexidine (an antiseptic) in human volunteers (Shayegh et al., 2008).

Peppermint: Peppermint and rosemary oils were each found to be more effective at preventing dental biofilm (plaque) formation than chlorhexidine (an antiseptic) (Rasooli et al., 2008).

Eucalyptus: Among several oils tested, tea tree (melaleuca), manuka, and eucalyptus demonstrated strong antibacterial activity against detrimental oral bacteria (Takarada et al., 2004).

Eucalyptus: Subjects using a mouthwash containing thymol, menthol, methyl salicylate, and eucalyptol for 6 months were found to not have developed oral bacteria that were resistant to the oils (Charles et al., 2000).

Cinnamon: Cinnamon oil exhibited a strong antimicrobial activity against two detrimental oral bacteria. Manuka, tea tree, and the component thymol also exhibited antimicrobial potency (Filoche et al., 2005).

Osteomyelitis
see **Bones:Osteomyelitis**

Osteoporosis
see **Bones:Osteoporosis**

Ovaries

Ovaries are the female reproductive organs in which eggs are produced and stored.

Oils: ⬤rosemary (regulates), ⬤geranium, ⬤Women's Blend, ⬤Digestive Blend

—**Ovarian Cyst:**

An ovarian cyst is a fluid-filled sac within the ovary. While ovarian cysts are common, and most cause no problems, they may cause feelings of aching or pressure and can cause pain, bleeding, and other problems if they become too large or become twisted or rupture.

Oils: ⬤basil

⬤: Dilute as recommended, and apply 1–2 drops on abdomen and reflex points on the feet. Add 1–2 drops to 1 Tbs. fractionated coconut oil, and massage into abdomen and lower back. Apply as a warm compress to the abdomen. Add 1–2 drops to 2 tsp. olive oil, insert into vagina, and retain overnight with a tampon.

⬤: Diffuse into the air. Inhale directly from bottle. Apply oil to hands, tissue, or cotton wick, and inhale.

Overeating
see **Eating Disorders:Overeating**

Overweight
see **Weight**

Oxygenating

The term "oxygenate" means to supply, to treat, or to infuse with oxygen. All of the cells in the body require oxygen to create the energy necessary to live and function correctly. The brain consumes 20% of the oxygen we inhale.

Oils: ⬤sandalwood, ⬤frankincense, ⬤oregano, ⬤fennel

⬤: Diffuse into the air. Inhale directly from bottle. Apply oil to hands, tissue, or cotton wick, and inhale.

⬤: Dilute as recommended, and apply 1–2 drops to forehead, chest, and sinuses.

Pain

Oils: ⬤lavender, ⬤eucalyptus, ⬤Soothing Blend, ⬤lemon, ⬤rosemary, ⬤clove, ⬤cypress, ⬤white fir, ⬤helichrysum, ⬤geranium, ⬤frankincense, ⬤lemongrass, ⬤marjoram, ⬤melaleuca, ⬤peppermint, ⬤rosemary, ⬤wintergreen

⬤=Aromatic, ⬤=Topical, ⬤=Internal *(See page 33 for further details.)*   205

Other Products: ○Soothing Rub to help soothe muscles and joints. ○Cellular Vitality Complex, ○Chewable Multivitamin to help relieve oxidation associated with inflammation that contributes to pain.

—Bone:

Bone pain is a gnawing, throbbing sensation in the bones and has many possible causes, including fractures, cancer, infection, injury, leukemia, and osteoporosis.

Oils: ○Soothing Blend, ○wintergreen, ○lavender, ○cypress, ○juniper berry, ○white fir, ○cedarwood, ○helichrysum, ○peppermint, ○sandalwood

—Chronic:

Chronic pain is generally defined as pain that lasts three months or longer.

Oils: ○Soothing Blend, ○wintergreen, ○cypress, ○white fir, ○juniper berry, ○helichrysum, ○cedarwood, ○ginger, ○peppermint, ○sandalwood

—General:

Oils: ○Soothing Blend, ○wintergreen, ○lavender, ○cypress, ○marjoram, ○white fir, ○helichrysum, ○peppermint, ○sandalwood

—Inflammation: *see also* **Inflammation**

Oils: ○rosemary○, ○eucalyptus○, ○lavender○, ○Soothing Blend

Other Products: ○Soothing Rub

—Joints:

Oils: ○Soothing Blend, ○wintergreen, ○Roman chamomile

Other Products: ○Soothing Rub

—Muscle:

Oils: ○Soothing Blend, ○white fir, ○clove, ○lavender, ○lemongrass (ligaments), ○cypress, ○marjoram, ○helichrysum, ○peppermint, ○sandalwood, ○wintergreen

Other Products: ○Soothing Rub

—Tissue:

Oils: ○Soothing Blend, ○helichrysum

Other Products: ○Soothing Rub

●: Dilute as recommended, and apply 1–2 drops on location. Combine with carrier oil, and massage into affected muscles and joints. Apply as a warm compress over affected areas.

○: Take capsules as directed on package.

○: Diffuse into the air. Inhale oil that is applied to a tissue or cotton wick.

○: **Additional Research:**

Lavender: Lavender oil was found to work as an anaesthetic (reducing pain) in a rabbit reflex test (Ghelardini et al., 1999).

Lavender: Oil from Lavandula angustifolia was found to reduce writhing in induced writhing in rats and to reduce edema (swelling) in carrageenan-induced paw edema, indicating an anti-inflammatory effect (Hajhashemi et al., 2003).

Lavender: The odor of lavender combined with relaxing music was found to lessen the intensity of pain following a vascular wound dressing change (Kane et al., 2004).

Lavender: In patients suffering from arthritis, it was found that a blend of lavender, marjoram, eucalyptus, rosemary, peppermint, and carrier oils reduced perceived pain and depression compared to a control (Kim et al., 2005).

Eucalyptus: A combination of peppermint oil and ethanol was found to have a significant analgesic effect with a reduction in sensitivity to headache; while a combination of peppermint, eucalyptus, and ethanol was found to relax muscles and to increase cognitive performance in humans (Göbel et al., 1994).

Eucalyptus: 1,8 cineole (eucalyptol) was found to have antinociceptive (pain-reducing) properties similar to morphine. Beta-pinene was found to reverse the effects of morphine in a degree similar to naloxone (a drug used to counter the effects of morphine overdose) (Liapi et al., 2007).

Eucalyptus: 1,8 cineole (eucalyptol) was found to display an anti-inflammatory effect on rats in several tests and was found to exhibit antinociceptive (pain-reducing) effects in mice, possibly by depressing the central nervous system (Santos et al., 2000).

Lemon: Inhaling the aroma of lemon essential oil was found to decrease pain response in rats and was also found to modulate the neuronal response to formalin-induced pain (Aloisi et al., 2002).

Lemon: Rats exposed long-term to lemon essential oil were found to demonstrate different anxiety and pain threshold levels than untreated rats. It was also found that exposure to lemon oil induced chemical changes in the neuronal circuits involved in anxiety and pain (Ceccarelli et al., 2004).

Rosemary: In patients suffering from arthritis, it was found that a blend of lavender, marjoram, eucalyptus, rosemary, peppermint, and carrier oils reduced perceived pain and depression compared to a control (Kim et al., 2005).

Rosemary: A combination of peppermint oil and ethanol was found to have a significant analgesic effect with a reduction in sensitivity to headache; while a combination of peppermint, eucalyptus, and ethanol was found to relax muscles and to increase cognitive performance in humans (Göbel et al., 1994).

Rosemary: 1,8 cineole (eucalyptol) was found to have antinociceptive (pain-reducing) properties similar to morphine. Beta-pinene was found to reverse the effects of morphine in a degree similar to naloxone (a drug used to counter the effects of morphine overdose) (Liapi et al., 2007).

Rosemary: An ethanol extract of rosemary was found to demonstrate antinociceptive (pain-blocking) and anti-inflammatory activity in mice and rats (González-Trujano et al., 2007).

Rosemary: Rosemary oil was found to have anti-inflammatory and peripheral antinociceptive (pain sensitivity–blocking) properties in mice (Takaki et al., 2008).

Clove: Beta-caryophyllene (found in clove oil) demonstrated anaesthetic (pain-reducing) activity in rats and rabbits (Ghelardini et al., 2001).

Rosemary: 1,8 cineole (eucalyptol) was found to display an anti-inflammatory effect on rats in several tests and was found to exhibit antinociceptive (pain-reducing) effects in mice, possibly by depressing the central nervous system (Santos et al., 2000).

Rosemary: An ethanol extract of rosemary was found to demonstrate antinociceptive (pain-blocking) and anti-inflammatory activity in mice and rats (González-Trujano et al., 2007).

Rosemary: Rosemary oil was found to have anti-inflammatory and peripheral antinociceptive (pain sensitivity–blocking) properties in mice (Takaki et al., 2008).

Coriander: Injection of coriander extract in mice was found to have a greater analgesic effect than dexamethasone (an anti-inflammatory drug) or stress, when mice were subjected to acute and chronic pain tests (Taherian et al., 2012).

Ginger: A double-blind, placebo-controlled study demonstrated that aroma massage with ginger and orange essential oils relieved knee joint pain in elderly subjects more than the placebo (massage with olive oil) or the control (conventional treatment without massage) (Yip et al., 2008).

Painting

Add one 15 ml bottle of your favorite essential oil (or oil blend) to any five gallon bucket of paint. Stir vigorously, mixing well, and then either spray paint or paint by hand. This should eliminate the paint fumes and after-smell.

Palpitations

see **Cardiovascular System:Palpitations**

Pancreas

The pancreas is a gland organ located behind the stomach. The pancreas is responsible for producing insulin and other hormones and for producing "pancreatic juices" that aid in digestion.

Oils: ⊖cypress, ⊖rosemary, ⊖⊘Respiratory Blend, ⊖⊘lemon, ⊖⊘Protective Blend

—Pancreatitis:

Pancreatitis is the term used to describe pancreas inflammation. Pancreatitis occurs when the pancreatic juices that are designed to aid in digestion in the small intestine become active while still inside the pancreas. When this occurs, the pancreas literally begins to digest itself. Acute pancreatitis lasts for only a short time and then resolves itself. Chronic pancreatitis does not resolve itself but instead gradually destroys the pancreas.

Oils: ⊖⊘lemon, ⊖⊘marjoram

—Stimulant For:

Oils: ⊖helichrysum

—Support:

Oils: ⊖⊘cinnamon, ⊖⊘geranium, ⊖⊘fennel

⊜: Dilute as recommended, and apply 1–2 drops over pancreas area or on reflex points on the feet.

⊘: Diffuse into the air. Inhale directly from bottle. Apply oil to hands, tissue, or cotton wick, and inhale.

Panic
see **Anxiety**

Paralysis
see **Nervous System:Paralysis**

Parasites

A parasite is an organism that grows on or in another organism at the host organism's expense. A parasite cannot live independently and is fed and sheltered by the host organism without making any helpful contribution itself.

Oils: O⊜oregano⊕, O⊜thyme, O⊜fennel, O⊜Roman chamomile, O⊜Digestive Blend, O⊜lavender⊕, ⊜melaleuca⊕, ⊜O clove

Other Products: O Digestive Softgels

—Intestinal:

Intestinal parasites are parasites that infect the intestinal tract. These parasites enter the intestinal tract through the mouth by unwashed or uncooked food, contaminated water, and unclean hands. Symptoms of intestinal parasites include diarrhea, abdominal pain, weight loss, fatigue, gas or bloating, nausea or vomiting, stomach pain, passing a worm in a stool, stools containing blood and mucus, and rash or itching around the rectum or vulva.

Oils: O⊜lemon, O⊜oregano⊕, O⊜Roman chamomile

—Worms:

Parasitic worms are worm-like organisms that live inside another living organism and feed off their host organism at the host organism's expense, causing weakness and disease. Parasitic worms can live inside of animals as well as humans.

Oils: O☺Digestive Blend, O☺lavender, ☺Orosemary, ☺Othyme, O☺peppermint, ☺❷Roman chamomile, O☺bergamot, ☺melaleuca

Blend 1: Combine 6 drops Roman chamomile, 6 drops eucalyptus, 6 drops lavender, and 6 drops lemon with 2 Tbs. fractionated coconut oil. Apply 10–15 drops over abdomen with a hot compress, and apply 1–2 drops on intestine and colon reflex points on the feet.

◯: Place 2–4 drops essential oil in empty capsule, and swallow. Add 1–2 drops to 4 oz. rice or almond milk; drink.

☺: Apply as warm compress over abdomen. Add 2–3 drops to 1 Tbs. fractionated coconut oil, and apply as rectal retention enema for 15 minutes or more. Dilute as recommended, and apply to abdomen and reflex points on the feet.

▭: **Additional Research:**

Oregano: Oregano oil administered orally was found to improve gastrointestinal symptoms in 7 of 11 patients who had tested positive for the parasite Blastocystis hominis and was found to cause disappearance of this parasite in 8 cases (Force et al., 2000).

Lavender: Essential oil from Lavandula angustifolia demonstrated ability to eliminate protozoal pathogens Giardia duodenalis, Trichomonas vaginalis, and Hexamita inflata at concentrations of 1% or less (Moon et al., 2006).

Melaleuca: Melaleuca oil was effective at killing *Anisakis simplex* larva in vitro. Data suggests that the mechanism of action against anisakis involves inhibition of acetylcholinesterase (Gómez-Rincón et al., 2014).

Parasympathetic Nervous System

see **Nervous System: Parasympathetic Nervous System**

Parkinson's Disease

Parkinson's disease is a progressive neurodegenerative disease marked by impairment of muscle movement and speech. Symptoms of Parkinson's disease include slowed motion, muscle stiffness, difficulty maintaining balance, impaired speech, loss of automatic movements (such as blinking, smiling, and swinging the arms while walking), and hand tremors.

Oils: O☺cinnamon▭, ☺marjoram, ☺lavender, ☺clary sage, ❷❷frankincense, ☺❷Grounding Blend, ❷☺sandalwood, ❷☺Calming Blend, ❷☺vetiver, ☺cypress (circulation), ☺❷bergamot, ☺❷geranium, ☺helichrysum, ☺juniper berry, ❷☺lemon, ❷☺orange, ☺❷peppermint, ☺❷rosemary, ☺❷thyme

Other Products: OEnergy & Stamina Complex to help support healthy nerve function. OCellular Vitality Complex, OChewable Multivitamin contain Coenzyme Q10, which has been studied for its potential benefits in alleviating Parkinson's disease▭. OEssential Oil Omega Complex or Vegan Essential Oil Omega Complex for essential omega fatty acids that help support healthy nerve cell function.

☺: Add 5–10 drops essential oil to 1 Tbs. fractionated coconut oil and massage on affected muscles, back, legs, and neck. Dilute as recommended and apply 1–2 drops to base of neck or reflex points on the feet. Add 3–5 drops to warm bathwater, and bathe.

○: Take capsules as directed on package.

⬢: Diffuse into the air. Inhale directly from bottle. Apply oil to hands, tissue, or cotton wick, and inhale.

▭: **Additional Research:**

> **Cinnamon:** The process of α-syn protein aggregation is a major component of Parkinson's disease. Preventing α-syn aggregation may help in the treatment of Parkinson's disease. Researchers have discovered that an aqueous cinnamon extract precipitation has a curative effect on α-syn aggregation in a Drosophila model of Parkinson's disease. Furthermore, in vitro tests have revealed that the cinnamon extract has an inhibitory effect on the process of α-syn fibrillation (Shaltiel-Karyo et al., 2012).

> **Eugenol (found in cassia, cinnamon, and clove):** Eugenol administration was found to prevent induced dopamine depression and lipid peroxidation inductivity in the mouse striatum model, suggesting that eugenol may be useful in the treatment of Parkinson's disease (Kabuto et al., 2007).

> **Coenzyme Q10:** A study of Parkinson's disease patients found that CoQ10 was significantly lower in the cortex region of their brains than in the brains of healthy patients (Hargreaves et al., 2008).

> **Coenzyme Q10:** Pretreatment of mice with CoQ10 was found to protect dopaminergic neurons from iron-induced oxidative stress that has been theorized to play a role in the development of Parkinson's disease (Kooncumchoo et al., 2006).

> **Coenzyme Q10:** A mitochondrial defect in fibroblast cells cultivated from 18 Parkinson's disease patients was found to be ameliorated in 50% of these cells treated with CoQ10 (Winkler-Stuck, 2004).

Pelvic Pain Syndrome

Pelvic pain syndrome is characterized by pain in the pelvis area that continues for several months. Symptoms include severe and steady pain, dull aching, a feeling of pressure deep in the pelvis, painful bowel movements, pain during intercourse, and pain when sitting down.

Oils: ⬢ginger, ⬢geranium, ⬢clove, ⬢bergamot, ⬢thyme, ⬢rose

🛁: Place 2–3 drops in warm bathwater, and soak for 10 minutes. Add 5–10 drops to 1 Tbs. fractionated coconut oil, and massage on pelvis and upper legs.

Periodontal Disease
see **Oral Conditions:Gum Disease**

Pests
see **Insects/Bugs, Mice**

Phlebitis
see **Cardiovascular System:Phlebitis**

Pimples
see **Acne**

Pink Eye
see **Eyes:Pink Eye**

Pineal Gland

The pineal gland is a tiny endocrine gland located close to the center of the brain. It is responsible for producing the hormone melatonin that regulates the sleep/wake cycle. The pineal gland also serves to regulate blood pressure, sexual development, growth, body temperature, and motor function.

Oils: ⬢frankincense, ⬢sandalwood, ⬢vetiver, ⬢ginger, ⬢cedarwood

⬢: Diffuse into the air. Inhale oil directly from bottle. Apply oil to hands, tissue, or cotton wick, and inhale.

Pituitary Gland

The pituitary gland is a small endocrine gland located at the base of the brain that secretes hormones directly into the bloodstream. It is composed of three different lobes, each responsible for producing a different set of hormones. The anterior lobe secretes the human growth hormone (stimulates overall body growth), adrenocorticotropic hormone (controls hormone secretion by the adrenal cortex), thyrotropic hormone (stimulates activity of the thyroid gland), and the gonadotropic hormones (control growth and reproductive activity of the ovaries and testes). The posterior lobe secretes antidiuretic hormone (causes water retention by the kidneys) and oxytocin (stimulates the mammary glands to release milk and causes uterine contractions). The pituitary gland is often referred to as the "master" endocrine gland because it controls the functioning of the other endocrine glands.

Oils: ⊘frankincense, ⊘sandalwood, ⊘vetiver, ⊘ginger

—Balances:

Oils: ⊘⊖ylang ylang, ⊘⊖geranium

—Increases Oxygen:

Oils: ⊘⊖frankincense, ⊘⊖sandalwood

⊘: Diffuse into the air. Inhale oil directly from bottle. Apply oil to hands, tissue, or cotton wick, and inhale.

⊖: Dilute as recommended, and apply 1–2 drops to forehead, back of neck, and reflex points on big toes.

Plague

see also **Antibacterial**

Plague is a potentially deadly bacterial disease that is caused by the *Yersinia pestis* bacteria, which is transmitted to humans and animals through close contact or through bites from fleas that have previously bitten infected animals. Symptoms include fever, headaches, and extremely swollen and hot lymph nodes. If left untreated, plague can quickly invade the lungs—causing severe pneumonia, high fever, bloody coughing, and death.

Oils: ⊖⊘clove, ⊘⊖Protective Blend, ⊖⊘frankincense, ⊖⊘oregano

⊖: Dilute as recommended, and apply to neck, chest, and reflex points on the feet.

⊘: Diffuse into the air.

Plaque

see **Antibacterial, Oral Conditions**

Pleurisy

see **Antibacterial, Respiratory System:Pleurisy**

PMS

see **Female Specific Conditions:PMS**

P

Personal Guide

Pneumonia

see also **Respiratory System, Antibacterial, Antifungal, Antiviral**

Pneumonia is an illness characterized by lung inflammation in which the lungs are infected by a bacteria, fungus, or virus. The result is a cough, chest pain, difficulty breathing, fever, shaking chills, headache, muscle pain, and fatigue. Pneumonia is a special concern for young children and individuals over the age of sixty-five. Pneumonia ranges in seriousness from mild to life threatening.

Oils: ⊘©Respiratory Blend, ⊘©Protective Blend, ⊘©thyme©, ⊘cinnamon©, ⊘©oregano©, ⊘©eucalyptus, ⊘©melaleuca, ⊘©lavender, ⊘lemon, O⊘tangerine©, ⊘©frankincense, ⊘©myrrh

Other Products: OProtective Softgels

⊘: Diffuse into the air. Place 4 drops in 1/2 cup hot water, and inhale steam deeply.

O: Take capsules as directed on package.

⊜: Dilute as recommended, and apply to chest, back, and reflex points on the feet. Apply as warm compress to the chest. Place 2–3 drops in 1 tsp. fractionated coconut oil; place oil in rectum, and retain overnight.

⊙: **Additional Research:**

Thyme: Oils with aldehyde or phenol as major components demonstrated a high level of antibacterial activity (Inouye et al., 2001).

Thyme: Cinnamon, thyme, and clove essential oils demonstrated an antibacterial effect on several respiratory tract pathogens (Fabio et al., 2007).

Cinnamon: Oils with aldehyde or phenol as major components demonstrated a high level of antibacterial activity (Inouye et al., 2001).

Cinnamon: Cinnamon, thyme, and clove essential oils demonstrated an antibacterial effect on several respiratory tract pathogens (Fabio et al., 2007).

Oregano: Oregano oil was found to kill antibiotic resistant strains of Staph, E. coli, Klebsiella pneumoniae, Helicobacter pylori, and Mycobacterium terrae (Preuss et al., 2005).

Tangerine: In rats with induced pulmonary fibrosis oral treatment of hydrodistilled tangerine essential oil suppressed body weight loss and significantly improved scores of alveolitis and fibrosis of lung tissue. The effects of tangerine essential oil on lung fibrosis were associated with free radical scavenging and antioxidant activity (Zhou et al., 2012).

Poison Ivy/Oak

Poison oak and poison ivy are plants with an oily sap called urushiol that causes an itchy rash when it comes into contact with the skin. Infection by poison oak or poison ivy is recognized by redness and itching of the skin, a rash, red bumps, and later oozing blisters. A rash caused by poison oak or by poison ivy usually lasts from 5–12 days.

Oils: ©rose, ©lavender, ©Joyful Blend, ©Roman chamomile

⊜: Dilute as recommended, and apply 1–2 drops on location. Add 2–3 drops to 1 tsp. fractionated coconut oil, and apply on location.

Pollution

see **Purification**

Polyps

see **Colon:Polyps, Nose:Nasal Polyp**

Pregnancy/Motherhood

Pregnancy is the period of time (generally nine months) in which a woman carries a developing fetus in her uterus.

Oils: ©©geranium, ©©ylang ylang, ©©lavender©, ©©grapefruit, ©©Roman chamomile

Other Products: ○Cellular Vitality Complex, ○Chewable Multivitamin, ○Essential Oil Omega Complex or Vegan Essential Oil Omega Complex, ○Food Nutrient Complex for nutrients essential to support cellular health and body function.

—Anxiety/Tension: *see Calming*

—Baby (Newborn):

> **Oils:** ©frankincense (1 drop on crown), ©myrrh (1 drop on umbilical cord and navel), ©Grounding Blend (1 drop on feet and spine)
>
> ©: Apply as indicated above.

—Breasts:

> In the first trimester of pregnancy, a woman's breasts become sore and tender as the body begins to prepare itself for breast-feeding. During pregnancy the breasts enlarge, the nipples grow larger and become darker, and the breasts may begin to leak colostrum—the first milk the body makes in preparation for the developing baby.
>
> **Oils:** ©lavender (soothes), ©geranium (soothes), ©Roman chamomile (sore nipples), ©fennel (tones)
>
> ©: Add 3–5 drops to 1 Tbs. fractionated coconut oil, and massage on location.

—Delivery:

> Delivery is the act or process of giving birth.
>
> **Oils:** ©©lavender (stimulates circulation, calming, antiseptic), ©clary sage, ©Grounding Blend
>
> ©: Dilute as recommended, and apply 1–2 drops on hips, bottoms of feet, or abdomen. Add 3–5 drops to 1 Tbs. fractionated coconut oil, and massage on hips, bottoms of feet, or abdomen.
>
> ©: Diffuse into the air. Inhale directly from bottle. Apply oil to hands, tissue, or cotton wick, and inhale.

> —Avoid Episiotomy:
>
> > **Oils:** ©geranium
> >
> > ©: Add 5–10 drops to 1/2 tsp. olive oil, and massage perineum.
>
> —Diffuse:
>
> > **Oils:** ©Calming Blend, ©Joyful Blend
> >
> > ©: Diffuse into the air.
>
> —Uterus:
>
> > **Oils:** ©clary sage
> >
> > ©: Apply 1–3 drops around the ankles to help tone uterus.

©=Aromatic, ©=Topical, ○=Internal *(See page 33 for further details.)*   213

–Transition:

Oils: ♥basil

🔗: Dilute as recommended, and apply 1–2 drops to temples or abdomen.

—Early Labor:

Preterm labor is labor that begins before the 37th week of pregnancy. Babies born before the 37th week are considered premature. Signs of preterm labor include contractions every 10 minutes or more often, cramps, low backache, pelvic pressure, and change in vaginal discharge (fluid or blood).

Oils: ♥lavender

🔗: Gently apply 1–3 drops on stomach or on heart area to help stop.

–Energy:

Blend 1: Combine 2 drops Roman chamomile, 2 drops geranium, and 2 drops lavender in 2 tsp. fractionated coconut oil, and massage into the skin.

—Hemorrhaging:

Postpartum Hemorrhaging is excessive bleeding following childbirth. It is commonly defined as losing 500 ml of blood after vaginal birth and 1000 ml of blood after a cesarean birth. Postpartum hemorrhaging generally occurs within 24 hours following the birth and can be life threatening if not stopped.

Oils: ♥helichrysum

🔗: Apply 1–3 drops on lower back to help prevent hemorrhaging.

—High Blood Pressure:

High blood pressure can potentially be dangerous in pregnancy. High blood pressure can cause a decreased flow of blood to the placenta, slowing down the baby's growth; premature placenta separation from the uterus, taking away the baby's oxygen and nutrients and causing heavy bleeding in the mother; premature birth; and the risk of future disease. Pregnancy can in some cases actually cause a woman's blood pressure to increase.

Oils: ♥♥ylang ylang♥, ♥♥eucalyptus♥, ♥♥lavender, ♥♥clove, ♥♥clary sage, ♥♥lemon. Note: Avoid rosemary, thyme, and possibly peppermint.

Bath 1: Place 3 drops ylang ylang in bathwater, and bathe in the evening twice a week.

Blend 2: Combine 5 drops geranium, 8 drops lemongrass, and 3 drops lavender in 1 oz. fractionated coconut oil. Rub over heart and on reflex points on left foot and hand.

🔗: Dilute as recommended, and apply on location, on reflex points on feet and hands, and over heart.

💨: Diffuse into the air. Apply oils to hands, and inhale oils from hands cupped over the nose. Inhale oil applied to a tissue or cotton wick.

—Labor (during):

Oils: ♥clary sage (may combine with fennel)

🔗: Apply 3 drops around ankles or on abdomen.

—Labor (post):

Oils: ᴑlavender, ᴑgeranium

ᴥ: Dilute as recommended, and apply 1–3 drops on abdomen, ankles, or bottoms of feet.

—Lactation (Milk Production):

Lactation is the production and secretion of milk from the mammary glands of females for the nourishment of their young offspring. Lactation is commonly referred to as "breast-feeding."

Oils: ᴑclary sage (start production), ᴑfennel or ᴑbasil (increase production), ᴑpeppermint (decrease production), ᴑWomen's Blend (contains jasmine◌ that may help decrease production)

ᴥ: Dilute as recommended, and apply 1–2 drops on breasts. Apply peppermint with cold compress to help reduce production. *Caution: Fennel should not be used for more than 10 days, as it will excessively increase flow through the urinary tract.*

—Mastitis: *see also* **Antibacterial**.

Mastitis is a breast infection occurring in women who are breast-feeding. Mastitis causes the breast to become red, swollen, and very painful. Symptoms of mastitis include breast tenderness, fever, general lack of well-being, skin redness, and a breast that feels warm to the touch. Mastitis generally occurs in just one breast, not in both.

Oils: ᴑlavender, ᴑInvigorating Blend (combine with lavender), ᴑpatchouli◌

ᴥ: Dilute as recommended, and apply 1–2 drops on breasts.

—Miscarriage (after):

A miscarriage is a pregnancy that ends on its own within the first 20 weeks. Signs of a miscarriage include vaginal bleeding, fluid or tissue being ejected from the vagina, and pain and cramping in the abdomen or lower back. Miscarriages occur before the baby is developed enough to survive. About half of all pregnancies end in miscarriage, but most happen too early for the mother to be aware that it has occurred. Women who miscarry after about 8 weeks of pregnancy should consult their doctor as soon as possible afterwards to prevent any future complications.

Oils: ᴑfrankincense, ᴑgrapefruit, ᴑgeranium, ᴑlavender, ᴑRoman chamomile

ᴥ: Dilute 5–6 drops in 1 Tbs. fractionated coconut oil, and massage on back, legs, and arms. Add 3–4 drops to warm bathwater, and bathe.

—Morning Sickness:

Morning sickness is the nauseated feeling accompanying the first trimester of pregnancy for many women. Morning sickness can often include vomiting. For most women, morning sickness begins around the sixth week of pregnancy and ends around the twelfth week. Although it is called "morning" sickness, the symptoms can occur at any time during the day.

Oils: ᴑᴥ◌ginger◌, ᴥᴑpeppermint, ᴑlemon◌

ᴥ: Dilute as recommended, and apply 1–3 drops on ears, down jaw bone, and on reflex points on the feet.

○: Place 1–3 drops in empty capsule; swallow capsule.

⊘: Diffuse into the air. Inhale directly from bottle. Apply oil to hands, tissue, or cotton wick, and inhale. Apply 1 drop on pillow to inhale at night.

—Placenta:

The placenta is the organ responsible for sustaining life in an unborn baby. The placenta attaches to the uterus wall and connects to the mother's blood supply to provide nutrients and oxygen for the fetus. The placenta plays other essential roles as well: It removes waste created by the fetus, triggers labor and delivery, and protects the fetus against infection.

Oils: ◒basil (to help retain)

⊜: Dilute as recommended, and apply 1–2 drops on lower abdomen and reflex points on the feet.

—Postpartum Depression:

Postpartum depression is depression sometimes experienced by mothers shortly after giving birth. New mothers may experience symptoms such as irritableness, sadness, uncontrollable emotions, fatigue, anxiety, difficulty sleeping, thoughts of suicide, hopelessness, and guilt. Postpartum depression is typically thought to result from a hormonal imbalance caused by the pregnancy and childbirth.

Oils: ⊘◒Joyful Blend, ⊘◒lemon◒, ⊘◒lavender◒, ⊘◒frankincense◒, ⊘◒clary sage, ⊘◒geranium, ⊘grapefruit, ⊘◒bergamot, ⊘◒Grounding Blend, ⊘◒myrrh, ⊘orange

⊘: Diffuse into the air. Inhale directly from bottle. Apply oil to hands, tissue, or cotton wick, and inhale.

⊜: Dilute as recommended, and apply 1–2 drops to temple or forehead. Add 5–10 drops to 1 Tbs. fractionated coconut oil, and use as massage oil. Add 1–3 drops to warm bathwater, and bathe.

—Preeclampsia: *see also Pregnancy/Motherhood: High Blood Pressure*

Preeclampsia, also known as toxemia, is pregnancy-induced high blood pressure. Symptoms include protein in the urine, elevated blood pressure levels, sudden weight gain, blurred vision, abdominal pains in the upper-right side, and swelling in the hands and face. Women suffering from preeclampsia are often put on bed rest for the remainder of the pregnancy to ensure the safety of the mother and baby.

Oils: ◒⊘cypress

⊜: Dilute 1:1 in fractionated coconut oil, and apply 1–2 drops on bottoms of feet and on abdomen.

⊘: Diffuse into the air. Inhale directly from bottle. Apply oil to hands, tissue, or cotton wick, and inhale.

—Self Love:

Oils: ⊘Joyful Blend

⊘: Diffuse into the air. Wear as perfume.

—Stretch Marks: *see Skin:Stretch Marks*

🔲: **Additional Research:**

Lavender: A triple blind randomized placebo-controlled trial, consisting of 60 subjects and evaluating the use of lavender oil for Cesarean postoperative pain management, found that inhalation of lavender (when compared to inhalation of a placebo) decreased postoperative pain and increased patient satisfaction. Furthermore, patients inhaling lavender oil required significantly lower dosages of Diclofenac suppository as a supplemental analgesic drug than the placebo group. The researchers state that lavender essential oil is not recommended as the sole analgesic treatment (Olapour et al., 2013).

Ylang ylang: Subjects who had ylang ylang oil applied to their skin had decreased blood pressure, increased skin temperature, and reported feeling more calm and relaxed compared to subjects in a control group (Hongratanaworakit et al., 2006).

Ylang ylang: Inhaled ylang ylang oil was found to decrease blood pressure and pulse rate and to enhance attentiveness and alertness in volunteers compared to an odorless control (Hongratanaworakit et al., 2004).

Eucalyptus: Treatment of rats with 1,8-cineole (or eucalyptol—found in eucalyptus, rosemary, and marjoram) demonstrated an ability to lower mean aortic pressure (blood pressure), without decreasing heart rate, through vascular wall relaxation (Lahlou et al., 2002).

Jasmine: Jasmine flowers applied to the breast were found to be as effective as the antilactation drug bromocriptine in reducing breast engorgement, milk production, and analgesic (pain-relieving drug) intake in women after giving birth. (Shrivastav et al., 1988).

Ginger: Ginger root given orally to pregnant women was found to decrease the severity of nausea and frequency of vomiting compared to control (Vutyavanich et al., 2001).

Lemon: A randomized clinical trial carried out on 100 pregnant women suffering from mild to moderate nausea found inhalation of lemon essential oil to be more effective at preventing nausea than inhalation of a carrier oil on days two and four of a four day trial (Yavari kia et al., 2014).

Patchouli: Patchouli alcohol (a tricyclic sesquiterpene and an essential oil of *Pogostemon cablin*) was found to inhibit chemically induced mastitis in a mouse model by inhibiting inflammation, suggesting patchouli may prevent mastitis (Li et al., 2014).

Lemon: Lemon oil vapor was found to have a strong antistress and antidepressant effects on mice subjected to several common stress tests (Komiya et al., 2006).

Lemon: Lemon oil and its component, citral, were found to decrease depressed behavior in a similar manner to antidepressant drugs in rats involved in several stress tests (Komori et al., 1995).

Lemon: In 12 patients suffering from depression, it was found that inhaling citrus aromas reduced the needed doses of antidepressants, normalized neuroendocrine hormone levels, and normalized immune function (Komori et al., 1995).

Lavender: Female students suffering from insomnia were found to sleep better and to have a lower level of depression during weeks they used a lavender fragrance when compared to weeks they did not use a lavender fragrance (Lee et al., 2006).

Laveder: Incensole acetate was found to open TRPV receptor in mice brain, a possible channel for emotional regulation (Moussaieff et al., 2008).

Prostate

The prostate gland is a small organ just beneath that bladder that is part of the male reproductive system. Its primary function is to create and store fluid that helps nourish and protect the sperm.

Oils: ◐helichrysum, ◐frankincense, ◐juniper berry

—Benign Prostatic Hyperplasia:

The size of the prostate begins at about the same size as a walnut but increases in size as a male ages. If the prostate grows too large, it can block passage of urine from the bladder through the urethra. This blockage can lead to increased risk for developing urinary tract stones, infections, or damaged kidneys.

Oils: ◐fennel

—Prostate Cancer: *see Cancer:Prostate*

—Prostatitis:

Prostatitis is an inflamed prostate, typically due to infection. This can cause pain in the lower back and groin area, painful urination, and the need to urinate frequently.

Oils: thyme, cypress, lavender

☝: Dilute as recommended, and apply to the posterior, scrotum, ankles, lower back, or bottoms of feet. Add 5 drops to 1 Tbs. fractionated coconut oil, insert into rectum, and retain throughout the night.

Psoriasis

Psoriasis is a skin condition characterized by patches of red, scaly skin that may itch or burn. The most commonly affected areas are the elbows, knees, scalp, back, face, palms, and feet. But other areas can be affected as well. Psoriasis doesn't have a known cure or cause, but it is thought an auto-immune disorder may play a role. Psoriasis tends to be less severe in the warmer months.

Oils: helichrysum, thyme, lavender, melaleuca, Roman chamomile, cedarwood, bergamot

Blend 1: Combine 2 drops Roman chamomile with 2 drops lavender, and apply on location.

☝: Dilute as recommended, and apply 1–2 drops on location.

Pulmonary

see **Respiratory System:Lungs**

Purification

Oils: Cleansing Blend, lemon, lemongrass, eucalyptus, melaleuca, cedarwood, orange, fennel

—Air:

Oils: lemon, peppermint, Cleansing Blend

—Cigarette Smoke:

Oils: Cleansing Blend

—Dishes:

Oils: lemon

—Water:

Oils: lemon, Cleansing Blend, peppermint

☝: Diffuse into the air. Add 10–15 drops to 1 oz. distilled water in a small spray bottle; shake well, and mist into the air.

☝: Add 1–2 drops to dishwater for sparkling dishes and a great smelling kitchen. Add 1–2 drops to warm bathwater, and bathe. Add 1–2 drops to bowl of water, and use to clean the outside of fruit and vegetables.

☝: Add 1 drop oil to 12–16 oz. of drinking water to help purify.

Pus

see **Infection**

Radiation

Radiation is energy emitted from a source and sent through space or matter. Different forms of radiation can include light, heat, sound, radio, micro-waves, gamma rays, or X-rays, among others. While many forms of radiation are around us every day and are perfectly safe (such as light, sound, and heat), frequent or prolonged exposure to high-energy forms of radiation can be detrimental to the body, possibly causing DNA mutation, damaged cellular structures, burns, cancer, or other damage.

Oils: O☻peppermint, O☻sandalwood

—**Gamma Radiation:**

Oils: O☻peppermint☺

—**Radiation Therapy:**

Radiation treatments can produce tremendous toxicity within the liver. Cut down on the use of oils with high phenol content to prevent increasing liver toxicity. Oils with high phenol content include wintergreen, birch, clove, basil, fennel, oregano, thyme, melaleuca, and cinnamon.

—**Ultraviolet Radiation:**

Oils: O☻sandalwood☺, ☻frankincense, ☻melaleuca☺, ☻thyme☺, ☻clove☺

—**Weeping Wounds From:**

Oils: ☻melaleuca, ☻thyme, ☻oregano

○: Place 1–2 drops under the tongue or place 2–3 drops in an empty capsule, and swallow.

☻: Dilute as recommended, and apply 1–2 drops on location.

☺: **Additional Research:**

Peppermint: In mice exposed to whole-body gamma irradiation, only 17% of mice who had been fed peppermint oil died; while 100% of mice who did not receive peppermint oil died. It was also found that the mice pre-fed peppermint oil were able to return blood cell levels to normal after 30 days, while control mice were not (and consequently died)—suggesting a protective or stimulating effect of the oil on blood stem cells (Samarth et al., 2004).

Peppermint: Peppermint extract fed orally to mice demonstrated the ability to protect the testis from gamma radiation damage (Samarth et al., 2009).

Peppermint: Peppermint oil fed to mice prior to exposure to gamma radiation was found to decrease levels of damage from oxidation, as compared to mice not pretreated with peppermint (Samarth et al., 2006).

Peppermint: Mice treated with oral administration of peppermint extract demonstrated a higher ability to tolerate gamma radiation than non-treated mice (Samarth et al., 2003).

Peppermint: Mice pretreated with peppermint leaf extract demonstrated less bone marrow cell loss than mice not pretreated with peppermint when exposed to gamma radiation (Samarth et al., 2007).

Sandalwood: Pretreatment with alpha-santalol before UVB (ultraviolet-b) radiation significantly reduced skin tumor development and multiplicity and induced proapoptotic and tumor-suppressing proteins (Arasada et al., 2008).

Sandalwood: A solution of 5% alpha-santalol (from sandalwood) was found to prevent skin-tumor formation caused by ultraviolet-b (UVB) radiation in mice (Dwivedi et al., 2006).

Melaleuca: Melaleuca alternifolia oil was found to mediate the reactive oxygen species (ROS) production of leukocytes (white blood cells), indicating a possible anti-inflammatory activity (Caldefie-Chézet et al., 2004).

Thyme: Various essential oils demonstrated an antioxidant effect toward skin lipid squalene oxidized by UV irradiation, with a blend of thyme and clove oil demonstrating the highest inhibitory effect (Wei et al., 2007).

Clove: Various essential oils demonstrated an antioxidant effect toward skin lipid squalene oxidized by UV irraditation, with a blend of thyme and clove oil demonstrating the highest inhibitory effect (Wei et al., 2007).

Rashes

see **Skin:Rashes**

Raynaud's Disease

see also **Arteries, Cardiovascular System:Circulation**

Raynaud's disease is a condition that causes the arteries supplying blood to the skin to suddenly narrow and inhibit blood circulation. As a result, specific areas of the body feel numb and cool. The most commonly affected areas are the toes, fingers, nose, and ears. During an attack, the skin turns white and then blue. As circulation returns and warms the affected areas, a prickling, throbbing, stinging, or swelling sensation often accompanies it. These attacks are often triggered by cold temperatures and by stress.

Oils: �cypress, �rosemary, �geranium, �helichrysum, �fennel, �clove, �lavender

⬤: Dilute as recommended, and apply 1–2 drops on the affected area, to carotid arteries, and on reflex points on the feet.

⬤: Diffuse into the air. Inhale oil directly from bottle, or inhale oil that is applied to hands, tissue, or cotton wick.

Relaxation

Relaxation is a state of rest and tranquility, free from tension and anxiety.

Oils: �lavender, �ylang ylang, �lemon, �Massage Blend, �Roman chamomile, �geranium, �frankincense, �sandalwood, �clary sage

⬤: Diffuse into the air. Inhale directly from bottle. Apply oil to hands, tissue, or cotton wick, and inhale. *See also Ions:Negative for oils that produce negative ions when diffused to help promote relaxation.*

⬤: Add 5–10 drops to 1 Tbs. fractionated coconut oil (or another carrier oil), and use as massage oil. Place 1–2 drops in warm bathwater, and bathe.

⬤: **Additional Research:**

Lavender: Nurses working in an ICU setting demonstrated decreased perception of stress when receiving a topical application of Lavandula angustifolia and Salvia sclarea essential oils (Pemberton et al., 2008).

Lavender: Subjects who smelled a cleansing gel with lavender aroma were more relaxed and able to complete math computations faster (Field et al., 2005).

Lavender: Subjects exposed to 3 minutes of lavender aroma were more relaxed and able to perform math computations faster and more accurately (Diego et al., 1998).

Lavender: Mice who inhaled lavender were found to have a decreased motility (natural movement) dependent on exposure time. Additionally, mice injected with caffeine (causing a hyperactivity) were found to reduce their movement to near normal levels after inhaling lavender (Buchbauer et al., 1991).

Ylang ylang: Subjects who had ylang ylang oil applied to their skin had decreased blood pressure, increased skin temperature, and reported feeling more calm and relaxed compared to subjects in a control group (Hongratanaworakit et al., 2006).

Lemon: Lemon oil was found to have an antistress effect in mice involved in several behavioral tasks (Komiya et al., 2006).

Respiratory System

The respiratory system's primary purposes are to supply the blood with oxygen that is then delivered to all parts of the body and to remove waste carbon dioxide from the blood and eliminate it from the body. The respiratory system consists of the mouth, nose, and pharynx (through which air is first taken in), larynx (voice box), trachea (airway leading from the larynx to the lungs), bronchi (which branch off from the trachea and into the lungs), bronchioles (smaller tubes that branch off from the bronchi), alveoli (tiny sacs filled with capillaries that allow inhaled oxygen to be transferred into the blood and carbon dioxide to be expelled from the blood into the air in the lungs), pleura (which covers the outside of the lungs and the inside of the chest wall), and diaphragm (a large muscle at the bottom of the chest cavity that moves to pull air into the lungs (inhale) and to push air out of the lungs (exhale)).

Oils: ⊘⊙Respiratory Blend, ⊘⊙eucalyptus⊙, ⊘⊙peppermint⊙, ⊘⊙white fir, ⊘⊙cinnamon⊙, ⊘⊙Protective Blend, ⊘⊙cardamom⊙, ⊘⊙melaleuca, ⊘⊙clary sage, ⊘⊙fennel, ⊘⊙helichrysum, ⊘⊙marjoram, ⊘⊙oregano, ⊘⊙bergamot⊙, ⊘⊙clove, ⊘⊙frankincense, ⊘⊙lemon, ⊘⊙rosemary, ⊘⊙lime

Blend 1: Combine 5 drops eucalyptus, 8 drops frankincense, and 6 drops lemon. Apply to bottoms of feet; or add to 1 oz. (2 Tbs.) fractionated coconut oil, and apply as a hot compress on chest.

Recipe 1: Combine 10 drops eucalyptus and 10 drops myrrh with 1 Tbs. fractionated coconut oil. Insert rectally for overnight retention enema.

Other Products: ○Respiratory Lozenge Drops, ○Seasonal Blend Softgels

—Asthma: *see Asthma*

—Breathing:

Oils: ⊘⊙Respiratory Blend, ⊘⊙cinnamon, ⊘⊙frankincense, ⊘⊙rosemary, ⊘⊙thyme, ⊘⊙marjoram, ⊘⊙juniper berry, ⊘⊙ginger

Other Products: ○Respiratory Lozenge Drops

—Bronchitis: *see Bronchitis*

—Cystic Fibrosis:

Cystic fibrosis is an inherited genetic condition that causes glands the lungs and other organs to secrete less hydrated, more sticky secretions. The stickiness of these secretions cause blockages and inflammation, damaging the lungs and other organs over time.

Oils: ⊘⊙bergamot⊙

—Hyperpnea:

Hyperpnea is rapid or heavy breathing that occurs normally as a result of strenuous physical exertion and abnormally in conjunction with fever and disorders.

Oils: ⊘⊙ylang ylang

—Lungs:

The lungs are paired organs located on either side of the heart. The lungs function to exchange oxygen and carbon dioxide (breathing). Oxygen passes into the blood by inhaling, and exhaling expels carbon dioxide. The lungs keep the body supplied with the oxygen necessary to keep cells alive. The lung on the right side of the body contains three lobes (sections) and is slightly larger than the lung on the left side of the body, which has two lobes.

Oils: ⓏⒸRespiratory Blend, ⓏⒸeucalyptus, ⓏⒸsandalwood, ⓏⒸfrankincense, ⓏⒸJoyful Blend, ⓏⒸProtective Blend (for infections)

Other Products: ⓄDetoxification Complex to help support healthy lung functioning.

—Oxygen:

Oils: Ⓩfrankincense, Ⓩsandalwood, Ⓩcedarwood

—Pleurisy:

Pleurisy is an inflammation of the moist membrane (pleura) that surrounds the lungs and lines the rib cage. Pleurisy is characterized by a dry cough, chest pain, and difficulty breathing. Viral infection is the most common cause of pleurisy; but lung infections, chest injuries, and drug reactions are also possible causes. Pleurisy usually lasts between a few days and a couple weeks.

Oils: ⓏⒸcypress, ⓏⒸthyme

—Pneumonia: *see Pneumonia*

Ⓩ: Diffuse into the air. Inhale directly from bottle. Apply oil to hands, tissue, or cotton wick, and inhale.

Ⓒ: Dilute as recommended, and apply to chest, sinuses, neck, or reflex points on the feet. Add 2–3 drops to water, and gargle. Apply to chest as warm compress. Add 20 drops to 1 Tbs. fractionated coconut oil, and insert rectally for overnight retention enema.

Ⓞ: Take supplements as directed on package.

Ⓣ: **Additional Research:**

Eucalyptus: Extracts from eucalyptus and thyme were found to have high nitrous oxide (NO) scavenging abilities and inhibited NO production in macrophage cells. This could possibly explain their role in aiding respiratory inflammatory diseases (Vigo et al., 2004).

Eucalyptus: Eucalyptus oil was found to have an anti-inflammatory and mucin-inhibitory effect in rats with lipopolysaccharide-induced bronchitis (Lu et al., 2004).

Eucalyptus: Therapy with 1,8 cineole (eucalyptol) in both healthy and bronchitis-afflicted humans was shown to reduce production of LTB4 and PGE2—both metabolites of arachidonic acid, a known chemical messenger involved in inflammation—in white blood cells (Juergens et al., 1998).

Peppermint: L-menthol was found to inhibit production of inflammation mediators in human monocytes (a type of white blood cell involved in the immune response) (Juergens et al., 1998).

Cinnamon: Vapor of cinnamon bark oil and cinnamic aldehyde was found to be effective against fungi involved in respiratory tract mycoses (fungal infections) (Singh et al., 1995).

Cinnamon: Cinnamon bark, lemongrass, and thyme oils were found to have the highest level of activity against common respiratory pathogens among 14 essential oils tested (Inouye et al., 2001).

Cardamom: Administration of cardamom to mice was found to have a protective effect against pan masala– (an herbal and tobacco blend sold in India) induced damage in the lungs of mice (Kumari et al., 2013).

Bergamot: Bergamot extract was found to display inhibitory activity on IL-8 gene expression (IL-8 is involved in the inflammatory processes associated with cystic fibrosis), indicating that bergamot may possess possible anti-inflammatory properties to reduce lung inflammation in cystic fibrosis patients (Borgatti et al., 2011).

Restlessness

see **calming**

Rheumatic Fever

see also **Antibacterial**

Rheumatic fever is the inflammation of the heart and joints in response to a strep throat or scarlet fever infection. This inflammation can cause permanent damage to the heart. Symptoms of rheumatic fever include painful and swollen joints, chest pain, fever, fatigue, the sensation of a pounding heartbeat, shortness of breath, rash, sudden jerky body movements, and unusual displays of emotion. Rheumatic fever is most common in children between ages 5 and 15.

Oils: ◐ginger (for pain)

◐: Dilute as recommended, and apply 1–2 drops on location.

Rheumatism

see **Arthritis:Rheumatoid Arthritis**

Rhinitis

see **Nose:Rhinitis**

Ringworm

see **Antifungal:Ringworm**

Sadness

see **Grief/Sorrow**

Salmonella

see **Antibacterial, Food Poisoning**

Scabies

see **Skin:Scabies**

Scarring

see **Skin:Scarring, Tissue:Scarring**

Schmidt's Syndrome

see **Adrenal Glands:Schmidt's Syndrome**

Sciatica

Sciatica is pain resulting from the irritation of the sciatic nerve. The sciatic nerve is the longest nerve in the body. It runs from the spinal cord through the buttock and hip area and down the back of each leg. When the sciatic nerve is pinched or irritated due to something such as a herniated disk, the pain experienced along the sciatic nerve is called "sciatica." Symptoms of sciatica include pain in the area, numbness and weakness along the sciatic nerve, tingling sensations, or a loss of bladder or bowel control.

Oils: ◐peppermint, ◐Roman chamomile, ◐helichrysum, ◐thyme, ◐Soothing Blend (for pain), ◐Grounding Blend, ◐white fir, ◐sandalwood, ◐lavender, ◐wintergreen

◐: Dilute as recommended, and apply 1–2 drops on lower back, buttocks, or legs. Add 5–10 drops to 1 Tbs. fractionated coconut oil, and massage on spine, back, legs, and bottoms of feet.

Scrapes

see **Wounds**

Scurvy

Scurvy is a disease caused by a deficiency of ascorbic acid (vitamin C). Some results of scurvy are general weakness, anemia, gum disease (gingivitis), skin hemorrhages, spots on the skin (usually the thighs and legs), and bleeding from the mucus membranes.

Oils: ⚬ginger

Other Products: ⃝Food Nutrient Complex contains vitamin C necessary for preventing scurvy.

⬮: Dilute as recommended, and apply 1–2 drops over kidneys, liver, and reflex points on the feet.

⬤: Take capsules as directed on package.

Sedative

see **Calming:Sedative**

Seizure

A seizure is an uncontrolled, abnormal electrical discharge in the brain which may produce a physical convulsion, minor physical signs, thought disturbances, or a combination of symptoms. The symptoms depend on what parts of the brain are involved.

Oils: ⚬clary sage, ⚬lavender⚬, ⚬rose⚬, ⚬⃝peppermint⚬, ⚬Grounding Blend, ⚬clove⚬, ⚬Calming Blend, ⚬Joyful Blend

Other Products: ⃝Energy & Stamina Complex to help support healthy nerve function. ⃝Essential Oil Omega Complex or Vegan Essential Oil Omega Complex, ⃝Food Nutrient Complex contain omega fatty acids, minerals, and other nutrients that support healthy brain function.

—Convulsions:

A convulsion is the repeated, rapid contracting and relaxing of muscles resulting in the uncontrollable shaking of the body. Convulsions usually last about 30 seconds to 2 minutes and are often associated with seizures.

Oils: ⚬lavender⚬, ⚬clary sage, ⚬Grounding Blend

—Epilepsy:

Epilepsy is a neurological condition where the person has recurring, unpredictable seizures. Epilepsy has many possible causes; although in many cases the cause is unknown. Possible causes may include illness, injury to the brain, or abnormal brain development.

Oils: ⚬clary sage

—Grand Mal Seizure:

The grand mal seizure, also known as the tonic-clonic seizure, is the most common seizure. The tonic phase lasts about 10–20 seconds. During this stage, the person loses consciousness, and the muscles contract—causing the person to fall down. During the clonic phase, the person experiences violent convulsions. This phase usually lasts less than two minutes.

Oils: ☁Grounding Blend (on feet), ☁⊘Calming Blend (around navel), ☁Joyful Blend (over heart)

Other Products: ◯Food Nutrient Complex contains zinc and copper—an imbalance of zinc and copper has been theorized to play a role in grand mal seizures.

☁: Dilute as recommended, and apply 1–2 drops to back of neck, navel, heart, or reflex points on the feet.

◯: Take capsules as directed on package.

⊘: Diffuse into the air.

⊕: **Additional Research:**

> **Lavender:** Linalool (found in several essential oils) was found to inhibit induced convulsions in rats by directly interacting with the NMDA receptor complex (Brum et al., 2001).

> **Rose:** Aqueous and ethanolic extracts of *Rosa damascena* were found to have potential anticonvulsant effect in drug-induced seizure model mice (Hosseini et al., 2011).

> **Rose:** Injection of rose essential oil before induction of amygdala kindling seizures in male rats significantly retarded the development of seizure stages and possessed the ability to counteract kindling stimulation when compared to the control group (Ramezani et al., 2008).

> **Peppermint:** Mice pretreated with an injection of peppermint essential oil demonstrated no seizures and 100% post-treatment survival after being injected with a lethal dose of pentylenetetrazol (PTZ) to cause seizures. Seven other essential oils were also tested, but peppermint was the most successful at preventing seizures and death. All tested essential oil treated mice (except oregano which caused complete fatality before administering PTZ) demonstrated increased seizure latency and intensity when compared to the control (Koutroumanidou et al., 2013).

> **Clove:** The aqueous and ethanolic extracts of clove were found to induce an anticonvulsive effect by increasing seizure latency in drug-induced seizure model mice, when compared to control (Hosseini et al., 2012).

> **Dill:** The aqueous extract of *Anethum graveolens* was shown to have an anticonvulsant effect in a mouse model of epilepsy (Arash et al., 2013).

Sexual Issues

—Arousing Desire: *see Aphrodisiac*

—Frigidity:

Female frigidity is a female's lack of sexual drive or her inability to enjoy sexual activities. This disorder has many possible physical and psychological causes, including stress, fatigue, guilt, fear, worry, alcoholism, or drug abuse.

Oils: ⊘☁clary sage, ⊘☁ylang ylang, ⊘☁Women's Blend, ⊘☁rose

—Impotence:

Impotence in men, also known as erectile dysfunction, is the frequent inability to have or sustain an erection. This may be caused by circulation problems, nerve problems, low levels of testosterone, medications, or psychological stresses.

Oils: ☁◯clary sage, ☁◯clove, ☁◯rose, ☁◯ginger, ☁◯sandalwood

—Libido (low):

Libido is a term used by Sigmund Freud to describe human sexual desire. Causes for a lack of sexual desire can be both physical and psychological. Some possible causes include anemia, alcoholism, drug abuse, stress, anxiety, past sexual abuse, and relationship problems.

Oils: ⊘☁ylang ylang, ⊘☁Joyful Blend

Other Products: ○Energy & Stamina Complex

—**Men:**

Oils: ⊘©cinnamon, ⊘©ginger, ⊘©myrrh

—**Women:**

Oils: ⊘©clary sage, ©geranium

⊘: Diffuse into the air. Dissolve 2–3 drops in 2 tsp. pure grain or perfumers alcohol, combine with distilled water in a 1 or 2 oz. spray bottle, and spray into the air or on clothes or bed linens.

©: Dilute as recommended, and wear on temples, neck, or wrists as perfume or cologne. Combine 3–5 drops of your desired essential oil with 1 Tbs. fractionated coconut oil to use as a massage oil. Combine 1–2 drops with 1/4 cup Therapeutic Bath Salts, and dissolve in warm bathwater for a romantic bath.

○: Take capsules as directed. Place 1–2 drops oil in an empty capsule, and swallow.

Sexually Transmitted Diseases (STD)
see AIDS/HIV, Herpes Simplex

Shingles
see also Antiviral, Childhood Diseases:Chickenpox, Nervous System:Neuralgia

Shingles is a viral infection caused by the same virus that causes chickenpox. After a person has had chickenpox, the virus lies dormant in the nervous system. Years later, that virus can be reactivated by stress, immune deficiency, or disease and cause shingles. Symptoms of shingles start with tingling, pain, neuralgia, or itching of an area of skin and become visually obvious as red blisters form in that same area along the nerve path, forming a red band on the skin. Blisters most commonly appear wrapping from the middle of the back to the middle of the chest but can form on the neck, face, and scalp as well. Another name for shingles is herpes zoster.

Oils: ©melaleuca, ©eucalyptus, ©lavender, ©lemon, ©geranium, ©bergamot

Blend 1: Combine 10 drops lavender, 10 drops melaleuca, and 10 drops thyme with 1 Tbs. fractionated coconut oil. Apply on feet and on location.

©: Dilute as recommended, and apply 1–2 drops on location. Add 5–10 drops essential oil to 1 Tbs. fractionated coconut oil, and massage on location and on bottoms of feet.

Shock
see also Cardiovascular System: Circulation, Cardiovascular System:Heart

Shock is a life-threatening condition where the body suffers from severely low blood pressure. This can be caused by low blood volume due to bleeding or dehydration, inadequate pumping of the heart, or dilation of the blood vessels due to head injury, medications, or poisons from bacterial infections. Shock can cause pale or bluish skin that feels cold or clammy to the touch, confusion, rapid breathing, and a rapid heartbeat. Without the needed oxygen being sent to the body's tissues and cells, the organs can shut down and, in severe cases, can lead to death. Shock often accompanies severe injuries or other traumatic situations. A person suffering from shock should be made to lie down with the feet elevated above the head, be kept warm, and have the head turned to the side in case of vomiting. Check breathing often, and ensure that any visible bleeding is stopped. Get emergency medical help as soon as possible.

Oils: ⊘⊘peppermint, ⊘Roman chamomile ⊘helichrysum (may help stop bleeding), ⊘me-laleuca, ⊘Joyful Blend, ⊘⊘ylang ylang, ⊘Grounding Blend, ⊘⊘myrrh, ⊘⊘melissa, ⊘⊘basil, ⊘rosemary

⊜: Dilute as recommended, and apply 1–2 drops on back of neck, feet, over heart, or on front of neck.

⊘: Diffuse into the air. Inhale directly from bottle. Apply oil to hands, tissue, or cotton wick, and inhale.

Shoulder
see **Joints:Shoulder**

Sinuses
Sinuses are several hollow cavities within the skull that allow the skull to be more lightweight without compromising strength. These cavities are connected to the nasal cavity through small channels. When the mucous membrane lining these channels becomes swollen or inflamed due to colds or allergies, these channels can become blocked—making it difficult for the sinuses to drain correctly. This can lead to infection and inflammation of the mucous membrane within the sinuses (sinusitis). There are sinus cavities behind the cheek bone and forehead and near the eyes and nasal cavity.

Oils: ⊘⊘helichrysum, ⊘⊘eucalyptus, ⊘⊘Respiratory Blend, ⊘⊘peppermint, ⊘⊘Protective Blend, ⊘cedarwood

—Sinusitis:
 Oils: ⊘⊘eucalyptus, ⊘⊘rosemary, ⊘⊘Respiratory Blend, ⊘Digestive Blend, ⊘⊘peppermint, ⊘⊘melaleuca, ⊘⊘white fir, ⊘⊘ginger

 Recipe 1: For chronic sinusitis, apply 1–2 drops Digestive Blend around navel four times daily; apply 2 drops peppermint under tongue two times daily.

⊘: Diffuse into the air. Inhale directly from bottle. Apply oil to hands, tissue, or cotton wick, and inhale. Place 1–2 drops in a bowl of hot water, and inhale vapors.

⊜: Dilute as recommended, and apply 1–2 drops along the sides of the nose or forehead (often clears out sinuses immediately).

Skeletal System
see **Bones**

Skin
see also Acne, Antibacterial, Antifungal, Boils, Burns, Foot, Cancer:Skin/Melanoma
The skin is the organ the covers the body, offering the first layer of protection to the internal organs and tissues from exposure to the environment and fungal, bacterial, and other types of infection. It helps regulate body heat and helps prevent evaporation of water from the body. The skin also carries nerve endings that allow the body to sense touch, heat, and pain. The skin is comprised of three layers. The upper layer is the epidermis, the middle layer is the dermis, and the deeper layer is the hypodermis (or subcutis layer).

Oils: ☺peppermint, ☺melaleuca, ☺Topical Blend, ☺Anti-Aging Blend, ☺sandalwood, ☺frankincense, ☺lavender, ☺myrrh, ☺geranium, ☺rosemary, ☺Grounding Blend, ☺ylang ylang, ☺marjoram, ☺cypress, ☺juniper berry, ☺cedarwood, O Detoxification Blend, ☺vetiver, ☺arborvitae, ☺helichrysum, ☺lemon, ☺orange, ☺lime, ☺patchouli

Other Products: ☺Anti-Aging Moisturizer, ☺Facial Cleanser, ☺Hydrating Cream, ☺Hydrating Serum, ☺Invigorating Scrub, ☺Skin Toner, ☺Two-Part Facial System, and ☺Skin Serum for vibrant, youthful-looking skin. ☺Face Wash to help improve tone and texture of the skin. ☺Protective Hand Wash to help protect against harmful microorganisms on the skin. ☺Invigorating and ☺Calming Bath Bars, or ☺Hand and Body Lotion to help cleanse and moisturize the skin. ☺Soothing Skin Ointment to help cleanse and support the skin's natural healing process. OEssential Oil Omega Complex or Vegan Essential Oil Omega Complex, OOmega-3 Fish Oil, OCellular Vitality Complex, OChewable Multivitamin, OFood Nutrient Complex contain omega fatty acids and other nutrients essential for healthy skin cell function. ODetoxification Complex to help support healthy cleansing and filtering of the skin.

☺: Dilute as recommended, and apply 1–2 drops on location. Add 5–10 drops to 2 Tbs. fractionated coconut oil, and use as massage oil. Add 1 drop essential oil to 1 tsp. unscented lotion, and apply on the skin. Add 1–2 drops to 1 Tbs. bath or shower gel, and apply to skin. Apply foaming hand wash to skin instead of soap, or use bath bars when washing hands or bathing.

O: Take capsules as directed on package. Add 3–5 drops of oil to an empty capsule; swallow capsule.

—**Acne:** *see* Acne

—**Boils:** *see* Boils

—**Burns:** *see* Burns

—**Callouses:**

A callous is a flat, thick growth of skin that develops on areas of the skin where there is constant friction or rubbing. Callouses typically form on the bottoms of the feet but can also form on the hands or other areas of the body exposed to constant friction.

Oils: ☺oregano, ☺Topical Blend, ☺Roman chamomile

☺: Dilute as recommended, and apply 1–2 drops on area.

—**Chapped/Cracked:**

Chapped or cracked skin is the result of the depletion of natural oils (sebum) in the skin, leading to dehydration of the skin beneath it. Some common causes for chapped skin include exposure to the cold or wind, repeated contact with soap or chemicals that break down oils, or a lack of essential fatty acids in the body.

Oils: ☺myrrh, ☺Topical Blend, ☺Anti-Aging Blend

Other Products: ☺Hand and Body Lotion and ☺Hydrating Cream and ☺Hydrating Serum to help moisturize and protect. ☺Soothing Skin Ointment to help cleanse and support the skin's natural healing process. OEssential Oil Omega Complex or Vegan Essential Oil Omega Complex or OOmega-3 Fish Oil to help supply essential omega fatty acids necessary for healthy skin. ⦿Invigorating and ⦿Calming Bath Bars contain natural oils that help moisturize and soften the skin.

⊜: Dilute as recommended, and apply 1–2 drops on location. Add 5–10 drops to 1 Tbs. fractionated coconut oil, and massage on location.

◯: Take capsules as directed on package.

—Corns: *see Foot:Corns*

—Dehydrated:

Oils: ⊜geranium, ⊜lavender, ⦿Anti-Aging Blend

Other Products: ⦿Hand and Body Lotion and ⦿Hydrating Cream and ⦿Hydrating Serum to help moisturize and protect. ⦿Invigorating and ⦿Calming Bath Bars contain natural oils that help moisturize and soften.

⊜: Dilute as recommended, and apply 1–2 drops on location. Add 5–10 drops to 2 Tbs. fractionated coconut oil, and use as massage oil. Add 1 drop essential oil to 1 tsp. unscented lotion, and apply on the skin. Add 1–2 drops to 1 Tbs. bath or shower gel, and apply to skin.

—Dermatitis/Eczema:

Dermatitis is any inflammation of the upper layers of the skin that results in redness, itching, pain, or possibly blistering. It can be caused by contact with an allergen or irritating substance, fungal infection, dehydration, or possibly another medical condition.

Oils: ⦿Topical Blend, ⦿helichrysum, ⦿juniper berry, ⦿thyme, ⦿geranium, ⦿arborvitae, ⦿melaleuca, ⦿lavender, ⦿patchouli, ⦿bergamot, ⦿rosemary

⊜: Add 5–10 drops to 1 Tbs. fractionated coconut oil, and apply on location. Dilute as recommended, and apply 1–2 drops on location.

—Diaper Rash: *see Children and Infants:Diaper Rash*

—Dry:

Oils: ⊜geranium, ⊜lavender, ⦿Roman chamomile, ⦿Anti-Aging Blend, ⊜sandalwood, ⊜lemon

Other Products: ⦿Anti-Aging Moisturizer and ⦿Hydrating Cream and ⦿Hydrating Serum to help relieve dryness and reduce the visible signs of aging. ⦿Hand and Body Lotion to help moisturize and protect. ⦿Reveal Facial System to help promote healthy skin matrix building and moisture retention.

⊜: Add 5–10 drops to 1 Tbs. fractionated coconut oil, and use as massage oil. Add 2–3 drops essential oil to 1 tsp. Hand and Body Lotion, and apply on the skin.

—Energizing:

Oils: ⊜bergamot, ⊜lemon

Other Products: ⦿Invigorating Scrub to polish and exfoliate the skin. ⦿Invigorating Bath Bar contains natural oatmeal kernels that help exfoliate.

⊜: Dilute as recommended, and apply 1–2 drops on location. Add 5–10 drops to 2 Tbs. fractionated coconut oil, and use as massage oil. Add 1 drop essential oil to 1 tsp. Hand

and Body Lotion, and apply on the skin. Add 1–2 drops to 1 Tbs. bath or shower gel, and apply to skin. Massage Invigorating Scrub over wet skin for up to one minute before rinsing with warm water.

—Facial Oils: *see also Dehydrated, Dry, Energizing, Oily/Greasy, and Revitalizing in this section for other oils that can be used for specific skin types/conditions.*

Oils: ⬥myrrh, ⬥sandalwood, ⬥vetiver

⬥: Add 5–10 drops to 1 Tbs. fractionated coconut oil, and apply to face. Add 1–2 drops essential oil to 1 tsp. unscented lotion, and apply on the skin.

—Fungal Infections: *see Antifungal:Athlete's Foot, Antifungal:Ringworm*

—Impetigo:

Impetigo is a bacterial skin infection that causes sores and blisters full of a yellowish fluid. These sores can be itchy and painful and can easily be spread to other areas of the skin or to another person.

Oils: ⬥geranium, ⬥lavender, ⬥Topical Blend, ⬥myrrh

⬥: Boil 4 oz. of water; cool; and add 5–10 drops essential oil: wash sores with this water, and then cover sores for an hour. Apply oils as a hot compress on location.

—Itching:

An itch is a tingling and unpleasant sensation that evokes the desire to scratch. Itching can be caused by various skin disorders or diseases, parasites such as scabies and lice, allergic reactions to chemicals or drugs, dry skin, insect bites, etc. Scratching the itching area too hard or too often can damage the skin.

Oils: ⬥peppermint, ⬥lavender, ⬥Calming Blend

Other Products: ⬥Invigorating Bath Bar contains natural oatmeal kernels that can help exfoliate skin and soothe itching.

⬥: Dilute as recommended, and apply 1–2 drops on location and on ears. Wash body with Bath Bar.

—Melanoma: *see Cancer:Skin/Melanoma*

—Moles:

Moles are small growths on the skin of pigment-producing skin cells that usually appear brown or black in color. Moles typically appear within a person's first 20 years of life and usually stay with a person throughout his or her life. While moles are not dangerous, melanoma (a type of skin cancer that develops in pigment cells) can resemble a mole at first. Moles that vary in color or that appear to change fairly quickly in size or shape could be cancerous and should be examined.

Oils: ⬥frankincense, ⬥sandalwood, ⬥geranium, ⬥lavender

⬥: Dilute as recommended, and apply 1 drop on location.

—Oily/Greasy:

Oils: ⬥lemon, ⬥Topical Blend, ⬥cypress, ⬥Topical Blend, ⬥frankincense, ⬥geranium, ⬥lavender, ⬥marjoram, ⬥orange, ⬥rosemary

Other Products: ⊘Face Wash to help balance skin sebum levels. ⊘Facial Cleanser to cleanse the skin and leave it feeling smooth and fresh.

⊘: Add 5–10 drops to 1 Tbs. fractionated coconut oil, and use as massage oil. Use Facial Cleanser as directed on package.

—Psoriasis: *see Psoriasis*

—Rashes:

A rash is an area of irritated skin, redness, or red bumps on the body. Rashes may be localized or may cover large patches of the body. A rash may be caused by a chemical or allergen irritating the skin or may occur as a symptom of another medical condition or infection.

Oils: ⊘melaleuca, ⊘lavender, ⊘Roman chamomile

⊘: Dilute as recommended, and apply 1–2 drops on location. Add 1–5 drops to 1 Tbs. fractionated coconut oil, and apply on location.

—Revitalizing:

Oils: ⊘cypress, ⊘lemon, ⊘Anti-Aging Blend, ⊘Topical Blend, ⊘fennel, ⊘lime

Other Products: ⊘Invigorating Scrub to polish and exfoliate the skin. ⊘Two-Part Facial System to help promote healthy skin matrix building and moisture retention. ⊘Invigorating Bath Bar contains natural oatmeal kernels that help exfoliate.

⊘: Add 5–10 drops to 1 Tbs. fractionated coconut oil, and use as massage oil. Add 2–3 drops essential oil to 1 tsp. unscented lotion, and apply on the skin. Massage Invigorating Scrub over wet skin for up to one minute before rinsing with warm water.

—Ringworm: *see Antifungal:Ringworm*

—Scabies:

Scabies is an infestation of the skin by mites (*Sarcoptes scabei*) that burrow into the upper layers of the skin, causing small, extremely itchy bumps.

Oils: ⊘Protective Blend, ⊘Topical Blend, ⊘melaleuca, ⊘peppermint, ⊘lavender, ⊘bergamot

⊘: Add 5–10 drops to 1 Tbs. fractionated coconut oil, and apply a small amount on location morning and night. Dilute as recommended, and apply 1–2 drops on location.

—Scarring:

Scars are fibrous connective tissue that is used to quickly repair a wound or injury in place of the regular skin or tissue.

Oils: ⊘lavender (burns), ⊘rose (helps prevent), ⊘frankincense (helps prevent), ⊘helichrysum (reduces), ⊘geranium, ⊘myrrh

Other Products: ⊘Soothing Skin Ointment to help cleanse and support the skin's natural healing process.

Blend 1: Combine 5 drops helichrysum and 5 drops lavender with 1 Tbs. sunflower oil or with liquid lecithin (an emulsifier extracted from eggs or soy), and apply on location.

Blend 2: Combine 1 drop lavender, 1 drop lemongrass, and 1 drop geranium; apply on location to help prevent scar formation.

🜄: Dilute as recommended, and apply 1–2 drops on location.

—**Sensitive**:

Oils: 🜂lavender, 🜂geranium

🜄: Dilute as recommended, and apply 1–2 drops on location.

—**Skin Ulcers**:

A skin ulcer is an open sore where the epidermis and possibly part or all of the dermis is missing, exposing the deeper layers of the skin. This can be caused by burns, pressure, friction, irritation, or infections damaging the upper layers of the skin.

Oils: 🜂lavender, 🜂myrrh, 🜂Topical Blend, 🜂helichrysum, 🜂Cleansing Blend

🜄: Dilute as recommended, and apply 1–2 drops on location.

—**Stretch Marks**:

Stretch marks are thin purple or red areas of the skin that appear as the skin is rapidly stretched over a short period of time, stretching and tearing the dermis layer (middle layer) of the skin. Many women notice the appearance of stretch marks in the last few months of pregnancy, but stretch marks can also appear on men or women during any period of rapid weight gain. These marks most often appear on the breasts, stomach, buttocks, thighs, and hips. Stretch marks tend to fade over time, but it is difficult to eliminate them completely.

Oils: 🜂lavender, 🜂myrrh

🜄: Add 5–10 drops to 1 Tbs. fractionated coconut oil or hazelnut oil, and apply on location.

—**Sunburn**: *see Burns:Sunburn*

—**Tones**:

Oils: 🜂lemon

🜄: Add 4–5 drops to 1 Tbs. fractionated coconut oil, and use as massage oil (avoid direct sunlight for 24 hours after application).

—**Vitiligo**:

Vitiligo is white patches of the skin caused by the death or dysfunction of pigment-producing cells in the area. While the exact cause is unknown, vitiligo may be caused by an immune or genetic disorder or may have a relationship to thyroid problems.

Oils: 🜂sandalwood, 🜂vetiver, 🜂frankincense, 🜂myrrh, 🜂Cleansing Blend

🜄: Dilute as recommended, and apply 1–2 drops behind ears and on back of neck or on reflex points on the feet; then cup hands together, and inhale the aroma from the hands.

—**Wrinkles**:

A wrinkle is a fold or crease in the skin that develops as part of the normal aging process. Wrinkles are thought to be caused by a breakdown of collagen (a protein that gives structure to cells and tissue) in the skin, causing the skin to become more fragile and loose.

Oils: ♻Anti-Aging Blend, ♻lavender, ♻myrrh◉, ♻fennel, ♻dill◉, ♻geranium, ♻frankincense, ♻rose, ♻rosemary, ♻clary sage, ♻cypress, ♻helichrysum, ♻lemon, ♻orange, ♻oregano, ♻sandalwood, ♻thyme, ♻ylang ylang

Other Products: ♻Anti-Aging Moisturizer to help relieve dryness and reduce the visible signs of aging. ♻Tightening Serum to help tighten the skin to eliminate fine line and wrinkles. ♻Hydrating Cream to help promote fuller, smoother looking skin. ♻Reveal Facial System to help promote healthy skin matrix building and moisture retention.

Blend 1: Combine 1 drop frankincense, 1 drop lavender, and 1 drop lemon. Rub on morning and night around the eyes (be careful not to get in eyes).

Blend 2: Combine 1 drop sandalwood, 1 drop helichrysum, 1 drop geranium, 1 drop lavender, and 1 drop frankincense. Add to 2 tsp. unscented lotion, and apply to skin.

⬤: Dilute as recommended, and apply 1–2 drops to skin. Add 5–10 drops to 1 Tbs. fractionated coconut oil or other carrier oil such as jojoba, apricot, hazelnut, or sweet almond, and apply on areas of concern. Add 3–5 drops to 1/2 cup Therapeutic Bath Salts, and dissolve in warm bathwater before bathing.

⬜: **Additional Research:**

Myrrh: Myrrh essential oil was shown to be an efficient quencher of singlet oxygen (a type of antioxidant action) by its ability to decrease formation of squalene peroxide in UV irradiated sebum on the facial skin of human subjects. These findings suggest that topical application of myrrh essential oil can help decrease sebum damage and in turn protect skin from aging (Auffray 2007).

Dill: An in vitro study using human fibroblast cells from adult skin showed that dill extract was able to stimulate LOXL gene expression to induce elastogenesis in adult skin cells. These findings suggest that dill extract may be able to increase skin elasticity and firming (Cenizo et al., 2006).

Cilantro: Cilantro extract was found to protect human keratinocytes (epidermis cells) against H2O2-induced oxidative stress, suggesting that cilantro may be useful at protecting skin cells from oxidative damage (Park et al., 2012).

Sleep

see also **Insomnia, Ions:Negative Ions**

Sleep is a regular period in which the body suspends conscious motor and sensory activity. Sleep is thought to play a role in restoring and healing the body and processing the memories of the day.

Oils: ♻⬤lavender◉, ♻⬤Calming Blend, ♻⬤Roman chamomile◉, ⬤marjoram

Recipe 1: Combine 5 drops geranium and 5 drops lavender with 1/4 cup Therapeutic Bath Salts; dissolve in warm bathwater, and bathe in the evening to help promote a good night's sleep.

⬤: Dilute as recommended, and apply 1–2 drops essential oil to spine, bottoms of feet, or back of neck. Add 1–2 drops to warm bathwater, and bathe before sleeping. Add 5–10 drops to 1 Tbs. fractionated coconut oil, and massage on back, arms, legs, and feet.

✿: Diffuse into the air. Add 1–2 drops to bottom of pillow before sleeping. Add 2–5 drops to 1 oz. distilled water in a small spray bottle, and mist into the air or on linens before sleeping.

⬜: **Additional Research:**

Lavender and Roman Chamomile: A study with 56 percutaneous coronary intervention patients in an intensive care unit found that an aromatherapy blend of lavender, Roman chamomile, and neroli decreased anxiety and improved sleep quality when compared to conventional nursing intervention (Cho et al., 2013).

Slimming and Toning Oils
see **Weight:Slimming/Toning**

Smell (loss of)
see **Nose:Olfactory loss**

Smoking
see **Addictions:Smoking, Purification:Cigarette Smoke**

Snake Bite
see **Bites/Stings:Snakes**

Sores
see **Wounds, Antibacterial, Antifungal, Antiviral**

Sore Throat
see **Throat:Sore, Antibacterial, Antiviral, Infection**

Spasms
see **Muscles/Connective Tissue, Digestive System**

Spina Bifida

Spina bifida is a birth defect in which the vertebrae of the lower spine do not form correctly, leaving a gap or opening between them. In the most severe cases, this can cause the meninges (the tissue surrounding the spinal cord), or even the spinal cord itself, to protrude through the gap. If the spinal cord protrudes through the gap, it can prevent the nerves from developing normally, causing numbness, paralysis, back pain, and loss of bladder and bowel control and function. This latter type often also develops with a defect in which the back part of the brain develops in the upper neck rather than within the skull, often causing a mental handicap.

Oils: ⊖⊘eucalyptus, ⊖⊘lavender, ⊖⊘Roman chamomile, ⊖⊘lemon, ⊖⊘orange, ⊖⊘rosemary

Other Products: ○Cellular Vitality Complex contains 400 mg of folic acid, which has been found to significantly reduce the chance of spina bifida developing in infants if taken as a daily supplement by their mothers before conception(Centers for Disease Control and Prevention, 2004).

○: Take capsules as directed on package

⊖: Dilute as recommended, and apply 1–2 drops to bottoms of feet, along spine, on forehead, and on back of neck.

⊘: Diffuse into the air.

Spine
see **Back**

Spleen
see also **Lymphatic System**

The spleen is a fist-sized spongy tissue that is part of the lymphatic system. Its purpose is to filter bacteria, viruses, fungi, and other unwanted substances out of the blood and to create lymphocytes (white blood cells that create antibodies).

Oils: ♥marjoram

🌀: Dilute as recommended and apply 1–2 drops over spleen or on reflex points on the feet. Apply as a warm compress over upper abdomen.

Sprains
see **Muscles/Connective Tissue:Sprains**

Spurs
See **Bones:Bone Spurs**

Stains
see **Housecleaning:Stains**

Staph Infection
See **Antibacterial:Staph Infection**

Sterility
see **Female Specific Conditions:Infertility, Male Specific Conditions:Infertility**

Stimulating

Oils: ♨♥peppermint, ♨♥Joyful Blend, ♨♥eucalyptus○, ♨♥orange, ♨♥ginger, ♨♥grapefruit, ♨♥rose, ♨♥rosemary○, ♨♥basil

🌿: Diffuse into the air. Inhale directly from bottle. Apply oil to hands, tissue, or cotton wick, and inhale.

🌀: Dilute as recommended, and apply 1–2 drops to forehead, neck, or bottoms of feet. Add 1–2 drops to an unscented bath gel, and add to warm bathwater while filling; bathe. Add 5–10 drops to 1 Tbs. fractionated coconut oil, and use as massage oil.

📖: **Additional Research:**

Eucalyptus: Imaging of the brain demonstrated that inhalation of 1,8-cineol (eucalyptol—a constituent of many essential oils, especially eucalyptus, rosemary, and marjoram) increased global cerebral blood flow after an inhalation-time of 20 minutes (Nasel et al., 1994).

Rosemary: Imaging of the brain demonstrated that inhalation of 1,8-cineol (eucalyptol—a constituent of many essential oils, especially eucalyptus, rosemary, and marjoram) increased global cerebral blood flow after an inhalation-time of 20 minutes (Nasel et al., 1994).

Stings
see **Bites/Stings**

Stomach
see **Digestive System:Stomach**

Strep Throat
see **Throat:Strep**

Stress

Stress is the body's response to difficult, pressured, or worrisome circumstances. Stress can cause both physical and emotional tension. Symptoms of stress include headaches, muscle soreness, fatigue, insomnia, nervousness, anxiety, and irritability.

S

Oils: ◎❸lavender◷, ❸❸Focus Blend, ❸❸lemon◷, ❸❸ylang ylang◷, ❸❸bergamot, ❸❸Joyful Blend, ❸❸Calming Blend, ❸❸grapefruit, ❸Massage Blend, ❸❸Roman chamomile, ❸❸geranium, ❸❸Grounding Blend, ❸❸frankincense, ❸❸marjoram

—Chemical:

Oils: ❸❸lavender, ❸❸rosemary, ❸❸grapefruit, ❸❸geranium, ❸❸clary sage, ❸❸lemon

—Emotional Stress:

Oils: ❸❸Joyful Blend, ❸❸clary sage, ❸❸bergamot, ❸❸geranium, ❸❸Roman chamomile, ❸❸sandalwood

—Environmental Stress:

Oils: ❸❸bergamot, ❸❸cypress, ❸❸geranium, ❸cedarwood

—Mental Stress:

Oils: ❸❸lavender◷, ❸❸Focus Blend, ❸❸grapefruit, ❸❸bergamot, ❸❸sandalwood, ❸❸geranium

—Performance Stress:

Oils: ❸❸grapefruit, ❸❸bergamot, ❸❸ginger, ❸❸rosemary

—Physical Stress:

Oils: ❸❸Calming Blend, ❸❸lavender, ❸❸bergamot, ❸❸geranium, ❸❸marjoram, ❸❸Roman chamomile, ❸❸rosemary, ❸❸thyme

—Stress Due to Tiredness or Insomnia:

Blend 1: Add 15 drops clary sage, 10 drops lemon, and 5 drops lavender to 2 Tbs. fractionated coconut oil. Massage on skin.

🖐: Diffuse into the air. Inhale directly from bottle. Apply oil to hands, tissue, or cotton wick, and inhale. Wear as perfume or cologne.

👄: Add 5–10 drops to 1 Tbs. fractionated coconut oil, and massage on skin. Add 1–2 drops to 1/4 cup Therapeutic Bath Salts, and dissolve in warm bathwater before bathing. Dilute as recommended, and apply 1–2 drops on neck, back, or bottoms of feet.

📖: **Additional Research:**

Lavender: Nurses working in an ICU setting demonstrated decreased perception of stress when receiving a topical application of Lavandula angustifolia and Salvia sclarea essential oils (Pemberton et al., 2008).

Lavender: Subjects placed in a small, soundproof room for 20 minutes were found to have reduced mental stress and increased arousal rate when exposed to the scent of lavender (Motomura et al., 2001).

Lemon: Lemon oil vapor was found to have strong antistress and antidepressant effects on mice subjected to several common behavioral stress tests (Komiya et al., 2006).

Ylang ylang: Subjects who had ylang ylang oil applied to their skin had decreased blood pressure, increased skin temperature, and reported feeling more calm and relaxed compared to subjects in a control group (Hongratanaworakit et al., 2006).

Stress Marks

see Skin:Stretch Marks

Stroke

see also **Brain, Blood:Clots, Cardiovascular System**

A stroke occurs when the blood supply to the brain is interrupted. Within a few minutes, brain cells begin to die. The affected area of the brain is unable to function, and one or more limbs on one side of the body become weak and unable to move. Strokes can cause serious disabilities, including paralysis and speech problems.

Oils: ⊘⊜cypress, ⊘⊜helichrysum, ⊙fennel⊙, ⊙cedarwood⊙, ⊙basil⊙

—Muscular Paralysis:

Oils: ⊜lavender

Blend 1: Combine 1 drop basil, 1 drop lavender, and 1 drop rosemary, and apply to spinal column and paralyzed area.

⊘: Inhale oil directly or applied to hands, tissue, or cotton wick. Diffuse into the air.

⊜: Dilute as directed, and apply 1–2 drops to the back of the neck and the forehead.

⊙: **Additional Research:**

Fennel: Both fennel oil and its constituent, anethole, were found to significantly reduce thrombosis (blood clots) in mice. They were also found to be free from the prohemorrhagic (increased bleeding) side effect that aspirin (acetylsalicylic acid) has (Tognolini et al., 2007).

Cedarwood: A chemical constituent, α-eudesmol, found in cedarwood oil demonstrated the ability to protect against brain injury after cerebral ischemia (stroke) in rats. Specifically, α-eudesmol was found to attenuate cerebral edema formation, reduce cerebral infarct size, and inhibit calcium-dependent glutamate release from synaptosomes (Asakura et al., 2000).

Basil: Oral pretreatment of basil extract was found to protect against brain damage induced by bilateral carotid artery occlusion in mice by reducing tissue death size and the oxidative degradation of lipids and restoring antioxidant content and motor functions. The researchers state that these results suggest that basil could be useful clinically in the prevention of stroke (Bora et al., 2011).

Sudorific

A sudorific is a substance that induces sweating.

Oils: ⊜thyme, ⊜rosemary, ⊜lavender, ⊜Roman chamomile, ⊜juniper berry

⊜: Add 5–10 drops to 1 Tbs. fractionated coconut oil, and apply to skin.

Suicidal Feelings

see **Depression**

Sunburn

see **Burns:Sunburn**

Sun Screen

Oils: ⊜helichrysum, ⊜arborvitae⊙, ⊜sandalwood

⊜: Add 5–10 drops to 1 Tbs. fractionated coconut oil, and apply to the skin.

⊙: **Additional Research:**

Sunscreen: Application of β-thujaplicin on mouse ear skin decreased sunburn cell formation by 40% as compared to untreated skin, suggesting that β-thujaplicin can inhibit ultraviolet B-induced apoptosis and skin damage (Baba et al., 1998).

Swelling

see **Edema, Inflammation**

Sympathetic Nervous System
see **Nervous System:Sympathetic Nervous System**

Tachycarida
see **Cardiovascular System:Tachycarida**

Taste (Impaired)
see also **Nose:Olfactory Loss**

Taste is the sensation of sweet, sour, salty, or bitter by taste buds on the tongue when a substance enters the mouth. This sensation, combined with the smell of the food, helps create the unique flavors we experience in food.

Oils: ⬤helichrysum, ⬤peppermint

⬤: Dilute as recommended, and apply 1 drop on the tongue or reflex points on the feet.

Teeth
see **Oral Conditions**

Temperature
See **Cooling Oils, Warming Oils**

Tendinitis
see **Muscles/Connective Tissue:Tendinitis**

Tennis Elbow
See **Joints:Tennis Elbow**

Tension

Oils: ⬤⬤Calming Blend, ⬤⬤lavender, ⬤Massage Blend, ⬤⬤cedarwood, ⬤⬤ylang ylang, ⬤⬤Roman chamomile, ⬤⬤frankincense, ⬤⬤basil (nervous), ⬤⬤bergamot (nervous), ⬤⬤grapefruit

⬤: Inhale oil applied to hands. Diffuse into the air.

⬤: Add 3–5 drops to 1/2 cup Therapeutic Bath Salts, and dissolve in warm bathwater before bathing. Add 5–10 drops to 1 Tbs. fractionated coconut oil, and use as massage oil.

Testes

Testes are the male reproductive organs. The testes are responsible for producing and storing sperm and male hormones such as testosterone. Hormones produced in the testes are responsible for the development of male characteristics: facial hair, wide shoulders, low voice, and reproductive organs.

Oils: ⬤⬤rosemary

—Regulation:

Oils: ⬤⬤clary sage, ⬤⬤sandalwood, ⬤⬤geranium

⬤: Dilute as recommended, and apply 1–2 drops on location or on reflex points on the feet.

⬤: Diffuse into the air. Inhale directly from bottle. Apply oil to hands, tissue, or cotton wick, and inhale.

Throat

see also **Respiratory System, Neck**

Oils: ◔cypress, ◔oregano

—**Congestion:**

    Oils: ◔◕peppermint, ◔◕myrrh

—**Cough:** *see* **Respiratory System**

—**Dry:**

    Oils: ○◔lemon, ○◔grapefruit

—**Infection In:**

    Oils: ◔◕○lemon, ○◔◕Protective Blend, ◔◕○peppermint, ◔◕oregano, ◔◕clary sage

Other Products: ○Protective Softgels

—**Laryngitis:** *see* **Laryngitis**

—**Sore:**

    Oils: ◔◕melaleuca, ○◔◕Protective Blend, ◔◕oregano, ◔◕sandalwood, ◔◕○lime, ◔◕bergamot, ◔◕geranium, ◔◕ginger, ◔◕myrrh

    Other Products: ○Protective Throat Drops to soothe irritated and sore throats.

—**Strep:**

    Strep throat is a throat infection caused by streptococci bacteria. This infection causes the throat and tonsils to become inflamed and swollen, resulting in a severe sore throat. Symptoms of strep throat include a sudden severe sore throat, pain when swallowing, high fever, swollen tonsils and lymph nodes, white spots on the back of the throat, skin rash, and sometimes vomiting. Strep throat should be closely monitored so that it doesn't develop into a more serious condition such as rheumatic fever or kidney inflammation.

    Oils: ○◔◕Protective Blend◔, ◔◕melaleuca, ◔◕ginger, ◔◕geranium, ◔◕oregano

—**Tonsillitis:**

    Tonsillitis is inflammation of the tonsils, typically due to infection. Tonsillitis causes the tonsils to become swollen and painful. Symptoms of tonsillitis include sore throat, red and swollen tonsils, painful swallowing, loss of voice, fever, chills, headache, and white patches on the tonsils.

    Oils: ◔◕melaleuca, ◔◕Protective Blend, ◔ginger, ◔◕lavender, ◔◕lemon, ◔◕bergamot, ◔◕clove, ◕thyme, ◔◕Roman chamomile

○:   Add 1 drop to 8 oz. water (32 oz. for Protective Blend), and drink. Place 1 drop oil under the tongue. Take supplement as directed.

◔:   Dilute as recommended, and apply 1–2 drops on throat or reflex points on the feet. Add 1–2 drops to 4 oz. (1/2 cup) water, and gargle.

◕:   Diffuse into the air. Inhale directly from bottle. Apply oil to hands, tissue, or cotton wick, and inhale.

Ⓘ: **Additional Research:**

Protective Blend: Cinnamon, thyme, and clove essential oils demonstrated an antibacterial effect on several respiratory tract pathogens including streptococci (Fabio et al., 2007).

Protective Blend: Eucalyptus globulus oil was found to inhibit several bacteria types, including strep (Cermelli et al., 2008).

Thrush

see **Antifungal:Candida, Antifungal:Thrush, Children and Infants:Thrush**

Thymus

see also **Immune System, Lymphatic System**

The thymus is an organ responsible for the development of T cells needed for immune system functioning. The thymus is located just behind the sternum in the upper part of the chest.

Oils: ⊘Protective Blend

🖐: Dilute as recommended, and apply over thymus or on bottoms of feet.

Thyroid

see also **Endocrine System**

The thyroid is a gland located in the front of the neck that plays a key role in regulating metabolism. The thyroid produces and secretes the hormones needed to regulate blood pressure, heart rate, body temperature, and energy production.

—**Dysfunction:**

Oils: ⊘⊘clove

—**Hyperthyroidism:** *see also* **Grave's Disease**

Hyperthyroidism is when the thyroid gland produces too much of its hormones, typically due to the thyroid becoming enlarged. This can result in a noticeably enlarged thyroid gland (goiter), sudden weight loss, sweating, a rapid or irregular heartbeat, shortness of breath, muscle weakness, nervousness, and irritability.

Oils: ⊘⊘myrrh, ⊘⊘lemongrass

Blend 1: Combine 1 drop myrrh and 1 drop lemongrass, and apply on base of throat and on reflex points on the feet.

—**Hypothyroidism:** *see also* **Hashimoto's Disease**

Hypothyroidism is the result of an underactive thyroid. Consequently, the thyroid gland doesn't produce enough of necessary hormones. Symptoms include fatigue, a puffy face, a hoarse voice, unexplained weight gain, higher blood cholesterol levels, muscle weakness and aches, depression, heavy menstrual periods, memory problems, and low tolerance for the cold.

Oils: ⊘⊘peppermint, ⊘⊘clove, ⊘⊘lemongrass

Blend 2: Combine 1 drop lemongrass with 1 drop of either peppermint or clove, and apply on base of throat and on reflex points on the feet.

—**Supports:**

Oils: ⊘myrrh

🜔: Dilute as recommended, and apply 1–2 drops on base of throat, hands, or reflex points on the feet.

📷: Diffuse into the air. Inhale oils applied to hands.

Tinnitus
see **Ears:Tinnitus**

Tired
see **Energy**

Tissue
Tissue refers to any group of similar cells that work together to perform a specific function in an organ or in the body. Some types of tissue include muscle tissue, connective tissue, nervous tissue, or epithelial tissue (tissue that lines or covers a surface, such as the skin or the lining of the blood vessels).

Oils: ♨lemongrass, ♨helichrysum, ♨basil, ♨marjoram, ♨sandalwood, ♨Roman chamomile, ♨lavender

Other Products: ○Soothing Rub to help soothe muscle and connective tissues.

—**Cleanses Toxins From:**
  Oils: ♨fennel

—**Connective Tissue:** *see* **Muscles/Connective Tissue**

—**Deep Tissue Pain:** *see* **Pain:Tissue**

—**Repair:**
  Oils: ♨lemongrass, ♨helichrysum, ♨orange

—**Regenerate:**
  Oils: ♨lemongrass, ♨helichrysum, ♨geranium, ♨patchouli

—**Scarring:**
  Scar tissue is the dense and fibrous tissue that forms over a healed cut or wound. The scar tissue serves as a protective barrier but is still inferior to the healthy, normal tissue. In an area of scar tissue, sweat glands are nonfunctional, hair does not grow, and the skin is not as protected against ultraviolet radiation. Scars fade and become less noticeable over time but cannot be completely removed.

  Oils: ♨lavender (burns), ♨rose (helps prevent), ♨frankincense (helps prevent), ♨helichrysum (reduces), ♨geranium, ♨myrrh

  Blend 1: Combine 5 drops helichrysum and 5 drops lavender with 1 Tbs. sunflower oil or with liquid lecithin (an emulsifier extracted from eggs or soy), and apply on location.

  Blend 2: Combine 1 drop lavender, 1 drop lemongrass, and 1 drop geranium, and apply on location to help prevent scar formation.

  🜔: Dilute as recommended, and apply 1–2 drops on location or on reflex points on the feet. Apply as warm compress. Add 5–10 drops to 1 Tbs. fractionated coconut oil, and massage on location.

Tonic

A tonic is a substance given to invigorate or strengthen an organ, tissue, or system or to stimulate physical, emotional, or mental energy and strength.

—General:

Oils: ⊝⊘lemongrass, ⊝⊘cinnamon, ⊝⊘sandalwood, ⊝⊘clary sage, ⊝⊘grapefruit, ⊝⊘ginger, ⊝⊘geranium, ⊝⊘marjoram, ⊝⊘myrrh, ⊝⊘orange, ⊝⊘Roman chamomile, ⊝⊘ylang ylang

—Heart:

Oils: ⊝⊘thyme, ⊝⊘lavender

—Nerve:

Oils: ⊝⊘clary sage, ⊝⊘melaleuca, ⊝⊘thyme

—Skin:

Oils: ⊝lemon

—Uterine:

Oils: ⊝⊘thyme

🔹: Add 5–10 drops to 1 Tbs. fractionated coconut oil, and massage on location. Dilute as recommended, and apply 1–2 drops to area or to reflex points on the feet. Add 1–2 drops to warm bathwater before bathing.

🔹: Diffuse into the air. Inhale directly from bottle. Apply oil to hands, tissue, or cotton wick, and inhale.

Tonsillitis
see **Throat:Tonsillitis**

Toothache
see **Oral Conditions:Toothache**

Toxemia
see also **Antibacterial, Pregnancy/Motherhood: Preeclampsia**

Toxemia is the general term for toxic substances in the bloodstream. This is typically caused by a bacterial infection in which bacteria release toxins into the blood.

Oils: ⊝⊘cypress

🔹: Dilute as recommended, and apply 1–2 drops on neck, over heart, or on bottoms of feet. Add 5–10 drops to 1 Tbs. fractionated coconut oil, and massage on neck, back, chest, and legs.

🔹: Diffuse into the air.

Toxins
see **Detoxification**

Travel Sickness
see **Nausea:Motion Sickness**

Tuberculosis (T.B.)

see also **Antibacterial, Respiratory System**

Tuberculosis is a bacterial disease spread through the air (via coughing, spitting, sneezing, etc.). Tuberculosis most commonly infects the lungs, but it can infect other bodily systems as well. Symptoms of tuberculosis include a chronic cough (often with blood), fever, chills, weakness and fatigue, weight loss, and night sweats. Tuberculosis is contagious and sometimes deadly.

Oils: ✿❄eucalyptus, ✿❄cypress, ✿❄Respiratory Blend, ✿❄thyme, ✿❄cedarwood, ✿❄Protective Blend, ✿lemon, ✿❄melissa, ✿❄vetiver○, ✿❄peppermint, ✿❄sandalwood

Other Products: ○Respiratory Lozenge Drops

—Airborne Bacteria:

Oils: ✿Protective Blend, ✿lemongrass○, ✿geranium○, ✿Cleansing Blend, ✿Respiratory Blend

—Pulmonary:

Oils: ✿❄oregano, ✿❄cypress, ✿❄eucalyptus, ✿❄frankincense

✿: Diffuse into the air. Inhale directly from bottle. Apply oil to hands, tissue, or cotton wick, and inhale. Add 2–3 drops to bowl of hot water, and inhale vapors.

❄: Dilute as recommended, and apply 1–2 drops on chest, back, or reflex points on the feet. Add 1–2 drops to 1 tsp. fractionated coconut oil, and apply as rectal implant. Add 5–10 drops to 1 Tbs. fractionated coconut oil, and massage on chest, back, and feet.

○: **Additional Research:**

Vetiver: The ethanolic extract of vetiver root was found to inhibit both virulent and avirulent strains of *M. tuberculosis*, suggesting that vetiver could be useful in treating tubercular infections (Saikia et al., 2012).

Lemongrass: A formulation of lemongrass and geranium oil was found to reduce airborne bacteria by 89% in an office environment after diffusion for 15 hours (Doran et al., 2009).

Geranium: A formulation of lemongrass and geranium oil was found to reduce airborne bacteria by 89% in an office environment after diffusion for 15 hours (Doran et al., 2009).

Tumor

see also **Cancer**

A tumor is an abnormal growth of cells in a lump or mass. Some tumors are malignant (cancerous) and some are benign (noncancerous). Benign tumors in most parts of the body do not create health problems. *For information on cancerous (malignant) tumors, see Cancer.*

Oils: ❄✿frankincense, ○Cellular Complex, ❄✿clove, ❄✿sandalwood

—Lipoma:

Lipoma is a benign tumor of the fatty tissues that most commonly forms just below the surface of the skin; but it can also form in any other area of the body where fatty tissue is present.

Oils: ❄frankincense, ❄clove, ○Cellular Complex, ❄grapefruit, ❄ginger

❄: Dilute as recommended, and apply 1–2 drops on location.

○: Take 3–5 drops in an empty capsule, or with food and beverage. Take up to twice per day as needed.

✿: Diffuse into the air. Inhale directly from bottle. Apply oil to hands, tissue, or cotton wick, and inhale.

Typhoid

see also **Antibacterial**

Typhoid fever is a bacterial infection caused by the bacteria *Salmonella typhi*. Typhoid is spread through food and water infected with the feces of typhoid carriers. Possible symptoms of typhoid include abdominal pain, severe diarrhea, bloody stools, chills, severe fatigue, weakness, chills, delirium, hallucinations, confusion, agitation, and fluctuating mood.

Oils: ☺☻cinnamon, ☺☻peppermint, ☺☻Cleansing Blend, ☺☻lemon, ☺☻Respiratory Blend

☺: Dilute as recommended, and apply over intestines or on reflex points on the feet.

☻: Diffuse into the air.

Ulcers

see also **Digestive System**

An ulcer is an open sore either on the skin or on an internal mucous membrane (such as that lining the stomach).

Oils: O☺frankincense, O☺myrrh, O☺marjoram☻, O☺lemon☻, O☺dill☻, O☺oregano, O☺rose, O☺thyme, O☺clove, O☺bergamot

—Duodenal:

A duodenal ulcer is an ulcer in the upper part of the small intestine.

Oils: O☺frankincense, O☺myrrh, O☺lemon, O☺oregano, O☺rose, O☺thyme, O☺clove, O☺bergamot

—Gastric: *see also* **Digestive System:Gastritis.**

A gastric ulcer is an ulcer in the stomach.

Oils: O☺geranium, O☺peppermint, O☺marjoram☻, O☺lemon☻, O☺dill☻, O☺frankincense, O☺orange, O☺bergamot

—Leg:

An ulcer on the leg may be due to a lack of circulation in the lower extremities or possibly due to a bacterial, fungal, or viral infection. *See also Circulatory System:Circulation, Antibacterial, Antifungal, Antiviral.*

Oils: ☺Cleansing Blend, ☺lavender, ☺Roman chamomile, ☺geranium

—Mouth: *see* **Canker Sores**

—Peptic:

A peptic ulcer is an ulcer that forms in an area of the digestive system where acid is present, such as in the stomach (gastric), esophagus, or upper part of the small intestine (duodenal). *See also Duodenal, Gastric in this section.*

Recipe 1: Flavor a quart of water with 1 drop cinnamon, and sip all day.

—Varicose Ulcer:

A varicose ulcer is an ulcer on the lower leg where varicose (swollen) veins are located.

Oils: ☺melaleuca, ☺geranium, ☺lavender, ☺eucalyptus, ☺thyme

◯: Add 1 drop oil to rice or almond milk, and drink. Place oil in an empty capsule and swallow. Add 1 drop or less as flavoring to food after cooking.

◔: Dilute as recommended, and apply 1–2 drops over area. Apply as warm compress.

▭: **Additional Research:**

Marjoram: Oral administration of marjoram extract was shown to significantly decrease the incidence of ulcers, basal gastric secretion, and acid output in rats (Al-Howiriny et al., 2009).

Lemon: Lemon essential oil and its majority compound (limonene) exhibited a gastroprotective effect against induced gastric ulcers in rats (Rozza et al., 2011).

Dill: Oral administration of dill seed extract was found to have effective antisecretory and anti-ulcer activity against HCl- and ethanol-induced stomach lesions in mice (Hosseinzadeh et al., 2002).

Unwind
see **Calming**

Uplifting

Oils: ⊘lemon☉, ⊘orange, ⊘Joyful Blend, ⊘Invigorating Blend, ⊘bergamot, ⊘grapefruit, ⊘Women's Blend, ⊘myrrh, ⊘wintergreen, ⊘lavender

⊘: Diffuse into the air. Inhale directly from bottle. Apply oil to hands, tissue, or cotton wick; inhale. Wear as perfume or cologne.

▭: **Additional Research:**

Lemon: Lemon odor was found to enhance the positive mood of volunteers exposed to a stressor (Kiecolt-Glaser et al., 2008).

Lemon: Lemon oil and its component, citral, were found to decrease depressed behavior in a similar manner to antidepressant drugs in rats involved in several stress tests (Komori et al., 1995).

Ureter
see **Urinary Tract**

Urinary Tract

The urinary tract is the collection of organs and tubes responsible for producing and excreting urine. The urinary tract is comprised of the kidneys, bladder, ureters, and urethra.

Oils: ◔⊘sandalwood, ◔⊘thyme, ◔⊘melaleuca, ◔⊘bergamot, ◔⊘lavender, ◔⊘rosemary

—**General Stimulant:**
  Oils: ◔⊘eucalyptus, ◔⊘bergamot

—**Infection:** *see also* **Bladder:Cystitis/Infection**
  Oils: ◔Cleansing Blend, ◔⊘lemongrass, ◔cedarwood, ◔⊘geranium, ◔bergamot, ◔⊘juniper berry

Blend 1: Combine 1 drop Protective Blend with 1 drop oregano; apply as a hot compress over abdomen and pubic area.

Other Products: ◯Protective Softgels

—**Stones In:** *see also* **Kidneys:Kidney Stones**

Stones are solid masses that form as minerals and other chemicals crystallize and adhere together. They can form in the bladder or kidneys. While small stones generally cause no problems, larger stones may block the ureters or urethra, causing intense pain and possibly injury.

  Oils: ◔fennel, ◔geranium

—Support:

Oils: ©@geranium, ©@cypress, ©@melaleuca

🖐: Dilute as recommended, and apply 1–2 drops over lower abdomen, lower back, or pubic area. Add 5–10 drops to 1 Tbs. fractionated coconut oil, and massage on abdomen, lower, back, or pubic area. Apply as a warm compress.

◐: Take supplement as directed.

🐾: Diffuse into the air.

Uterus

see also Endometriosis, Female Specific Conditions

The uterus is the female reproductive organ in which a fetus is formed and develops until birth.

Oils: ©frankincense, ©lemon, ©myrrh, ©cedarwood, ©geranium

—Regeneration of Tissue:

Oils: ©frankincense

—Uterotonic:

An uterotonic is a medication used to stimulate uterus contractions. Uterotonics should be avoided or used with extreme caution during pregnancy as they may be abortive. Uterotonics are used to start or speed up labor, to reduce hemorrhaging, and to cause contractions after a miscarriage.

Oils: ©thyme

—Uterine Cancer: *See Cancer:Uterine*

🖐: Dilute as recommended, and apply 1–2 drops on lower abdomen or on reflex points on the feet and ankles. Add 2–5 drops essential oil to 1 tsp. fractionated coconut oil, and insert into vagina for overnight retention (a tampon may be used if necessary to help retain the oil). Apply as a warm compress.

Vaginal

—Candida: *see also Antifungal:Candida*

Candida refers to a genus of yeast that are normally found in the digestive tract and on the skin of humans. These yeast are typically symbiotically beneficial to humans. However, several species of *Candida*, such as *Candida albicans*, can cause infections, such as vaginal candidiasis, that cause localized itching, soreness, and redness.

Oils: ©melaleuca©, ©Ooregano©, ©clove©, ©Protective Blend, ©bergamot, ©peppermint©, ©thyme©, ©lavender©, ©eucalyptus, ©rosemary, ©ODigestive Blend

—Infection: *see also Candida (above), Antibacterial, Antifungal, Antiviral*

Vaginal infections occur when there is a disruption in the normal balance of vaginal organisms, such as the sudden presence of yeast, bacteria, or viruses. Common signs of vaginal infection include redness, swelling, itching, pain, odor, change in discharge color or amount, a burning sensation when urinating, and pain or bleeding during intercourse. The most common vaginal infections are yeast infection, trichomoniasis, and bacterial vaginosis.

Oils: ©rosemary, ©cinnamon (dilute heavily), ©melaleuca, ©oregano, ©thyme, ©myrrh, ©clary sage, ©cypress, ©juniper berry, ©eucalyptus, ©lavender

—Vaginitis:

Vaginitis is vaginal inflammation, typically due to infection, characterized by redness, swelling, itching, irritation, discharge, and pain of the vaginal area.

Oils: ⊘rosemary, ⊘cinnamon (dilute heavily), ⊘eucalyptus, ⊘melaleuca, ⊘lavender

Recipe 1: Valerie Worwood suggests combining 1 drop lavender, 1 drop melaleuca, 1 tsp. vinegar, 1/2 tsp. lemon juice, and 2–1/2 cups of warm water for a douche that can be used three days a week.

⊜: Dilute oils as recommended, and apply 1–2 drops on location. Add 2–3 drops to 1 tsp. fractionated coconut oil, insert using vaginal syringe, and retain using tampon overnight. Add 2–3 drops to 1 tsp. fractionated coconut oil, soak tampon in mixture, insert, and leave in all day or overnight. Add 1–2 drops to warm water, and use in a douche. Add 1–2 drops to warm bathwater, and bathe.

◯: Place 1–2 drops under the tongue, or place 2–3 drops in an empty capsule, and swallow.

⊟: **Additional Research:**

Melaleuca: Tea tree oil was found to inhibit 301 different types of yeasts isolated from the mouths of cancer patients suffering from advanced cancer, including 41 strains that are known to be resistant to antifungal drugs (Bagg et al., 2006).

Melaleuca: Eleven types of Candida were found to be highly inhibited by tea tree oil (Banes-Marshall et al., 2001).

Melaleuca: Tea tree oil was found to disrupt the cellular membrane and to inhibit respiration in Candida albicans (Cox et al., 2000).

Melaleuca: Melaleuca oil at concentrations of .16% was found to inhibit the transformation of C. albicans from single-cell yeast to the pathogenic mycelial (multi-cellular strands) form (D'Auria et al., 2001).

Melaleuca: Tea Tree oil was found to alter the membrane properties and functions of Candida albicans cells, leading to cell inhibition or death (Hammer et al., 2004).

Melaleuca: Terpinen-4-ol, a constituent of tea tree oil, and tea tree oil were found to be effective against several forms of vaginal Candida infections in rats, including azole-resistant forms (Mondello et al., 2006).

Melaleuca: Melaleuca: Melaleuca oil inhibited several Candida species in vitro (Vazquez et al., 2000).

Oregano: Mice infected with Candida albicans who were fed origanum oil or carvacrol diluted in olive oil had an 80% survival rate after 30 days, while infected mice fed olive oil alone all died after 10 days (Manohar et al., 2001).

Clove: Clove oil was found to have very strong radical scavenging activity (antioxidant). It was also found to display an antifungal effect against tested Candida strains (Chaieb et al., 2007).

Peppermint: Peppermint oil was found to have a higher fungistatic and fungicidal activity against various fungi (including Candida) than the commercial fungicide bifonazole (Mimica-Dukić et al., 2003).

Thyme: Thyme oil was found to inhibit Candida species by causing lesions in the cell membrane and inhibiting germ tube (an outgrowth that develops when the fungi is preparing to replicate) formation (Pina-Vaz et al., 2004).

Lavender: Lavender oil demonstrated both fungistatic (stopped growth) and fungicidal (killed) activity against Candida albicans (D'Auria et al., 2005).

Varicose Ulcers

see Ulcers:Varicose Ulcer

Varicose Veins

Varicose veins are twisted, enlarged, blue and purple veins most often found on the legs and ankles. They have several possible causes, including weakened valves causing blood to pool around the vein. In some cases, varicose veins are merely a cosmetic problem because of their appearance, but in other cases they can be quite painful. *See also Hemorrhoids for varicose veins of the anus or rectum.*

Oils: ⊘cypress, ⊘lemongrass, ⊘lemon, ⊘peppermint, ⊘helichrysum, ⊘Invigorating Blend, ⊘geranium, ⊘lavender, ⊘rosemary, ⊘juniper berry, ⊘orange

🜁: Dilute as recommended, and apply oils gently from ankles up the legs. *Consistent application of oils for an extended period of time is the key.* Add 3–5 drops to 1 Tbs. fractionated coconut oil, and massage above the veins towards the heart. Wearing support hose and elevating the feet can also help keep blood from pooling in the legs.

Vascular System
see **Cardiovascular System;** *see also* **Arteries, Capillaries, Veins**

Vasodilator
see **Arteries:Arterial Vasodilator**

Veins

A vein is a blood vessel that carries blood from the capillaries back to the heart. Veins may also have one-way valves on the inside that help keep blood from flowing backwards and pooling in the lower extremities due to gravity.

Oils: ⊘lemongrass, ⊘cypress, ⊘lemon, ⊘helichrysum

—Blood Clot in Vein:

Blend 1: Apply 1 drop cypress and 1 drop helichrysum on location of clot to help dissolve.

🜁: Dilute as recommended, and apply 1–2 drops on location. Add 5–10 drops to 1 Tbs. fractionated coconut oil, and massage on location.

Vertigo
see also **Ears, Nausea:Motion Sickness**

Vertigo refers to the sensation that the environment and objects around an individual are moving or spinning, usually causing a loss of balance or feelings of nausea. Vertigo may be caused by ear infections, ear disorders, or motion sickness.

Oils: ⊘⊛ginger, ⊘helichrysum, ⊘geranium, ⊘basil, ⊘lavender

Recipe 1: Apply 1–2 drops each of helichrysum, geranium, and lavender to the tops of each ear (massaging slightly); then apply the oils behind each ear, pulling your hands down behind the jaw bone to just below the jaw. Finish by applying 1–2 drops of basil behind and down each ear. This can be performed multiple times a day until symptoms decrease.

🜁: Dilute as recommended, and apply 1–2 drops around ears and on reflex points on the feet.

🜂: Inhale oil directly from bottle. Apply oil to hands, tissue, or cotton wick, and inhale.

Viral Disease/Viruses
see **Antiviral**

Vitiligo
see **Skin:Vitiligo**

Voice (Hoarse)
see also **Laryngitis**

A hoarse voice is typically caused by laryngitis (inflammation of the larynx due to infection), but it can also be caused by other problems such as an ulcer, sore, polyp, or tumor on or near the vocal cords.

Oils: Ⓞbergamot

Recipe 1: Add 1 drop melaleuca, 1 drop rosemary, 1 drop clove, and 1 drop lemon to 1 tsp. honey. Swish around in the mouth for a couple of minutes to liquefy with saliva; then swallow.

Ⓞ: Add 1 drop to 1 tsp. honey, and swallow.

Vomiting
see **Nausea:Vomiting**

Warming Oils
Oils: Ⓣcinnamon, Ⓣoregano, Ⓣthyme, Ⓣmarjoram, Ⓣrosemary, Ⓣjuniper berry

Ⓣ: Add 5–10 drops to 1 tsp. fractionated coconut oil, and massage briskly into skin.

Warts
A wart is a small, firm, hard growth on the skin, usually located on the hands and feet, that is typically caused by a virus.

Oils: Ⓣfrankincense, ⓉProtective Blend, Ⓣmelaleuca, Ⓣoregano (layer with Protective Blend), Ⓣclove, Ⓣcypress, Ⓣarborvitae, Ⓣcinnamon, Ⓣlemon, Ⓣlavender

Recipe 1: Combine 5 drops cypress, 10 drops lemon, and 2 Tbs. apple cider vinegar. Apply on location twice daily; bandage. Keep a bandage on until wart is gone.

—Genital:
A genital wart is a small, painful wart or cluster of warts located in the genital area or in the mouth or throat. This type of wart is typically spread by contact with the skin through sexual activity.

Oils: Ⓣfrankincense, ⓉProtective Blend, Ⓣmelaleuca, Ⓣoregano, Ⓣthyme

—Plantar:
Plantar warts are painful warts that grow on the bottoms of the feet. They are usually flattened and embedded into the skin due to the pressure caused by walking on them.

Oils: Ⓣoregano

Ⓣ: Dilute as recommended, or dilute 1–2 drops of oil in a few drops fractionated coconut oil; then apply 1–2 drops on location daily.

Water Purification
Oils: ⓄⓉlemon, ⓄⓉCleansing Blend, Ⓞpeppermint, Ⓞorange

Ⓞ: Add 1 drop of oil to 12–16 oz. of drinking water to help purify.

Ⓣ: Add 1–2 drops to dishwater for sparkling dishes and a great smelling kitchen. Add 1–2 drops to warm bathwater, and bathe. Add 1–2 drops to a bowl of water, and use the water to clean the outsides of fruits and vegetables.

Water Retention
see **Edema, Diuretic**

Weakness
see **Energy**

Weight

Proper exercise and nutrition are the most critical factors for maintaining a healthy weight. Other factors that may influence weight include an individual's metabolism, level of stress, hormonal imbalances, low or high thyroid function, or the level of insulin being produced by the body.

—Obesity:

Obesity is the condition of being overweight to the extent that it effects health and lifestyle. By definition, obesity is considered as a body mass index (BMI) of 30 kg/m² or greater.

Oils: ⊘Ograpefruit⊕ ⊘OMetabolic Blend, ⊘Ooregano⊕, ⊘Othyme⊕, ⊘Oorange⊕, ⊘rosemary, ⊘⊘juniper berry, ⊘fennel

Other Products: OTrim Shakes, OEnergy & Stamina Complex for enhanced cellular energy. OFruit & Veggie Drink Mix for a whole food source of essential nutrients and antioxidants. OCellular Vitality Complex contains polyphenols resveratrol and epigallocatechin-3-gallate (EGCG), which have been studied for their abilities to help prevent obesity.

—Slimming/Toning:

Oils: ⊘Ograpefruit⊕, O⊘Metabolic Blend, ⊘Oorange, ⊘lemongrass, ⊘rosemary, ⊘thyme, ⊘lavender

Other Products: OTrim Shakes.

—Weight Loss:

Oils: ⊘OMetabolic Blend, ⊘Joyful Blend, ⊘⊘patchouli

Other Products: OTrim Shakes. OFruit & Veggie Drink Mix for a whole food source of essential nutrients.

Recipe 1: Add 5 drops lemon and 5 drops grapefruit to 1 gallon of water, and drink throughout the day.

🜁: Diffuse oil into the air. Inhale oil directly from bottle; or inhale oil that is applied to hands, tissue, or cotton wick.

🜔: Add 8 drops of Metabolic Blend to 16 oz. of water, and drink throughout the day between meals. Add 1 drop of oil to 12–16 oz. of water, and drink. Drink Trim or V Shake 1–2 times per day as a meal alternative. Take capsules as directed on package.

📖: **Additional Research:**

Grapefruit: The scent of grapefruit oil and its component, limonene, was found to affect the autonomic nerves and to reduce appetite and body weight in rats exposed to the oil for 15 minutes three times per week (Shen et al., 2005).

Grapefruit: Grapefruit essential oil was found to directly inhibit adipogenesis of adipocytes, indicating that grapefruit has an antiobesity effect (Haze et al., 2010).

Carvacrol (found in oregano and thyme essential oils): After 10 weeks of feeding, the body weight gain, visceral fat-pad weights, and final body weights of mice fed a high-fat diet and carvacrol were significantly lower than that of mice fed a high-fat diet without carvacrol (specifically a 24% decrease in final body weight, a 43% decrease in body weight gain, and a 36% decrease in total visceral fat-pad weight was observed when carvacrol was ingested)(Cho et al., 2012). Interestingly, the food intake during the 10-week feeding period did not differ among the groups and mRNA expressions were different among the two groups (Cho et al., 2012).

D-Limonene (found in lime, lemon, bergamot, dill, grapefruit, lavender, lemongrass, Roman chamomile, tangerine, and wild orange essential oils): Oral intake of D-limonene effectively protects against the development of hyperglycemia and dyslipidemia in mice fed a high-fat diet (Jing et al., 2013). This study also found evidence suggesting that D-limonene may prevent lipid accumulation in the livers of mice fed a high-fat diet and improve metabolic dysfunctions by ameliorating glucose tolerance in obese mice (Jing et al., 2013).

Lime: Injection of lime essential oil prevented weight gain by suppressing the appetite of mice even when administered ketotifen, an antihistamine with the undesirable side effects of decreased metabolism and increased appetite (Asnaashari et al., 2010).

Cinnamon: When compared to six other plant extracts, cinnamon and apple polyphenolic plant extracts were found to be anti-obesogenic due to their body fat-lowering effect in diet-induced obesity model rats (Boque et al., 2013).

Whiplash

Whiplash is the over-stretching or tearing of the muscles, ligaments, and/or tendons in the neck and head. This is typically caused by a sudden collision or force pushing the body in one direction, while the head's tendency to remain in the same place causes the head to quickly rock in the opposite direction the body is going.

Oils: Soothing Blend, lemongrass (ligaments), marjoram (muscles), birch, basil, juniper berry, helichrysum, vetiver, clove, peppermint, Roman chamomile

: Dilute as recommended, and apply 1–2 drops on back of neck. Add 5–10 drops to 1 Tbs. fractionated coconut oil, and massage on back of neck, on shoulders, and on upper back.

Whooping Cough
see Childhood Diseases: Whooping Cough

Withdrawal
see Addictions:Withdrawal

Women
see Female Specific Conditions

Workaholic
see Addictions:Work

Worms
see Antifungal:Ringworm, Parasites:Worms

Wounds
see also Antibacterial, Blood:Bleeding

A wound is a general term for an injury that involves tissue (typically the skin or underlying skeletal muscles) being torn, cut, punctured, scraped, or crushed.

Oils: clove, melaleuca, helichrysum, lavender, lemongrass, Cleansing Blend, basil, cypress, eucalyptus, frankincense, Roman chamomile, peppermint (after wound has closed), myrrh, rose, sandalwood, thyme, juniper berry, bergamot

Recipe 1: Place 1–3 drops of helichrysum on fresh wound to help stop bleeding. Add 1 drop clove to help reduce pain. Once bleeding has stopped, apply a drop of lavender (to help start healing), a drop of melaleuca (to help fight infection), and a drop of lemongrass (for possible ligament damage). Bandage the wound. When changing the bandage, apply 1 drop basil or sandalwood to help promote further healing. Add 1 drop Cleansing Blend or Protective Blend to help prevent infection.

Other Products: Soothing Skin Ointment to help cleanse and support the skin's natural healing process.

Blend 1: Add 1 drop lavender to 1 drop Cleansing Blend and apply to wound.

—Children/Infants:

   Oils: ⊘Roman chamomile

   Recipe 2: Add 1–3 drops each of helichrysum and lavender to 1 tsp. fractionated coconut oil, and apply a small amount to wound.

—Bleeding:

   Oils: ⊘helichrysum, ⊘rose, ⊘lavender, ⊘lemon

   Blend 2: Combine 1 drop Roman chamomile, 1 drop geranium, and 1 drop lemon, and apply with a warm compress 2–3 times a day for 3–4 days, then reduce to once a day until healed.

—Disinfect:

   Oils: ⊘melaleuca, ⊘thyme, ⊘lavender

—Healing:

   Oils: ⊘basil⊕, ⊘helichrysum, ⊘melaleuca, ⊘lavender, ⊘myrrh, ⊘sandalwood

—Inflammation: *see Inflammation*

—Scarring: *see Skin:Scarring, Tissue:Scarring*

—Surgical:

   Oils: ⊘peppermint, ⊘melaleuca

   Blend 2: Add 3 drops helichrysum, 3 drops frankincense, and 4 drops lavender to 2 tsp. fractionated coconut oil. Apply a few drops when changing bandages.

—Weeping:

   Oils: ⊘myrrh, ⊘patchouli

⊝: Dilute as recommended, and apply 1–2 drops on location.

▥: **Additional Research:**

   Basil: Basil (Ocimum gatissimum) oil was found to facilitate the healing process of wounds in rabbits to a greater extent than two antibacterial preparations, Cicatrin and Cetavlex (Orafidiya et al., 2003)

   Clove: Beta-caryophyllene (found in clove and copal oils) demonstrated anaesthetic (pain reducing) activity in rats and rabbits (Ghelardini et al., 2001).

   Cinnamon: A topically applied cinnamon oil based microemulsion showed increased wound healing ability in rats by preventing sepsis of the excised wound (Ghosh et al., 2013).

Wrinkles
see Skin:Wrinkles

Yeast
see Antifungal:Candida

Yoga

Oils: ⊘sandalwood, ⊘cedarwood

⊘: Diffuse into the air.

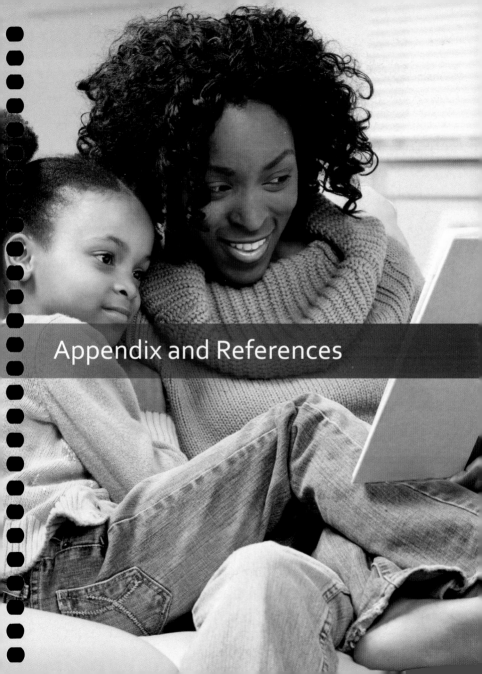

Appendix and References

Appendix A: Body Systems Chart

The following chart lists all of the products discussed within this book and indicates which body systems they primarily affect. While this chart does not include every system that could possibly be affected by each product, it attempts to list the primary systems that are most often affected. It is provided to give the beginning aromatherapy student a starting point for personal use and analysis.

Product Name	Cardiovascular System	Digestive System	Emotional Balance	Hormonal System	Immune System	Muscles and Bones	Nervous System	Respiratory System	Skin and Hair
Arborvitae			•					•	•
Basil	•					•			
Bergamot		•	•						•
Birch						•			
Bone Nutrient Complex						•	•		•
Calming Bath Bar			•				•		•
Calming Blend			•				•		
Cardamom		•						•	
Cassia					•				
Cedarwood							•	•	
Cellular Complex	•				•	•		•	
Cellular Vitality Complex	•				•	•	•	•	•
Chewable Multivitamin	•	•		•	•	•	•	•	•
Cinnamon Bark					•				
Clary Sage			•						
Cleansing Blend		•	•		•				•
Clove	•	•			•			•	
Coriander		•		•					
Cypress	•						•		
Detoxification Blend		•		•	•			•	•
Dill	•	•							
Digestive Blend		•							
Digestive Enzyme Complex		•							
Energy & Stamina Complex	•				•	•	•		
Essential Oil Omega Complex	•	•			•		•		•
Eucalyptus								•	•
Face Wash					•				•
Fennel		•		•					
Focus Blend			•	•	•		•		
Food Nutrient Complex	•	•	•	•	•	•	•	•	•
Frankincense			•		•		•		•
Geranium			•						•
GI Cleansing Formula		•			•				
Ginger		•					•		
Grapefruit	•								

Product Name	Cardiovascular System	Digestive System	Emotional Balance	Hormonal System	Immune System	Muscles and Bones	Nervous System	Respiratory System	Skin and Hair
Grounding Blend			●			●	●		●
Hair Care Products									●
Hand & Body Lotion									●
Helichrysum	●				●				
Invigorating Bath Bar			●		●		●		●
Invigorating Blend			●		●		●		
Joyful Blend			●	●					
Juniper Berry		●	●				●		●
Lavender	●		●				●		●
Lemon		●			●			●	
Lemongrass					●	●			
Lime		●			●			●	
Marjoram	●					●			
Massage Blend			●	●	●	●	●		
Melaleuca					●	●		●	●
Melissa			●						●
Metabolic Blend		●	●						
Myrrh				●	●		●		●
Omega-3 Fish Oil	●	●			●		●		●
Orange		●	●		●				●
Oregano					●	●		●	
Patchouli									●
Peppermint		●			●	●		●	●
Phytoestrogen Complex			●	●		●			●
Protective Blend					●				●
Repellent Blend									●
Respiratory Blend								●	
Roman Chamomile			●				●		●
Rose			●						●
Rosemary					●		●	●	
Sandalwood			●			●	●		●
Soothing Blend						●	●		
Spearmint		●	●						
Tension Blend						●	●		
Thyme					●	●			
Topical Blend					●				●
Trim and V Shake		●		●		●			
Vetiver			●	●			●		●
White Fir								●	
Wintergreen						●			
Women's Blend			●	●			●		
Women's Monthly Blend			●	●					●
Ylang Ylang	●		●	●					

255

Appendix B: Single Essential Oils Property Chart

The following chart presents some of the properties of each of the single oils. An attempt has been made to indicate the effectiveness of the oils for each property, where supporting information existed. However, this information should not be considered conclusive. It is provided to give the beginning aromatherapy student a starting point for personal use and analysis. Also, keep in mind the applicable safety data when applying an oil for its property. For example, cinnamon bark is one of the best known antiseptics, but it is also extremely irritating to the skin. It may work well to sanitize the bathroom with, but it should be used with extreme caution on the skin.

Properties of Essential Oils

Antibacterial: an agent that prevents the growth of (or destroys) bacteria.

Anticatarrhal: an agent that helps remove excess catarrh from the body. Expectorants help promote the removal of mucus from the respiratory system.

Antidepressant: an agent that helps alleviate depression.

Antifungal: an agent that prevents and combats fungal infection.

Anti-infectious: an agent that prevents and combats the spread of germs.

Anti-inflammatory: an agent that alleviates inflammation.

Antimicrobial: an agent that resists or destroys pathogenic microorganisms.

Antiparasitic: an agent that prevents and destroys parasites.

Antirheumatic: an agent that helps prevent and relieve rheumatism.

Antiseptic: an agent that destroys and prevents the development of microbes.

Antispasmodic: an agent that prevents and eases spasms or convulsions.

Antiviral: a substance that inhibits the growth of a virus.

Analgesic: a substance that relieves pain.

Immune-stimulant: an agent that stimulates the natural defense mechanism of the body.

Single Oil Name	Antibacterial	Anticatarrhal	Antidepressant	Antifungal	Anti-infectious	Anti-inflammatory	Antimicrobial	Antiparasitic	Antirheumatic	Antiseptic	Antispasmodic	Antiviral	Analgesic	Immune-stimulant
Arborvitae	++			+++			++	++		++				
Basil	++	+	+		+	+++				+	+	+		
Bergamot					+	+++		+		+	+		+	
Birch						+		+	+++	+				
Cardamom	++				+	++	+			+	+			
Cassia	+		+	+	+	+	++	+		++++	+	+		
Cedarwood			+	+	+					++				
Cinnamon	+		+	+	+	+	++	+		++++	+	+		
Clary Sage	+		+		+					+	+			
Clove	+++	+		++	+			++	+	+		+++		
Coriander	++		++		++			+		+			+	
Cypress	+				+			+	+	+	+			
Dill	+			+		+				++				
Eucalyptus	++	++			+	+						+++	++	+
Fennel	+	++				+	+	+		+	+			
Frankincense		++	++			+++	+				+			+++
Geranium	+++		++	++	+	+				+				
Ginger		++								++			++	
Grapefruit	++									++				
Helichrysum	++	+++		+		++	++			+	+++			
Juniper Berry										++	+		+	
Lavender			++		+	++	+	+	+	+	++		++	
Lemon	++				+		++		+	+++	+			++
Lemongrass	+		+	+		++	+			+			++	
Lime	++									++		+		
Marjoram	+	+		+	+					++	++	+	++	
Melissa	+		++				+				++	++		
Melaleuca	+++			++++	+	+		+		+		+++		++
Myrrh		+		+	+	+++	++	+		+		+++		
Orange	++		++	+		+				++				
Oregano	+++	+		+++	+++			+++	++	+	+	++	++	++
Patchouli	+		+	+	+	+	+			+		+		
Peppermint	+	+		+	+	++	+			+	+	+	++	
Roman Chamomile	+		+		+	+++				+	++		++	
Rose					+									
Rosemary	+++	+		+++	+	+++							+++	
Sandalwood	+	+++	++	+						++	+			
Spearmint	++			+		+				+	+			+
Thyme	+	+		+++			++	+	++		+	+		++
Vetiver					+					+	+			+
White Fir		+								++			+	
Wintergreen						+++			+	+	+		+	
Ylang Ylang			+		+					+	+			

Research References

Aalinkeel R et al. (2008 Aug 25). "The dietary bioflavonoid, quercetin, selectively induces apoptosis of prostate cancer cells by down-regulating the expression of heat shock protein 90," Prostate.

Abdel-Sattar E, Zaitoun AA, Farag MA, El Gayed SH, Harraz FM (2009 Feb 25). "Chemical composition, insecticidal and insect repellent activity of Schinus molle L. leaf and fruit essential oils against Trogoderma granarium and Tribolium castaneum," Nat Prod Res. Epub ahead of print: 1-10.

Abdullah, D., Ping, Q. N., & Liu, G. J. (1996 Jan). Enhancing effect of essential oils on the penetration of 5-fluorouracil through rat skin. Yao Xue Xue Bao, 31(3), 214-221.

Abebe, W. (2002). Herbal medication: potential for adverse interactions with analgesic drugs. Journal of Clinical Pharmacy and Therapeutics, 27(6), 391-401.

Abedon, B (2008). "Essentra - a patented extract that reduces stress and enhances sleep," (http://www.nutragenesisnutrition.com/images/stories/pdf/ess_stress_wp.pdf):1-4.

Abenavoli L, Capasso R, Milic N, Capasso F (2010 Jun 7). "Milk thistle in liver diseases: past, present, future," Phytother Res. Epub ahead of print.

Adam B, Liebregts T, Best J, Bechmann L, Lackner C, Neumann J, Koehler S, Holtmann G (2006 Feb). "A combination of peppermint oil and caraway oil attenuates the post-inflammatory visceral hyperalgesia in a rat model," Scand J Gastroenterol. 41(2):155-60.

Agrawal, P., Rai, V., & Singh, R. B. (1996 Sep). Randomized placebo-controlled, single blind trial of holy basil leaves in patients with noninsulin-dependent diabetes mellitus. Int J Clin Pharmacol Ther, 34(9), 406-409.

Akha, O., Rabiei, K., Kashi, Z., Bahar, A., Zaeif-Khorasani, E., Kosaryan, M., . . . Emadian, O. (2014). The effect of fennel (Foeniculum vulgare) gel 3% in decreasing hair thickness in idiopathic mild to moderate hirsutism, A randomized placebo controlled clinical trial. Caspian J Intern Med, 5(1), 26-29.

Al-Ali, K. H., El-Beshbishy, H. A., El-Badry, A. A., & Alkhalaf, M. (2013 Dec). Cytotoxic activity of methanolic extract of Mentha longifolia and Ocimum basilicum against human breast cancer. Pak J Biol Sci, 16(23), 1744-1750.

Al-Anati L, Essid E, Reinehr R, Petzinger E (2009 Apr). "Silibinin protects OTA-mediated TNF-alpha release from perfused rat livers and isolated rat Kupffer cells," Mol Nutr Food Res. 53(4):460-6.

Alberts, B., Bray, D., Hopkin, K., Johnson, A., Lewis, J., Raff, M., . . . Walter, P. (2013). Essential cell biology. New York, NY: Garland Science.

Alexandrovich I, Rakovitskaya O, Kolmo E, Sidorova T, Shushunov S (2003 Jul-Aug). "The effect of fennel (Foeniculum Vulgare) seed oil emulsion in infantile colic: a randomized, placebo-controlled study," Altern Ther Health Med. 9(4):58-61.

al-Hader AA, Hasan ZA, Aqel MB (1994 Jul 22). "Hyperglycemic and insulin release inhibitory effects of Rosmarinus officinalis," J Ethnopharmacol. 43(3):217-21.

Al-Howiriny, T., Alsheikh, A., Alqasoumi, S., Al-Yahya, M., ElTahir, K., & Rafatullah, S. (2009 Aug). Protective Effect of Origanum majorana L. 'Marjoram' on various models of gastric mucosal injury in rats. Am J Chin Med, 37(3), 531-545.

Ali, S. A., Rizk, M. Z., Ibrahim, N. A., Abdallah, M. S., Sharara, H. M., & Moustafa, M. M. (2010 Dec). Protective role of Juniperus phoenicea and Cupressus sempervirens against CCl(4). World J Gastrointest Pharmacol Ther, 1(6), 123-131.

Almela L, Sánchez-Muñoz B, Fernández-López JA, Roca MJ, Rabe V (2006 Jul). "Liquid chromatograpic-mass spectrometric analysis of phenolics and free radical scavenging activity of rosemary extract from different raw material," J Chromatogr A. 1120(1-2):221-9.

Aloisi AM, Ceccarelli I, Masi F, Scaramuzzino A (2002 Oct 17). "Effects of the essential oil from citrus lemon in male and female rats exposed to a persistent painful stimulation," Behav Brain Res. 136(1):127-35.

Alqareer A, Alyahya A, Andersson L (2006 Nov). "The effect of clove and benzocaine versus placebo as topical anesthetics," J Dent. 34(10):747-50.

al-Zuhair H, el-Sayeb B, Ameen HA, al-Shoora H (1996 Jul-Aug). "Pharmacological studies of cardamom oil in animals," Pharmacol Res. 34(1-2):79-82.

Amano S, Akutsu N, Ogura Y, Nishiyama T (2004 Nov). "Increase of laminin 5 synthesis in human keratinocytes by acute wound fluid, inflammatory cytokines and growth factors, and lysophospholipids," Br J Dermatol. 151(5):961-70.

Amantea D, Fratto V, Maida S, Rotiroti D, Ragusa S, Nappi G, Bagetta G, Corasaniti MT (2009). "Prevention of Glutamate Accumulation and Upregulation of Phospho-Akt may Account for Neuroprotection Afforded by Bergamot Essential Oil against Brain Injury Induced by Focal Cerebral Ischemia in Rat," Int Rev Neurobiol. 85:389-405.

Ambrosone CB, McCann SE, Freudenheim JL, Marshall JR, Zhang Y, Shields PG (2004 May). "Breast cancer risk in premenopausal women is inversely associated with consumption of broccoli, a source of isothiocyanates, but is not modified by GST genotype," J Nutr. 134(5):1134-8.

American Cancer Society (2008). "Cancer Facts and Figures." Downloaded at http://www.cancer.org/downloads/STT/2008CAFFfinalsecured.pdf.

Ammon HP (2002). "Boswellic acids (components of frankincense) as the active principle in treatment of chronic inflammatory diseases," Wien Med Wochenschr. 152(15-16):373-8.

Anderson KJ, Teuber SS, Gobeille A, Cremin P, Waterhouse AL, Steinberg FM (2001 Nov). "Walnut polyphenolics inhibit in vitro human plasma and LDL oxidation," J Nutr. 131(11):2837-42.

Andradea, E. H. A., Alves, C. N., Guimarães, E. F., Carreira, L. M. M., & Maia, J. G. S. (2011 Sep). Variability in essential oil composition of Piper dilatatum L.C. Rich. Biochemical Systematics and Ecology, 39, 669-675.

Andrews R.E., Parks L.W., Spence K.D. (1980) Some Effects of Douglas Fir Terpenes on Certain Microorganisms. Applied and Environmental Microbiology. 40: 301-304.

Andrian E., Grenier D., Rouabhia M. (2006) Porphyromonas gingivalis-Epithelial Cell Interactions in Periodontitis. Journal of Dental Research. 85: 392-403.

Antimutagenic effects of extracts from sage (Salvia officinalis) in mammalian system in vivo. (2006 Jul 19). "Relaxant effects of Rosa damascena on guinea pig tracheal chains and its possible mechanism(s)," J Ethnopharmacol. 106(3):377-82.

Appendino G, Ottino M, Marquez N, Bianchi F, Giana A, Ballero M, Sterner O, Fiebich BL, Munoz E (2007 Apr). "Arzanol, an anti-inflammatory and anti-HIV-1 phloroglucinol alpha-Pyrone from Helichrysum italicum ssp. microphyllum," J Nat Prod. 70(4):608-12.

Aqel MB (1991 May-Jun). "Relaxant effect of the volatile oil of Rosmarinus officinalis on tracheal smooth muscle," J Ethnopharmacol. 33(1-2):57-62.

Arasada BL, Bommareddy A, Zhang X, Bremmon K, Dwivedi C. (2008 Jan-Feb). "Effects of alpha-santalol on proapoptotic caspases and p53 expression in UVB irradiated mouse skin," Anticancer Res. 28(1A):129-32.

Arash, A., Mohammad, M. Z., Jamal, M. S., Mohammad, T. A., & Azam, A. (2013 Oct). Effects of the Aqueous Extract of Anethum graveolens Leaves on Seizure Induced by Pentylenetetrazole in Mice. Malays J Med Sci, 20(5), 23-30.

Archana R, Namasivayam A (1999 Jan). "Antistressor effect of Withania somnifera," J Ethnopharmacol. 64(1):91-3.

Arima, Y., Nakai, Y., Hayakawa, R., & Nishino, T. (2003 Jan). Antibacterial effect of beta-thujaplicin on staphylococci isolated from atopic dermatitis: relationship between changes in the number of viable bacterial cells and clinical improvement in an eczematous lesion of atopic dermatitis. J Antimicrob Chemother, 51(1), 113-122.

Asakura, K., Matsuo, Y., Oshima, T., Kihara, T., Minagawa, K., Araki, Y., . . . Ninomiya, M. (2000 Apr). omega-agatoxin IVA-sensitive Ca(2+) channel blocker, alpha-eudesmol, protects against brain injury after focal ischemia in rats. Eur J Pharmacol, 394(1), 57-65.

Asao T, Kuwano H, Ide M, Hirayama I, Nakamura JI, Fujita KI, Horiuti R (2003 Apr). "Spasmolytic effect of peppermint oil in barium during double-contrast barium enema compared with Buscopan," Clin Radiol. 58(4):301-5.

Asensio, C. M., Nepote, V., & Grosso, N. R. (2011 Sep). Chemical stability of extra-virgin olive oil added with oregano essential oil. J Food Sci, 76(7), S445-450.

Asnaashari, S., Delazar, A., Habibi, B., Vasfi, R., Nahar, L., Hamedeyazdan, S., & Sarker, S. D. (2010 Dec). Essential oil from Citrus aurantifolia prevents ketotifen-induced weight-gain in mice. Phytother Res, 24(12), 1893-1897.

Auffray, B. (2007 Feb). Protection against singlet oxygen, the main actor of sebum squalene peroxidation during sun exposure, using Commiphora myrrha essential oil. Int J Cosmet Sci, 29(1), 23-29.

Awale, S., Tohda, C., Tezuka, Y., Miyazaki, M., & Kadota, S. (2011). Protective Effects of Rosa damascena and Its Active Constituent on Abeta(25-35)-Induced Neuritic Atrophy. Evid Based Complement Alternat Med, 2011, 1-8.

Baba, T., Nakano, H., Tamai, K., Sawamura, D., Hanada, K., Hashimoto, I., & Arima, Y. (1998 Jan). Inhibitory effect of beta-thujaplicin on ultraviolet B-induced apoptosis in mouse keratinocytes. J Invest Dermatol, 110(1), 24-28.

Babu, K. G., Singh, B., Joshi, V. P., & Singh, V. (2002). Essential oil composition of Damask rose (Rosa damascena Mill.) distilled under different pressures and temperatures. Flavour and Fragrance Journal, 17(2), 136-140.

Badia P, Wesensten N, Lammers W, Culpepper J, Harsh J (1990 Jul). "Responsiveness to olfactory stimuli presented in sleep," Physiol Behav. 48(1):87-90.

Bagchi D, Hassoun EA, Bagchi M, Stohs SJ (1993 Aug). "Protective effects of antioxidants against endrin-induced hepatic lipid peroxidation, DNA damage, and excretion of urinary lipid metabolites," Free Radic Biol Med. 15(2):217-22.

Bagchi D, Sen CK, Ray SD, Das DK, Bagchi M, Preuss HG, Vinson JA (2003 Feb-Mar). "Molecular mechanisms of cardioprotection by a novel grape seed proanthocyanidin extract," Mutat Res. 523-24:87-97.

Bagg J, Jackson MS, Petrina Sweeney M, Ramage G, Davies AN (2006 May). "Susceptibility to Melaleuca alternifolia (tea tree) oil of yeasts isolated from the mouths of patients with advanced cancer," Oral Oncol. 42(5):487-92.

Bahramikia, S., & Yazdanparast, R. (2009 Aug). Efficacy of different fractions of Anethum graveolens leaves on serum lipoproteins and serum and liver oxidative status in experimentally induced hypercholesterolaemic rat models. Am J Chin Med, 37(4), 685-699.

Bakirel T, Bakirel U, Keleş OU, Ulgen SG, Yardibi H (2008 Feb 28). "In vivo assessment of antidiabetic and antioxidant activities of rosemary (Rosmarinus officinalis) in alloxan-diabetic rabbits," J Ethnopharmacol. 116(1):64-73.

Balazs L, Okolicany J, Ferrebee M, Tolley B, Tigyi G (2001 Feb). "Topical application of the phospholipid growth factor lysophosphatidic acid promotes wound healing in vivo," Am J Physiol Regul Integr Comp Physiol. 280(2):R466-72.

Balestrieri, E., Pizzimenti, F., Ferlazzo, A., Giofre, S. V., Iannazzo, D., Piperno, A., . . . Macchi, B. (2011 Mar). Antiviral activity of seed extract from Citrus bergamia towards human retroviruses. Bioorg Med Chem, 19(6), 2084-2089.

Balick, MJ, Cox PA. (1996). Plants, People and Culture: The Science of Ethnobotany. Scientific American Library, New York.

Ballard CG, O'Brien JT, Reichelt K, Perry EK (2002 Jul). "Aromatherapy as a safe and effective treatment for the management of agitation in severe dementia: the results of a double-blind, placebo-controlled trial with Melissa," J Clin Psychiatry. 63(7):553-8.

Ballabeni V, Tognolini M, Bertoni S, Bruni R, Guerrini A, Rueda GM, Barocelli E (2007 Jan). "Antiplatelet and antithrombotic activities of essential oil from wild Ocotea quixos (Lam.) Kosterm. (Lauraceae) calices from Amazonian Ecuador," Pharmacol Res. 55(1):23-30.

Ballabeni V, Tognolini M, Giorgio C, Bertoni S, Bruni R, Barocelli E (2009 Oct 13). "Ocotea quixos Lam. essential oil: In vitro and in vivo investigation on its anti-inflammatory properties," Fitoterapia. Epub ahead of print.

Banerjee S, Ecavade A, Rao AR (1993 Feb). "Modulatory influence of sandalwood oil on mouse hepatic glutathione S-transferase activity and acid soluble sulphydryl level," Cancer Lett. 68(2-3):105-9.

Banes-Marshall L, Cawley P, Phillips CA (2001). "In vitro activity of Melaleuca alternifolia (tea tree) oil against bacterial and Candida spp. isolates from clinical specimens," Br J Biomed Sci. 58(3):139-45.

Bani, S., Hasanpour, S., Mousavi, Z., Mostafa Garehbaghi, P., & Gojazadeh, M. (2014 Jan). The Effect of Rosa Damascena Extract on Primary Dysmenorrhea: A Double-blind Cross-over Clinical Trial. Iran Red Crescent Med J, 16(1), 1-6.

Banno N, Akihisa T, Yasukawa K, Tokuda H, Tabata K, Nakamura Y, Nishimura R, Kimura Y, Suzuki T (2006 Sep 19). "Anti-inflammatory activities of the triterpene acids from the resin of Boswellia carteri," J Ethnopharmacol. 107(2):249-53.

Bao L, Yao XS, Tsi D, Yau CC, Chia CS, Nagai H, Kurihara H (2008 Jan 23). "Protective effects of bilberry (Vaccinium myrtillus L.) extract on KbrO3-induced kidney damage in mice," J Agric Food Chem. 56(2):420-5.

Baqui, A. A., Kelley, J. I., Jabra-Rizk, M. A., Depaola, L. G., Falkler, W. A., & Meiller, T. F. (2001 Jul). In vitro effect of oral antiseptics on human immunodeficiency virus-1 and herpes simplex virus type 1. J Clin Periodontol, 28(7), 610-616.

Barthelman M., Chen W., Gensler H.L., Huang C., Dong Z., Bowden G.T. (1998) Inhibitory Effects of Perillyl Alcohol on UVB-induced Murine Skin Cancer and AP-1 Transactivation. Cancer Research. 58: 711-716.

Bassett IB, Pannowitz DL, Barnetson RS (1990 Oct 15). "A comparative study of tea-tree oil versus benzoylperoxide in the treatment of acne," Med J Aust. 153(8):455-8.

Bastiaens M, Hoefnagel J, Westendorp R, Vermeer BJ, Bouwes Bavinck JN (2004 Jun). "Solar lentigines are strongly related to sun exposure in contrast to ephelides," Pigment Cell Res. 17(3).

Bastos J.F.A., Moreira I.J.A., Ribeiro T.P., Medeiros I.A., Antoniolli A.R., De Sousa D.P., Santos M.R.V. (2009) Hypotensive and Vasorelaxant Effects of Citronellol, a Monoterpene Alcohol, in Rats. Basic & Clinical Pharmacology & Toxicology. 106: 331-337.

Basu A, Lucas EA (2007 Aug). "Mechanisms and effects of green tea on cardiovascular health," Nutr Rev. 65(8 Pt 1):361-75.

Behnam S, Farzaneh M, Ahmadzadeh M, Tehrani AS (2006). "Composition and antifungal activity of essential oils of Mentha piperita and Lavendula angustifolia on post-harvest phytopathogens," Commun Agric Appl Biol Sci. 71(3 Pt B):1321-6.

Belardinelli R, Mucaj A, Lacalaprice F, Solenghi M, Principi F, Tiano L, Littarru GP (2005). "Coenzyme Q10 improves contractility of dysfunctional myocardium in chronic heart failure," Biofactors. 25(1-4):137-45.

Benencia F, Courrèges MC (2000 Nov). "In vitro and in vivo activity of eugenol on human herpes virus," Phytother Res. 14(7):495-500.

Benencia, F., & Courreges, M. C. (1999 May). Antiviral activity of sandalwood oil against herpes simplex viruses-1 and -2. Phytomedicine, 6(2), 119-123.

Berić T, Nikolić B, Stanojević J, Vuković-Gacić B, Knezević-Vukević J (2008 Feb). "Protective effect of basil (Ocimum basilicum L.) against oxidative DNA damage and mutagenesis," Food Chem Toxicol. 46(2):724-32.

Bezanilla F. (2006) The action potential: From voltage-gated conductances to molecular structures. Biological Research. 39: 425-435.

Bhattacharya SK, Goel RK (1987 Mar). "Anti-stress activity of sitoindosides VII and VIII, new acylsterylglucosides from Withania somnifera, Phytother Res. 1(1):32-7.

Bhattacharya SK, Kumar A, Ghosal S (1995). "Effects of glycowithanolides from Withania somnifera on animal model of Alzheimer's disease and perturbed central cholinergic markers of cognition in rats," Phytother. Res. 9:110-3.

Bhushan S, Kumar A, Malik F, Andotra SS, Sethi VK, Kaur IP, Taneja SC, Qazi GN, Singh J (2007 Oct). "A triterpenediol from Boswellia serrata induces apoptosis through both the intrinsic and extrinsic apoptotic pathways in human leukemia HL-60 cells," Apoptosis. 12(10):1911-26.

Blain EJ, Ali AY, Duance VC (2010 Jun). "Boswellia frereana (frankincense) supresses cytokine-induced matrix metalloproteinase expression and production of pro-inflammatory molecules in articular cartilage," Phytother Res. 24(6):905-12.

Blanes-Mira C, Clemente J, Jodas G, Gil A, Fernandez-Ballester G, Ponsati B, Gutierrez J, Perez-Paya E, Ferrer-Montiel A (2002 Oct). "A synthetic hexapeptide (Argireline) with antiwrinkle activity," Int J Cosmet Sci. 24(5):303-10.

Bobe G et al. (2008 Mar). "Flavonoid intake and risk of pancreatic cancer in male smokers (Finland)," Cancer Epidemiol Biomarkers Prev. 17(3):553-62.

Modern Essentials Usage Guide

Bone ME, Wilkinson DJ, Young JR, McNeil J, Charlton S (1990 Aug). "Ginger root--a new antiemetic. The effect of ginger root on postoperative nausea and vomiting after major gynaecological surgery," Anaesthesia. 45(8):669-71.

Boots AW, Wilms LC, Swennen EL, Kleinjans JC, Bast A, Haenen GR (2008 Jul-Aug). "In vitro and ex vivo anti-inflammatory activity of quercetin in healthy volunteers," Nutrition. 24(7-8):703-10.

Boque, N., Campion, J., de la Iglesia, R., de la Garza, A. L., Milagro, F. I., San Roman, B., . . . Martinez, J. A. (2013 Mar). Screening of polyphenolic plant extracts for anti-obesity properties in Wistar rats. J Sci Food Agric, 93(5), 1226-1232.

Bora, K. S., Arora, S., & Shri, R. (2011 Oct). Role of Ocimum basilicum L. in prevention of ischemia and reperfusion-induced cerebral damage, and motor dysfunctions in mice brain. J Ethnopharmacol, 137(3), 1360-1365.

Borgatti, M., Mancini, I., Bianchi, N., Guerrini, A., Lampronti, I., Rossi, D., . . . Gambari, R. (2011 Apr). Bergamot (Citrus bergamia Risso) fruit extracts and identified components alter expression of interleukin 8 gene in cystic fibrosis bronchial epithelial cell lines. BMC Biochem, 12, 15.

Bose M, Lambert JD, Ju J, Reuhl KR, Shapses SA, Yang CS (2008 Sep). "The major green tea polyphenol, (-)-epigallocatechin-3-gallate, inhibits obesity, metabolic syndrome, and fatty liver disease in high-fat-fed mice," J Nutr. 138(9):1677-83.

Boudier D, Perez E, Rondeau D, Bordes S, Closs B (2008 Mar). "Innovatory approach fights pigment disturbances," Personal Care.

Boussetta T, Raad H, Lettéron P, Gougerot-Pocidalo MA, Marie JC, Driss F, El-Benna J (2009 Jul 31). "Punicic acid a conjugated linolenic acid inhibits TNFalpha-induced neutrophil hyperactivation and protects from experimental colon inflammation in rats," PLoS One. 4(7):e6458.

Bouwstra J.A., Gooris G.S., Dubbelaar F.E.R., Weeheim A.M., Ijzerman A.P., Ponec M. (1998) Role of ceramide 1 in the molecular organization of the stratum corneum lipids. Journal of Lipid Research. 39: 186-196.

Bowen, R. (2006). The gastrointestinal barrier. In W.E. Wingfield & M.R. Raffe (Eds.), The veterinary ICU book (40-46). Alpine, WY: Teton NewMedia.

Bowles, E. J. (2003). The chemistry of aromatherapeutic oils (3rd ed.). Australia: Allen & Unwin.

Bradley BF, Brown SL, Chu S, Lea RW (2009 Jun). "Effects of orally administered lavender essential oil on responses to anxiety-provoking film clips," Hum Psychopharmacol. 24(4):319-30.

Bradley BF, Starkey NJ, Brown SL, Lea RW (2007 May 22). "Anxiolytic effects of Lavandula angustifolia odour on the Mongolian gerbil elevated plus maze," J Ethnopharmacol. 111(3):517-25.

Brady A, Loughlin R, Gilpin D, Kearney P, Tunney M (2006 Oct). "In vitro activity of tea-tree oil against clinical skin isolates of methicillin-resistant and -sensitive Staphylococcus aureus and coagulase-negative staphylococci growing planktonically and as biofilms," J Med Microbiol. 55(Pt 10):1375-80.

Brand C, Ferrante A, Prager RH, Riley TV, Carson CF, Finlay-Jones JJ, Hart PH. (2001 Apr). "The water-soluble components of the essential oil of Melaleuca alternifolia (tea tree oil) suppress the production of superoxide by human monocytes, but not neutrophils, activated in vitro.," Inflamm Res. 50(4):213-9.

Brand C, Grimbaldeston MA, Gamble JR, Drew J, Finlay-Jones JJ, Hart PH (2002 May). "Tea tree oil reduces the swelling associated with the efferent phase of a contact hypersensitivity response," Inflamm Res. 51(5):236-44.

Brand C, Townley SL, Finlay-Jones JJ, Hart PH (2002 Jun). "Tea tree oil reduces histamine-induced oedema in murine ears," Inflamm Res. 51(6):283-9.

Brass EP, Adler S, Sietsema KE, Hiatt WR, Orlando AM, Amato A; CHIEF Investigators (2001 May). "Intravenous L-carnitine increases plasma carnitine, reduces fatigue, and may preserve exercise capacity in hemodialysis patients," Am J Kidney Dis. 37(5):1018-28.

Brenner, G. M., & Stevens, C. (2009). Pharmacology (3rd ed.). Philadelphia, PA: Saunders Elsevier.

Brien S, Lewith G, Walker A, Hicks SM, Middleton D (2004 Dec). "Bromelain as a Treatment for Osteoarthritis: a Review of Clinical Studies," Evid Based Complement Alternat Med. 1(3):251-257.

Brown AL et al. (2008 Aug). "Effects of dietary supplementation with the green tea polyphenol epigallocatechin-3-gallate on insulin resistance and associated metabolic risk factors: randomized controlled trial," Br J Nutr. 19:1-9.

Brown T.L., LeMay H.E., Bursten B.E. Chemistry: The Central Science. 10th ed. Upper Saddle River: Pearson Prentice Hall, 2006.

Brum LF, Elisabetsky E, Souza D (2001 Aug). "Effects of linalool on [(3)H]MK801 and [(3)H] muscimol binding in mouse cortical membranes," Phytother Res. 15(5):422-5.

Buchbauer G, Jirovetz L, Jäger W, Dietrich H, Plank C (1991 Nov-Dec). "Aromatherapy: evidence for sedative effects of the essential oil of lavender after inhalation," Z Naturforsch C. 46(11-12):1067-72.

Bucheli P., Vidal, K., Shen, L., Gu, Z., Zhang, C., Miller, L. E., & Wang, J. (2011 Feb). Goji berry effects on macular characteristics and plasma antioxidant levels. Optom Vis Sci, 88(2), 257-262.

Bucher HC, Hengstler P, Schindler C, Meier G (2002 Mar). "N-3 polyunsaturated fatty acids in coronary heart disease: a meta-analysis of randomized controlled trials," Am J Med. 112(4):298-304.

Buck DS, Nidorf DM, Addino JG (1994 Jun). "Comparison of two topical preparations for the treatment of onychomycosis: Melaleuca alternifolia (tea tree) oil and clotrimazole," J Fam Pract. 38(6):601-5.

Bukovska, A., Cikos, S., Juhas, S., Il'kova, G., Rehak, P., & Koppel, J. (2007 Feb). Effects of a combination of thyme and oregano essential oils on TNBS-induced colitis in mice. Mediators Inflamm, 2007, 23296.

Bulbring E. (1946) Observations on the Isolated Phrenic Nerve Diaphragm Preparation of the Rat. British Journal of Pharmacology. 1: 38-61.

Burke BE, Baillie JE, Olson RD (2004 May). "Essential oil of Australian lemon myrtle (Backhousia citriodora) in the treatment of molluscum contagiosum in children," Biomed Pharmacother. 58(4):245-7.

Bushra, R., Aslam, N., & Khan, A. Y. (2011 Mar). Food-drug interactions. Oman Med J, 26(2), 77-83.

Cabrera-Vique C, Marfil R, Gimenez R, Martinez-Augustin O (2012 May). "Bioactive compounds and nutritional significance of virgin argan oil—an edible oil with potential as a functional food," Nutr Rev. 70(5):266-79.

Caccioni DR, Guizzardi M, Biondi DM, Renda A, Ruberto G (1998 Aug 18). "Relationship between volatile components of citrus fruit essential oils and antimicrobial action on Penicillium digitatum and penicillium italicum," Int J Food Microbiol. 43(1-2):73-9.

Caldefie-Chézet F, Fusillier C, Jarde T, Laroye H, Damez M, Vasson MP, Guillot J (2006 May). "Potential anti-inflammatory effects of Melaleuca alternifolia essential oil on human peripheral blood leukocytes," Phytother Res. 20(5):364-70.

Caldefie-Chézet F, Guerry M, Chalchat JC, Fusillier C, Vasson MP, Guillot J (2004 Aug). "Anti-inflammatory effects of Melaleuca alternifolia essential oil on human polymorphonuclear neutrophils and monocytes," Free Radic Res. 38(8):805-11.

Campelo, L. M., Goncalves, F. C., Feitosa, C. M., & de Freitas, R. M. (2011 Jul). Antioxidant activity of Citrus limon essential oil in mouse hippocampus. Pharm Biol, 49(7), 709-715.

Candan F, Unlu M, Tepe B, Daferera D, Polissiou M, Sökmen A, Akpulat HA (2003 May). "Antioxidant and antimicrobial activity of the essential oil and methanol extracts of Achillea millefolium subsp. millefolium Afan. (Asteraceae)," J Ethnopharmacol. 87(2-3):215-20.

Canyon DV, Speare R (2007 Apr). "A comparison of botanical and synthetic substances commonly used to prevent head lice (Pediculus humanus var. capitis) infestation," Int J Dermatol. 46(4):422-6.

Capasso R, Savino F, Capasso F (2007 Oct). "Effects of the herbal formulation ColiMil on upper gastrointestinal transit in mice in vivo," Phytother Res. 21(10):999-1101.

Cappello G, Spezzaferro M, Grossi L, Manzoli L, Marzio L. (2007 Jun). "Peppermint oil (Mintoil) in the treatment of irritable bowel syndrome: a prospective double blind placebo-controlled randomized trial," Dig Liver Dis. 39(6):530-6.

Carnesecchi S., Bradaia A., Fischer B., Coelho D., Scholler-Guinard M., Gosse F., Raul F. (2002) Perturbation by Geraniol of Cell Membrane Permeability and Signal Transduction Pathways in Human Colon Cancer Cells. The Journal of Pharmacology and Experimental Therapeutics. 303: 711-715.

Appendix & Research References

Carnesecchi S., Bras-Goncalves R., Bradaia A., Zeisel M., Gosse F., Poupon M-F., Raul F. (2004) Geraniol, a component of plant essential oils, modulates DNA synthesis and potentiates 5-fluorouracil efficacy on human colon tumor xenografts. Cancer Letters. 215: 53-59.

Carnesecchi S., Langley K., Exinger F., Gosse F., Raul F. (2002) Geraniol, a Component of Plant Essential Oils, Sensitizes Human Colonic Cancer Cells to 5-Fluorouracil Treatment. The Journal of Pharmacology and Experimental Therapeutics. 301: 625-630.

Carnesecchi S, Schneider Y, Ceraline J, Duranton B, Gosse F, Seiler N, Raul F (2001 Jul). "Geraniol, a component of plant essential oils, inhibits growth and polyamine biosynthesis in human colon cancer cells," J Pharmacol Exp Ther. 298(1):197-200.

Carson CF, Cookson BD, Farrelly HD, Riley TV (1995 Mar). "Susceptibility of methicillin-resistant Staphylococcus aureus to the essential oil of Melaleuca alternifolia," J Antimicrob Chemother. 35(3):421-4.

Carvalho-Freitas MI, Costa M (2002 Dec). "Anxiolytic and sedative effects of extracts and essential oil from Citrus aurantium L," Biol Pharm Bull. 25(12):1629-33.

Catalán A, Pacheco JG, Martínez A, Mondaca MA (2008 Mar). "In vitro and in vivo activity of Melaleuca alternifolia mixed with tissue conditioner on Candida albicans," Oral Surg Oral Med Oral Pathol Oral Radiol Endod. 105(3):327-32.

Ceccarelli I, Lariviere WR, Fiorenzani P, Sacerdote P, Aloisi AM (2004 Mar 19). "Effects of long-term exposure of lemon essential oil odor on behavioral, hormonal and neuronal parameters in male and female rats," Brain Res. 1001(1-2):78-86.

Cenizo, V., Andre, V., Reymermier, C., Sommer, P., Damour, O., & Perrier, E. (2006 Aug). LOXL as a target to increase the elastin content in adult skin: a dill extract induces the LOXL gene expression. Exp Dermatol, 15(8), 574-581.

Centers for Disease Control and Prevention (CDC) (2004 May 7). "Spina bifida and anencephaly before and after folic acid mandate--United States, 1995-1996 and 1999-2000," MMWR Morb Mortal Wkly Rep. 53(17):362-5.

Ceriotti G, Spandrio L, Gazzaniga A (1967 Jul-Aug). "[Demonstration, isolation and physical and chemical characteristics of narciclasine, a new antimitotic of plant origin]," Tumori. 53(4):359-71.

Cermelli C, Fabio A, Fabio G, Quaglio P (2008 Jan). "Effect of eucalyptus essential oil on respiratory bacteria and viruses," Curr Microbiol. 56(1):89-92.

Cháfer, M., Sanchez-Gonzalez, L., Gonzalez-Martinez, C., & Chiralt, A. (2012 Aug). Fungal decay and shelf life of oranges coated with chitosan and bergamot, thyme, and tea tree essential oils. J Food Sci, 77(8), E182-187.

Chaieb K, Zmantar T, Ksouri R, Hajlaoui H, Mahdouani K, Abdelly C, Bakhrouf A (2007 Sep). "Antioxidant properties of the essential oil of Eugenia caryophyllata and its antifungal activity against a large number of clinical Candida species," Mycoses. 50(5):403-6.

Chaiyakunapruk N, Kitikannakorn N, Nathisuwan S, Leeprakobboon K, Leelasettagool C (2006 Jan). "The efficacy of ginger for the prevention of postoperative nausea and vomiting: a meta-analysis," Am J Obstet Gynecol. 53(17):362-5.

Chakraborty PK, Mustafi SB, Raha S (2008 Sep). "Pro-survival effects of repetitive low-grade oxidative stress are inhibited by simultaneous exposure to resveratrol," Pharmacol Res. 2).

Chambers H.F. (2001) The Changing Epidemiology of Staphylococcus aureus?. Emerging Infectious Diseases. 7: 178-182.

Chang, K. S., Tak, J. H., Kim, S. I., Lee, W. J., & Ahn, Y. J. (2006 Nov). Repellency of Cinnamomum cassia bark compounds and cream containing cassia oil to Aedes aegypti (Diptera: Culicidae) under laboratory and indoor conditions. Pest Manag Sci, 62(11), 1032-1038.

Chang WC, Yu YM, Chiang SY, Tseng CY (2008 Apr). "Ellagic acid supresses oxidised low-density lipoprotein-induced aortic smooth muscle cell proliferation: studies on the activation of extracellular signal-regulated kinase ½ and proliferating cell nuclear antigen expression," Br J Nutr. 99(4):709-14.

Chapman A.G. (1998) Glutamate receptors in epilepsy. Progress in Brain Research. 116: 371-383.

Chapman A.G. (2000) Glutamate and Epilepsy. The Journal of Nutrition. 130: 1043S-1045S.

Charles CH, Vincent JW, Borycheski L, Amatnieks Y, Sarina M, Qaqish J, Proskin HM (2000 Sep). "Effect of an essential oil-containing dentifrice on dental plaque microbial composition," Am J Dent. 13(2):26C-30C.

Charrouf Z, Guillaume D (2010 May). "Should the amazigh diet (regular and moderate argan-oil consumption) have a beneficial impact on human health?," Crit Rev Food Sci Nutr. 50(5):473-7.

Checker R, Chatterjee S, Sharma D, Gupta S, Variyar P, Sharma A, Poduval TB (2008 May). "Immunomodulatory and radioprotective effects of lignans derived from fresh nutmeg mace (Myristica fragrans) in mammalian splenocytes," Int Immunopharmacol. 8(5):661-9.

Chen M, Zhang J, Yu S, Wang S, Zhang Z, Chen J, Xiao J, Wang Y (2012). "Anti-lung-cancer activity and liposome-based delivery systems of beta-elemene," Evid Based Complement Alternat Med. 2012:259523.

Chen YC, Chiu WT, Wu MS (2006 Jul). "Therapeutic effect of topical gamma-linolenic acid on refractory uremic pruritus," Am J Kidney Dis. 48(1):69-76.

Chen, Y., Zeng, H., Tian, J., Ban, X., Ma, B., & Wang, Y. (2014 Apr). Dill (Anethum graveolens L.) seed essential oil induces Candida albicans apoptosis in a metacaspase-dependent manner. Fungal Biol, 118(4), 394-401.

Cheung S, Tai J (2007 Jun). "Anti-proliferative and antioxidant properties of rosemary Rosmarinus officinalis," Oncol Rep. 17(6):1525-31.

Chevrier MR, Ryan AE, Lee DY, Zhongze M, Wu-Yan Z, Via CS (2005 May). "Boswellia carterii extract inhibits TH1 cytokines and promotes TH2 cytokines in vitro," Clin Diagn Lab Immunol. 12(5):575-80.

Chien, L. W., Cheng, S. L., & Liu, C. F. (2012 Aug). The effect of lavender aromatherapy on autonomic nervous system in midlife women with insomnia. Evid Based Complement Alternat Med, 2012.

Chinou IB, Roussis V, Perdetzoglou D, Loukis A (1996 Aug). "Chemical and biological studies on two Helichrysum species of Greek origin," Planta Med. 62(4):377-9.

Cho, M. Y., Min, E. S., Hur, M. H., & Lee, M. S. (2013 Feb). Effects of aromatherapy on the anxiety, vital signs, and sleep quality of percutaneous coronary intervention patients in intensive care units. Evid Based Complement Alternat Med, 2013, 1-6.

Cho, S., Choi, Y., Park, S., & Park, T. (2012 Feb). Carvacrol prevents diet-induced obesity by modulating gene expressions involved in adipogenesis and inflammation in mice fed with high-fat diet. J Nutr Biochem, 23(2), 192-201.

Choi, H. Y., Yang, Y. C., Lee, S. H., Clark, J. M., & Ahn, Y. J. (2010 May). Efficacy of spray formulations containing binary mixtures of clove and eucalyptus oils against susceptible and pyrethroid/ malathion-resistant head lice (Anoplura: Pediculidae). J Med Entomol, 47(3), 387-391.

Choi, U. K., Lee, O. H., Yim, J. H., Cho, C. W., Rhee, Y. K., Lim, S. I., & Kim, Y. C. (2010 Feb). Hypolipidemic and antioxidant effects of dandelion (Taraxacum officinale) root and leaf on cholesterol-fed rabbits. Int J Mol Sci, 11(1), 67-78.

Chung, M. J., Cho, S. Y., Bhuiyan, M. J., Kim, K. H., & Lee, S. J. (2010 Jul). Anti-diabetic effects of lemon balm (Melissa officinalis) essential oil on glucose- and lipid-regulating enzymes in type 2 diabetic mice. Br J Nutr, 104(2), 180-188.

Ciacci C, Peluso G, Iannoni E, Siniscalchi M, Iovino P, Rispo A, Tortora R, Bucci C, Zingone F, Margarucci S, Calvani M (2007 Oct). "L-Carnitine in the treatment of fatigue in adult celiac disease patients: a pilot study," Dig Liver Dis. 39(10):922-8.

Ciftci O., Ozdemir I., Tanyildizi S., Yildiz S., Oguzturk H. (2011) Antioxidative effects of curcumin, β-myrcene and 1,8-cineole against 2,3,7,8-tetracholorodibenzo-p-dioxin - induced oxidative stress in rats liver. Toxicology and Industrial Health. 27: 447-453.

Cioanca, O., Hritcu, L., Mihasan, M., Trifan, A., & Hancianu, M. (2014 May). Inhalation of coriander volatile oil increased anxiolytic-antidepressant-like behaviors and decreased oxidative status in beta-amyloid (1-42) rat model of Alzheimer's disease. Physiol Behav, 131, 68-74.

Cioanca, O., Hritcu, L., Mihasan, M., & Hancianu, M. (2013 Aug). Cognitive-enhancing and antioxidant activities of inhaled coriander volatile oil in amyloid beta(1-42) rat model of Alzheimer's disease. Physiol Behav, 120, 193-202.

Coderch L., Lopez O., de la Maza A., Parra J.L. (2003) Ceramides and Skin Function. American Journal of Clinical Dermatology. 4: 107-129.

Cooley K, Szczurko O, Perri D, Mills EJ, Bernhardt B, Zhou Q, Seely D (2009 Aug 31). "Naturopathic care for anxiety: a randomized controlled trial IS-RCTN78958974," PLoS One. 4(8):e6628.

Modern Essentials Usage Guide

Corasaniti, M. T., Maiuolo, J., Maida, S., Fratto, V., Navarra, M., Russo, R., . . . Bagetta, G. (2007 Jun). Cell signaling pathways in the mechanisms of neuroprotection afforded by bergamot essential oil against NMDA-induced cell death in vitro. Br J Pharmacol, 151(4), 518-529.

Couse JF, Lindzey J, Grandien K, Gustafsson JA, Korach KS (1997 Nov). "Tissue distribution and quantitative analysis of estrogen reseptor-alpha (ERalpha) and estrogen receptor-beta (ERbeta) messenger ribonucleic acid in the wild-type and ERalpha-knockout mouse," Endocrinology. 138"11):4613-21.

Cowan M.K., Talaro K.P. Microbiology: A Systems Approach. 2nd ed. New York: McGraw Hill, 2009.

Cox SD, Mann CM, Markham JL, Bell HC, Gustafson JE, Warmington JR, Wyllie SG (2000 Jan). "The mode of antimicrobial action of the essential oil of Melaleuca alternifolia (tea tree oil)," J Appl Microbiol. 88(1):170-5.

Cross SE, Russell M, Southwell I, Roberts MS (2008 May). "Human skin penetration of the major components of Australian tea tree oil applied in its pure form and as a 20% solution in vitro," Eur J Pharm Biopharm. 69(1):214-22.

Crowell P.L., Chang R.R., Ren Z., Elson C.E., Gould M.N. (1991) Selective Inhibition of Isoprenylation of 21-26kDa Proteins by the Anticarcinogen d-Limonene and Its Metabolites. J. Biol. Chem. 266: 17679-17685.

Cuellar, M. J., Giner, R. M., Recio, M. C., Manez, S., & Rios, J. L. (2001 Mar). Topical anti-inflammatory activity of some Asian medicinal plants used in dermatological disorders. Fitoterapia, 72(3), 221-229.

Cui Y et al. (2008 May 15). "Dietary flavonoid intake and lung cancer—a population-based case-control study," Cancer. 112(10):2241-8.

Curi R, Alvarez M, Bazotte RB, Botion LM, Godoy JL, Bracht A (1986). "Effect of Stevia rebaudiana on glucose tolerance in normal adult humans," Braz J Med Biol Res. 19(6):771-4.

Curio M, Jacone H, Perrut J, Pinto AC, Filho VF, Silva RC (2009 Aug). "Acute effect of Copaifera reticulata Ducke copaiba oil in rats tested in the elevated plus-maze: an ethological analysis," J Pharm Pharmacol. 61(8):1105-10.

Dai ZJ, Tang W, Lu WF, Gao J, Kang HF, Ma XB, Min WL, Wang XJ, Wu WY (2013 Mar 14). "Antiproliferative and apoptotic effects of beta-elemne on human hepatoma HepG2 cells," Cancer Cell Int. 13(1):27.

Darmstadt GL, Mao-Qiang M, Chi E, Saha SK, Ziboh VA, Black RE, Santosham M, Elias PM (2002). "Impact of topical oils on the skin barrier: possible implications for neonatal health in developing countries," Acta Paediatr. 91(5):546-54.

Darmstadt GL, Saha SK, Ahmed AS, Chowdhury MA, Law PA, Ahmed S, Alam MA, Black RE, Santosham M (2005 Mar 19-25). "Effect of topical treatment with skin barrier-enhancing emollients on nosocomial infections in preterm infants in Bangladesh: a randomised controlled trial," Lancet. 365(9464):1039-45.

Damiani C.E.N., Rossoni L.V., Vassallo D.V. (2003) Vasorelaxant effects of eugenol on rat thoracic aorta. Vascular Pharmacology. 40: 59-66.

Das, I., Acharya, A., Berry, D. L., Sen, S., Williams, E., Permaul, E., . . . Saha, T. (2012 Sep). Antioxidative effects of the spice cardamom against non-melanoma skin cancer by modulating nuclear factor erythroid-2-related factor 2 and NF-kappaB signalling pathways. Br J Nutr, 108(6), 984-997.

D'Auria FD, Laino L, Strippoli V, Tecca M, Salvatore G, Battinelli L, Mazzanti G (2001 Aug). "In vitro activity of tea tree oil against Candida albicans mycelial conversion and other pathogenic fungi," J Chemother. 13(4):377-83.

D'Auria FD, Tecca M, Strippoli V, Salvatore G, Battinelli L, Mazzanti G (2005 Aug). "Antifungal activity of Lavandula angustifolia essential oil against Candida albicans yeast and mycelial form," Med Mycol. 43(5):391-6.

Davaatseren, M., Hur, H. J., Yang, H. J., Hwang, J. T., Park, J. H., Kim, H. J., . . . Sung, M. J. (2013 Aug). Taraxacum official (dandelion) leaf extract alleviates high-fat diet-induced nonalcoholic fatty liver. Food Chem Toxicol, 58, 30-36.

Davies K (1995). "Oxidative stress: the paradox of aerobic life," Biochem Soc Symp. 61:1–31.

de Almeida R.N., Araujo D.A.M., Goncalvevs J.C.R., Montenegro F.C., de Sousa D.P., Leite J.R., Mattei R., Benedito M.A.C., de Carvalho J.G.B., Cruz J.S., Maia J.G.S. (2009) Rosewood oil induces sedation and inhibits compound action potential in rodents. Journal of Ethanopharmacology. 124: 440-443.

de Almeida R.N., de Sousa D.P., Nobrega F.F.F., Claudino F.S., Araujo D.A.M., Leite J.R., Mattei R. (2008) Anticonvulsant effect of a natural compound α,β-epoxy-carvone and its actioin on the nerve excitability. Neuroscience Letters. 443: 51-55.

Debersac P, Heydel JM, Amiot MJ, Goudonnet H, Artur Y, Suschetet M, Siess MH (2001 Sep). "Induction of cytochrome P450 and/or detoxication enzymes by various extracts of rosemary: description of specific patterns," Food Chem Toxicol. 39(9):907-18.

Deeptha K, Kamaleeswari M, Sengottuvelan M, Nalini N (2006 Nov). "Dose dependent inhibitory effect of dietary caraway on 1,2-dimethylhydrazine induced colonic aberrant crypt foci and bacterial enzyme activity in rats," Invest New Drugs. 24(6):479-88.

de la Garza, A. L., Etxeberria, U., Lostao, M. P., San Roman, B., Barrenetxe, J., Martinez, J. A., & Milagro, F. I. (2013 Dec). Helichrysum and grapefruit extracts inhibit carbohydrate digestion and absorption, improving postprandial glucose levels and hyperinsulinemia in rats. J Agric Food Chem, 61(49), 12012-12019.

Delaquis, P. J., Stanich, K., Girard, B., & Mazza, G. (2002 Mar). Antimicrobial activity of individual and mixed fractions of dill, cilantro, coriander and eucalyptus essential oils. Int J Food Microbiol, 74(1–2), 101-109.

DeLeo F.R., Otto M., Kreiswirth B.N., Chambers H.F. (2010) Community-associated meticillin-resistant Staphylococcus aureus. The Lancet. 375: 1557-1568.

Department of Environmental Medicine, Odense University, Denmark (1992 Dec). "Ginger (Zingiber officinale) in rheumatism and musculoskeletal disorders," Med Hypotheses. 39(4):342-8.

de Rapper, S., Kamatou, G., Viljoen, A., & van Vuuren, S. (2013 Jun). The in vitro antimicrobial activity of lavandula angustifolia essential oil in combination with other aroma-therapeutic oils. Evid Based Complement Alternat Med, 2013, 1-10.

De S. Aguiar, R. W., Ootani, M. A., Ascencio, S. D., Ferreira, T. P., dos Santos, M. M., & dos Santos, G. R. (2014 Jan). Fumigant antifungal activity of Corymbia citriodora and Cymbopogon nardus essential oils and citronellal against three fungal species. Scientific World Journal, 2014, 1-8.

De Spirt S, Stahl W, Tronnier H, Sies H, Bejot M, Maurette JM, Heinrich U (2009 Feb). "Intervention with flaxseed and borage oil supplements modulates skin condition in women," Br J Nutr. 101(3):440-5.

de Sousa D.P., Goncalves J.C.R., Quintanas-Junior L., Cruz J.S., Araujo D.A.M., de Almeida R.N. (2006) Study of anticonvulsant effect of citronellol, a monoterpene alcohol, in rodents. Neuroscience Letters. 401: 231-235.

Deters A, Zippel J, Hellenbrand N, Pappai D, Possemeyer C, Hensel A (2010 Jan 8). "Aqueous extracts and polysaccharides from Marshmallow roots (Althea officinalis L.): cellular internalisation and stimulation of cell physiology of human epithelial cells in vitro," J Ethnopharmacol. 127(1):62-9.

Devika PT, Mainzen Prince PS (2008 Jan). "(-) Epigallocatechin gallate (EGCG) prevents isoprenaline-induced cardiac marker enzymes and membrane-bound ATPases," J Pharm Pharmacol. 60(1):125-33.

De Vriendt T, Moreno LA, De Henauw S (2009 Sep). "Chronic stress and obesity in adolescents: scientific evidence and methodological issues for epidemiological research," Nutr Metab Cardiovasc Dis. 19(7):511-9.

Dias, F. M., Leffa, D. D., Daumann, F., Marques Sde, O., Luciano, T. F., Possato, J. C., . . . de Lira, F. S. (2014 Feb). Acerola (Malpighia emarginata DC.) juice intake protects against alterations to proteins involved in inflammatory and lipolysis pathways in the adipose tissue of obese mice fed a cafeteria diet. Lipids Health Dis, 13, 1-9.

Díaz C, Quesada S, Brenes O, Aguilar G, Cicció JF (2008). "Chemical composition of Schinus molle essential oil and its cytotoxic activity on tumour cell lines," Nat Prod Res. 22(17):1521-34.

Diego MA, Jones NA, Field T, Hernandez-Reif M, Schanberg S, Kuhn C, McAdam V, Galamaga R, Galamaga M (1998 Dec). "Aromatherapy positively affects mood, EEG patterns of alertness and math computations," Int J Neurosci. 96(3-4):217-24.

Diggins K.C. (2008) Treatment of mild to moderate dehydration in children with oral rehydration therapy. Journal of the American Academy of Nurse Practitioners. 20: 402-406.

Dikshit A, Naqvi AA, Husain A. (1986 May). "Schinus molle: a new source of natural fungitoxicant," Appl Environ Microbiol. 51(5):1085-8.

Dimas K, Kokkinopoulos D, Demetzos C, Vaos B, Marselos M, Malamas M, Tzavaras T (1999 Mar). "The effect of sclareol on growth and cell cycle progression of human leukemic cell lines," Leuk Res. 23(3):217-34.

Dimpfel W, Pischel I, Lehnfeld R (2004 Sep 29). "Effects of lozenge containing lavender oil, extracts from hops, lemon balm and oat on electrical brain activity of volunteers," Eur J Med Res. 9(9):423-31.

Ding XF, Shen M, Xu LY, Dong JH, Chen G (2013 May). "13,14-bis(cis-3,5-dimethyl-1-piperazinyl)-beta-elemene, a novel beta-elemene derivative, shows potent antitumor activities via inhibition of mTOR in human breast cancer cells," Oncol Lett. 5(5):1554-1558.

Domitrović R, Jakovac H, Romić Z, Rahelić D, Tadić Z (2010 Aug 9). "Antifibrotic activity of Taraxacum officinale root in carbon tetrachloride-induced liver damage in mice," J Ethnopharmacol. 130(3):569-77.

Doran AL, Morden WE, Dunn K, Edwards-Jones V (2009 Apr). "Vapour-phase activities of essential oils against antibiotic sensitive and resistant bacteria including MRSA," Lett Appl Microbiol. 48(4):387-92.

Drobiova H, Thomson M, Al-Qattan K, Peltonen-Shalaby R, Al-Amin Z, Ali M (2009 Feb 20). "Garlic increases antioxidant levels in diabetic and hypertensive rats determined by a modified peroxidase method," Evid Based Complement Alternat Med. Epub ahead of print.

Duarte MC, Leme EE, Delarmelina C, Soares AA, Figueira GM, Sartoratto A (2007 May 4). "Activity of essential oils from Brazilian medicinal plants on Escherichia coli," J Ethnopharmacol. 111(2):197-201

Dudai N, Weinstein Y, Krup M, Rabinski T, Ofir R (2005 May). "Citral is a new inducer of caspase-3 in tumor cell lines," Planta Med. 71(5):484-8.

Dunn C, Sleep J, Collett D (1995 Jan). "Sensing an improvement: an experimental study to evaluate the use of aromatherapy, massage and periods of rest in an intensive care unit," J Adv Nurs. 21(1):34-40.

Dunstan JA, Mori TA, Barden A, Beilin LJ, Taylor AL, Holt PG, Prescott SL (2003 Dec). "Fish oil supplementation in pregnancy modifies neonatal allergen-specific immune responses and clinical outcomes in infants at high risk of atopy: a randomized, controlled trial," J Allergy Clin Immunol. 112(6):1178-84.

Duwiejua M, Zeitlin IJ, Waterman PG, Chapman J, Mhango GJ, Provan GJ (1993 Feb). "Anti-inflammatory activity of resins from some species of the plant family Burseraceae," Planta Med. 59(1):12-6.

Dwivedi C, Abu-Ghazaleh A (1997 Aug). "Chemopreventive effects of sandalwood oil on skin papillomas in mice," Eur J Cancer Prev. 6(4):399-401.

Dwivedi C, Guan X, Harmsen WL, Voss AL, Goetz-Parten DE, Koopman EM, Johnson KM, Valluri HB, Matthees DP (2003 Feb). "Chemopreventive effects of alpha-santalol on skin tumor development in CD-1 and SENCAR mice," Cancer Epidemiol Biomarkers Prev. 12(2):151-6.

Dwivedi C, Maydew ER, Hora JJ, Ramaeker DM, Guan X. (2005 Oct). "Chemopreventive effects of various concentrations of alpha-santalol on skin cancer development in CD-1 mice," Eur J Cancer Prev. 14(5):473-6.

Dwivedi C, Valluri HB, Guan X, Agarwal R (2006 Sep). "Chemopreventive effects of alpha-santalol on ultraviolet B radiation-induced skin tumor development in SKH-1 hairless mice," Carcinogenesis. 27(9):1917-22.

Ebihara T, Ebihara S, Maruyama M, Kobayashi M, Itou A, Arai H, Sasaki H (2006 Sep). "A randomized trial of olfactory stimulation using black pepper oil in older people with swallowing dysfunction," J Am Geriatr Soc. 54(9):1401-6.

Edwards-Jones V, Buck R, Shawcross SG, Dawson MM, Dunn K (2004 Dec). "The effect of essential oils on methicillin-resistant Staphylococcus aureus using a dressing model," Burns. 30(8):772-7.

Elson CE, Underbakke GL, Hanson P, Shrago E, Wainberg RH, Qureshi AA (1989 Aug). "Impact of lemongrass oil, an essential oil, on serum cholesterol," Lipids. 24(8):677-9.

Elwakeel HA, Moneim HA, Farid M, Gohar AA (2007 Jul). "Clove oil cream: a new effective treatment for chronic anal fissure," Colorectal Dis. 9(6):549-52.

Enan E (2001 Nov). "Insecticidal activity of essential oils: octopaminergic sites of action," Comp Biochem Physiol C Toxicol Pharmacol. 130(3):325-37.

Enshaieh S, Jooya A, Siadat AH, Iraji F (2007 Jan-Feb). "The efficacy of 5% topical tea tree oil gel in mild to moderate acne vulgaris: a randomized, double-blind placebo-controlled study," Indian J Dermatol Venereol Leprol. 73(1):22-5.

Eriksson K., Levin J.O. (1996) Gas chromatographic-mass spectrometric identification of metabolites from α-pinene in human urine after occupational exposure to sawing fumes. J. Chromatography B. 677: 85-98.

Erkkilä AT, Lichtenstein AH, Mozaffarian D, Herrington DM (2004 Sep). "Fish intake is associated with a reduced progression of coronary artery atherosclerosis in postmenopausal women with coronary artery disease," Am J Clin Nutr. 80(3):626-32.

Erkkilä AT, Schwab US, de Mello VD, Lappalainen T, Mussalo H, Lehto S, Kemi V, Lamberg-Allardt C, Uusitupa MI (2008 Sep). "Effects of fatty and lean fish intake on blood pressure in subjects with coronary heart disease using multiple medications," Eur J Nutr. 47(6):319-28.

Esfandiary, E., Karimipour, M., Mardani, M., Alaei, H., Ghannadian, M., Kazemi, M., . . . Esmaeili, A. (2014 Apr). Novel effects of Rosa damascena extract on memory and neurogenesis in a rat model of Alzheimer's disease. J Neurosci Res, 92(4), 517-530.

Evandri MG, Battinelli L, Daniele C, Mastrangelo S, Bolle P, Mazzanti G (2005 Sep). "The antimutagenic activity of Lavandula angustifolia (lavender) essential oil in the bacterial reverse mutation assay," Food Chem Toxicol. 43(9):1381-7.

Evans J.D., Martin S.A. (2000) Effects of Thymol on Ruminal Microorganisms. Current Microbiology. 41: 336-340.

Fabio A, Cermelli C, Fabio G, Nicoletti P, Quaglio P (2007 Apr). "Screening of the antibacterial effects of a variety of essential oils on microorganisms responsible for respiratory infections," Phytother Res. 21(4):374-7.

Fan AY, Lao L, Zhang RX, Zhou AN, Wang LB, Moudgil KD, Lee DY, Ma ZZ, Zhang WY, Berman BM (2005 Oct 3). "Effects of an acetone extract of Boswellia carterii Birdw. (Burseraceae) gum resin on adjuvant-induced arthritis in lewis rats," J Ethnopharmacol. 101(1-3):104-9.

Fang, J. Y., Leu, Y. L., Hwang, T. L., & Cheng, H. C. (2004 Nov). Essential oils from sweet basil (Ocimum basilicum) as novel enhancers to accelerate transdermal drug delivery. Biol Pharm Bull, 27(11), 1819-1825.

Fang, Y.-Z., Yang, S., & Wu, G. (2002). Free radicals, antioxidants, and nutrition. Nutrition, 18(10), 872-879.

Fathiazad, F., Matlobi, A., Khorrami, A., Hamedeyazdan, S., Soraya, H., Hammami, M., . . . Garjani, A. (2012 Jan). Phytochemical screening and evaluation of cardioprotective activity of ethanolic extract of Ocimum basilicum L. (basil) against isoproterenol induced myocardial infarction in rats. Daru, 20(1), 87.

Faturi C, Leite, J. R., Alves, P. B., Canton, A. C., & Teixeira-Silva, F. (2010 May). Anxiolytic-like effect of sweet orange aroma in Wistar rats. Prog Neuropsychopharmacol Biol Psychiatry, 34(4), 605-609.

Feinblatt HM (1960 Jan). "Cajeput-type oil for the treatment of furunculosis," J Natl Med Assoc. 52:32-4.

Fernandez, L. F., Palomino, O. M., & Frutos, G. (2014 Jan). Effectiveness of Rosmarinus officinalis essential oil as antihypotensive agent in primary hypotensive patients and its influence on health-related quality of life. J Ethnopharmacol, 151(1), 509-516.

Ferrara, L., Naviglio, D., & Armone Caruso, A. (2012). Cytological aspects on the effects of a nasal spray consisting of standardized extract of citrus lemon and essential oils in allergic rhinopathy. ISRN Pharm, 2012, 1-6.

Ferrini AM, Mannoni V, Aureli P, Salvatore G, Piccirilli E, Ceddia T, Pontieri E, Sessa R, Oliva B (2006 Jul-Sep). "Melaleuca alternifolia essential oil possesses potent anti-staphylococcal activity extended to strains resistant to antibiotics," Int J Immunopathol Pharmacol. 19(3):539-44.

Field T, Diego M, Hernandez-Reif M, Cisneros W, Feijo L, Vera Y, Gil K, Grina D, Claire He Q (2005 Feb). "Lavender fragrance cleansing gel effects on relaxation," Int J Neurosci. 115(2):207-22.

Filoche SK, Soma K, Sissons CH (2005 Aug). "Antimicrobial effects of essential oils in combination with chlorhexidine digluconate," Oral Microbiol Immunol. 20(4):221-5.

Fine DH, Furgang D, Barnett ML, Drew C, Steinberg L, Charles CH, Vincent JW (2000 Mar). "Effect of an essential oil-containing antiseptic mouthrinse on plaque and salivary Streptococcus mutans levels," J Clin Periodontol. 27(3):157-61.

263

Modern Essentials Usage Guide

Fitzhugh DJ, Shan S, Dewhirst MW, Hale LP (2008 Jul). "Bromelain treatment decreases neutrophil migration to sites of inflammation," Clin Immunol. 128(1):66-74.

Flor-Weiler, L. B., Behle, R. W., & Stafford, K. C., 3rd. (2011 Mar). Susceptibility of four tick species, Amblyomma americanum, Dermacentor variabilis, Ixodes scapularis, and Rhipicephalus sanguineus (Acari: Ixodidae), to nootkatone from essential oil of grapefruit. J Med Entomol, 48(2), 322-326.

Force M, Sparks WS, Ronzio RA (2000 May). "Inhibition of enteric parasites by emulsified oil of oregano in vivo," Phytother Res. 14(3):213-4.

Fowke JH, Morrow JD, Motley S, Bostick RM, Ness RM (2006 Oct). "Brassica vegetable consumption reduces urinary F2-isoprostane levels independent of micronutrient intake," Carcinogenesis. 27(10):2096-102.

Franek KJ, Zhou Z, Zhang WD, Chen WY (2005 Jan). "In vitro studies of baicalin alone or in combination with Salvia miltiorrhiza extract as a potential anti-cancer agent," Int J Oncol. 26(1):217-24.

Frangou S, Lewis M, McCrone P (2006 Jan). "Efficacy of ethyl-eicosapentaenoic acid in bipolar depression: randomised double-blind placebo-controlled study," Br J Psychiatry. 188:46-50.

Freires Ide, A., Murata, R. M., Furletti, V. F., Sartoratto, A., Alencar, S. M., Figueira, G. M., . . . Rosalen, P. L. (2014 Jun). Coriandrum sativum L. (Coriander) Essential Oil: Antifungal Activity and Mode of Action on Candida spp., and Molecular Targets Affected in Human Whole-Genome Expression. PLoS ONE, 9(6), 1-13.

Freise J, Köhler S (1999 Mar). "Peppermint oil-caraway oil fixed combination in non-ulcer dyspepsia--comparison of the effects of enteric preparations," Pharmazie. 54(3):210-5.

Freitas F.P., Freitas S.P., Lemos G.C.S., Vieira I.J.C., Gravina G.A., Lemos F.J.A. (2010) Comparative Larvicidal Activity of Essential Oils from Three Medicinal Plants against Aedes aeypti L. Chemistry & Biodiversity. 7: 2801-2807.

Frydman-Marom, A., Levin, A., Farfara, D., Benromano, T., Scherzer-Attali, R., Peled, S., . . . Ovadia, M. (2011 Feb). Orally administered cinnamon extract reduces beta-amyloid oligomerization and corrects cognitive impairment in Alzheimer's disease animal models. PLoS ONE, 6(1), 1-11.

Fukumoto S, Sawasaki E, Okuyama S, Miyake Y, Yokogoshi H (2006 Feb-Apr). "Flavor components of monoterpenes in citrus essential oils enhance the release of monoamines from rat brain slices," Nutr Neurosci. 9(1-2):73-80.

Furuhjelm C, Warstedt K, Larsson J, Fredriksson M, Böttcher MF, Fälth-Magnusson K, Duchén K (2009 Sep). "Fish oil supplementation in pregnancy and lactation may decrease the risk of infant allergy," Acta Paediatr. 98(9):1461-7.

Gaetani G.F., Ferraris A.M., Rolfo M., Mangerini R., Arena S., Kirkman H.N. (1996) Predominant role of catalase in the disposal of hydrogen peroxide within human erythrocytes. Blood. 87: 1595-1599.

Ganesan B, Buddhan S, Anandan R, Sivakumar R, AnbinEzhilan R. (2010 Mar). "Antioxidant defense of betaine against isoprenaline-induced myocardial infarction in rats," Mol Biol Rep. 37(3):1319-27.

Gaunt L.F., Higgins S.C., Hughes J.F. (2005) Interaction of air ions and bactericidal vapours to control micro-organisms. Journal of Applied Microbiology. 99: 1324-1329.

Gayathri B, Manjula N, Vinaykumar KS, Lakshmi BS, Balakrishnan A (2007 Apr). "Pure compound from Boswellia serrata extract exhibits anti-inflammatory property in human PBMCs and mouse macrophages through inhibition of TNFalpha, IL-1beta, NO and MAP kinases," Int Immunopharmacol. 7(4):473-82.

Ghelardini C, Galeotti N, Di Cesare Mannelli L, Mazzanti G, Bartolini A (2001 May-Jul). "Local anaesthetic activity of beta-caryophyllene," Farmaco. 56(5-7):387-9.

Ghelardini C, Galeotti N, Mazzanti G (2001 Aug). "Local anaesthetic activity of monoterpenes and phenylpropanes of essential oils," Planta Med. 67(6):564-6.

Ghelardini C, Galeotti N, Salvatore G, Mazzanti G (1999 Dec). "Local anaesthetic activity of the essential oil of Lavandula angustifolia," Planta Med. 65(8):700-3.

Ghersetich I, Lotti T, Campanile G, Grappone C, Dini G (1994 Feb). "Hyaluronic acid in cutaneous intrinsic aging," Int J Dermatol. 33(2):119-22.

Ghosh, V., Saranya, S., Mukherjee, A., & Chandrasekaran, N. (2013 May). Antibacterial microemulsion prevents sepsis and triggers healing of wound in wistar rats. Colloids Surf B Biointerfaces, 105, 152-157.

Gibriel, A., Al-Sayed, H., Rady, A., & Abdelaleem, M. (2013 Jun). Synergistic antibacterial activity of irradiated and nonirradiated cumin, thyme and rosemary essential oils. Journal of Food Safety, 33(2), 222-228.

Gilani, A. H., Jabeen, Q., Khan, A. U., & Shah, A. J. (2008 Feb). Gut modulatory, blood pressure lowering, diuretic and sedative activities of cardamom. J Ethnopharmacol, 115(3), 463-472.

Göbel H, Schmidt G, Soyka D (1994 Jun). "Effect of peppermint and eucalyptus oil preparations on neurophysiological and experimental algesimetric headache parameters," Cephalalgia. 14(3):228-34.

Goel A, Ahmad FJ, Singh RM, Singh GN (2010 Feb). "3-Acetyl-11-keto-beta-boswellic acid loaded-polymeric nanomicelles for topical anti-inflammatory and anti-arthritic activity," J Pharm Pharmacol. 62(2):273-8.

Goes, T. C., Antunes, F. D., Alves, P. B., & Teixeira-Silva, F. (2012 Aug). Effect of sweet orange aroma on experimental anxiety in humans. J Altern Complement Med, 18(8), 798-804.

Golab M, Skwarlo-Sonta K (2007 Mar). "Mechanisms involved in the anti-inflammatory action of inhaled tea tree oil in mice," Exp Biol Med (Maywood). 232(3):420-6.

Gomes NM, Rezende CM, Fontes SP, Matheus ME, Fernandes PD. (2007 Feb 12). "Antinociceptive activity of Amazonian Copaiba oils," J Ethnopharmacol. 109(3):486-92.

Gómez-Rincón, C., Langa, E., Murillo, P., Valero, M. S., Berzosa, C., & López, V. (2014 May). Activity of Tea Tree (Melaleuca alternifolia) Essential Oil against L3 Larvae of Anisakis simplex. 2014, 1-6.

Goncalves J.C.R., Alves A.M.H., de Araujo A.E.V., Cruz J.S., Araujo D.A.M. (2010) Distinct effects of carvone analogues on the isolated nerve of rats. European Journal of Pharmacology. 645: 108-112.

Goncalves J.C.R., Oliveira F.S., Benedito R.B., de Sousa D.P., de Almeida R.N., Araujo D.A.M. (2008) Antinociceptive Activity of (-)-Carvone: Evidence of Association with Decreased Peripheral Nerve Excitability. Biological and Parmaceutical Bulletin. 31: 1017-1020.

Gonzalez-Castejon, M., Garcia-Carrasco, B., Fernandez-Dacosta, R., Davalos, A., & Rodriguez-Casado, A. (2014 May). Reduction of adipogenesis and lipid accumulation by Taraxacum officinale (Dandelion) extracts in 3T3L1 adipocytes: an in vitro study. Phytother Res, 28(5), 745-752.

González-Trujano ME, Peña EI, Martínez AL, Moreno J, Guevara-Fefer P, Déciga-Campos M, López-Muñoz FJ (2007 May 22). "Evaluation of the antinociceptive effect of Rosmarinus officinalis L. using three different experimental models in rodents," J Ethnopharmacol. 111(3):476-82.

Goodwin J.S., Atluru D., Sierakowski S., Lianos E.A. (1986) Mechanism of Action of Glucocorticosteroids: Inhibition of T Cell Proliferation and Interleukin 2 Production by Hydrocortisones Is Reversed by Leukotriene B4. Journal of Clinical Investigation. 77: 1244-1250.

Gorwitz R.J., Kruszon-Moran D., McAllister S.K., McQuillan G., McDougal L.K., Fosheim G.E., Jensen B.J., Killgore G., Tenover F.C., Kuehnert M.J. (2008) Changes in the Prevalence of Nasal Colonization with Staphylococcus aureusin the United States, 2001-2004. Journal of Infectious Diseases. 197: 1226-1234.

Gossell-Williams M, Hyde C, Hunter T, Simms-Stewart D, Fletcher H, McGrowder D, Walters CA (2011 Oct). "Improvement in HDL cholesterol in postmenopausal women supplemented with pumpkin seed oil: pilot study," Climacteric. 14(5):558-64.

Goswami, S. K., Inamdar, M. N., Jamwal, R., & Dethe, S. (2014 Jun). Effect of Cinnamomum cassia Methanol Extract and Sildenafil on Arginase and Sexual Function of Young Male Wistar Rats. J Sex Med, 11(6), 1475-1483.

Goswami, S. K., Inamdar, M. N., Jamwal, R., & Dethe, S. (2013 Dec). Efficacy of Cinnamomum cassia Blume. in age induced sexual dysfunction of rats. J Young Pharm, 5(4), 148-153

Grassmann J, Hippeli S, Dornisch K, Rohnert U, Beuscher N, Elstner EF (2000 Feb). "Antioxidant properties of essential oils. Possible explanations for their anti-inflammatory effects," Arzneimittelforschung. 50(2):135-9.

Grassmann J, Schneider D, Weiser D, Elstner EF (2001 Oct). "Antioxidative effects of lemon oil and its components on copper induced oxidation of low density lipoprotein," Arzneimittelforschung. 51(10):799-805.

Grespan, R., Paludo, M., Lemos Hde, P., Barbosa, C. P., Bersani-Amado, C. A., Dalalio, M. M., & Cuman, R. K. (2012 Oct). Anti-arthritic effect of eugenol on collagen-induced arthritis experimental model. Biol Pharm Bull, 35(10), 1818-1820.

Grether -Beck, S., Muhlberg, K., Brenden, H., & Krutmann, J. (2008 Jul). [Topical application of vitamins, phytosterols and ceramides. Protection against increased expression of interstitial collagenase and reduced collagen-I expression after single exposure to UVA irradiation]. Hautarzt, 59(7), 557-562.

Grigoleit HG, Grigoleit P (2005 Aug). "Peppermint oil in irritable bowel syndrome," Phytomedicine. 12(8):601-6.

Gross, M., Nesher, E., Tikhonov, T., Raz, O., & Pinhasov, A. (2013 Mar). Chronic food administration of Salvia sclarea oil reduces animals' anxious and dominant behavior. J Med Food, 16(3), 216-222.

Guillemain J, Rousseau A, Delaveau P (1989). "Neurodepressive effects of the essential oil of Lavandula angustifolia Mill," Ann Pharm Fr. 47(6):337-43.

Gumral, N., Doguc Kumbul, D., Aylak, F., Saygin, M., & Savik, E. (2013 Jan). Juniperus communis Linn oil decreases oxidative stress and increases antioxidant enzymes in the heart of rats administered a diet rich in cholesterol. Toxicol Ind Health.

Gundidza M (1993 Nov). "Antimicrobial activity of essential oil from Schinus molle Linn," Cent Afr J Med. 39(11):231-4.

Guo X., Longnecker M.P., Michalek J.E. (2001) Relation of serum tetrachlorodibenzo-p-dioxin concentration to diet among veterans in the Air Force health study with background-level exposure. Journal of Toxicology and Environmental Health, Part A. 63: 159-172.

Gupta A., Myrdal P.B. (2004) Development of perillyl alcohol topical cream formulation. International Journal of Pharmaceutics. 269: 373-383.

Gurney A.M. (1994) Mechanisms of Drug-induced Vasodilation. Journal of Pharmacy and Pharmacology. 46: 242-251.

Haag J.D., Lindstrom M.J., Gould M.N. (1992) Limonene-induced Regression of Mammary Carcinomas. Cancer Research. 52: 4021-4026.

Habashy, R. R., Abdel-Naim, A. B., Khalifa, A. E., & Al-Azizi, M. M. (2005 Feb). Anti-inflammatory effects of jojoba liquid wax in experimental models. Pharmacol Res, 51(2), 95-105.

Hadley SK, Gaarder SM (2005 Dec 15). "Treatment of irritable bowel syndrome," Am Fam Physician. 72(12):2501-6.

Hagen TM, Liu J, Lykkesfeldt J, Wehr CM, Ingersoll RT, Vinarsky V, Bartholomew JC, Ames BN. "Feeding acetyl-L-carnitine and lipoic acid to old rats significantly improves metabolic function while decreasing oxidative stress," Proc Natl Acad Sci U S A. 99(4):1870-5.

Hager K, Kenklies M, McAfoose J, Engel J, Münch G (2007). "Alpha-lipoic acid as a new treatment option for Alzheimer's disease--a 48 months follow-up analysis," J Neural Transm Suppl. (72):189-93.

Hajhashemi V, Abbasi N (2008 Mar). "Hypolipidemic activity of Anethum graveolens in rats," Phytother Res. 22(3):372-5.

Hajhashemi V, Ghannadi A, Sharif B (2003 Nov). "Anti-inflammatory and analgesic properties of the leaf extracts and essential oil of Lavandula angustifolia Mill," J Ethnopharmacol. 89(1):67-71.

Hajhashemi V, Zolfaghari B, Yousefi A (2012). "Antinociceptive and anti-inflammatory activities of Satureja hortensis seed essential oil, hydroalcoholic and polyphenolic extracts in animal models," Med Princ Pract. 21(2):178-82.

Hakim IA, Harris RB, Ritenbaugh C (2000). "Citrus peel use is associated with reduced risk of squamous cell carcinoma of the skin," Nutr Cancer. 37(2):161-8.

Halder, S., Mehta, A. K., Kar, R., Mustafa, M., Mediratta, P. K., & Sharma, K. K. (2011 May). Clove oil reverses learning and memory deficits in scopolamine-treated mice. Planta Med, 77(8), 830-834.

Halder, S., Mehta, A. K., Mediratta, P. K., & Sharma, K. K. (2011 Aug). Essential oil of clove (Eugenia caryophyllata) augments the humoral immune response but decreases cell mediated immunity. Phytother Res, 25(8), 1254-1256.

Hammer KA, Carson CF, Riley TV (2008 Aug). "Frequencies of resistance to Melaleuca alternifolia (tea tree) oil and rifampicin in Staphylococcus aureus, Staphylococcus epidermidis and Enterococcus faecalis," Int J Antimicrob Agents. 32(2):170-3.

Hammer KA, Carson CF, Riley TV (1996 Jun). "Susceptibility of transient and commensal skin flora to the essential oil of Melaleuca alternifolia (tea tree oil)," J Antimicrob Chemother. 24(3):186-9.

Hammer KA, Carson CF, Riley TV (2004 Jun). "Antifungal effects of Melaleuca alternifolia (tea tree) oil and its components on Candida albicans, Candida glabrata and Saccharomyces cerevisiae," J Antimicrob Chemother. 53(6):1081-5.

Han, S. H., Hur, M. H., Buckle, J., Choi, J., & Lee, M. S. (2006 Aug). Effect of aromatherapy on symptoms of dysmenorrhea in college students: A randomized placebo-controlled clinical trial. J Altern Complement Med, 12(6), 535-541.

Hargreaves IP, Lane A, Sleiman PM (2008 Dec 5). "The coenzyme Q10 status of the brain regions of Parkinson's disease patients," Neurosci Lett. 447(1):17-9.

Hart PH, Brand C, Carson CF, Riley TV, Prager RH, Finlay-Jones JJ (2000 Nov). "Terpinen-4-ol, the main component of the essential oil of Melaleuca alternifolia (tea tree oil), suppresses inflammatory mediator production by activated human monocytes," Inflamm Res. 49(11):619-26.

Hay IC, Jamieson M, Ormerod AD (1998 Nov). "Randomized trial of aromatherapy. Successful treatment for alopecia areata," Arch Dermatol. 135(5):1349-52.

Hayes AJ, Markovic B (2002 Apr). "Toxicity of Australian essential oil Backhousia citriodora (Lemon myrtle). Part 1. Antimicrobial activity and in vitro cytotoxicity," Food Chem Toxicol. 40(4):535-43.

Hayflick L (1979 Jul). "The cell biology of aging," J Invest Dermatol. 73(1):8-14.

Haze S, Sakai K, Gozu Y (2002 Nov). "Effects of fragrance inhalation on sympathetic activity in normal adults," Jpn J Pharmacol 90(3):247-53.

Haze, S., Sakai, K., Gozu, Y., & Moriyama, M. (2010 Jul). Grapefruit oil attenuates adipogenesis in cultured subcutaneous adipocytes. Planta Med, 76(10), 950-955.

Hazgui S et al. (2008 Apr). "Epigallocatechin-3-gallate (EGCG) inhibits the migratory behavior of tumor bronchial epithelial cells," Respir Res. 9:33.

Helland IB, Smith L, Saarem K, Saugstad OD, Drevon CA (2003 Jan). "Maternal supplementation with very-long-chain n-3 fatty acids during pregnancy and lactation augments children's IQ at 4 years of age," Pediatrics. 111(1):e39-44.

Herz, R. S., & Engen, T. (1996 Sep). Odor memory: Review and analysis. Psychon Bull Rev, 3(3), 300-313.

Heuberger, E., Hongratanaworakit, T., & Buchbauer, G. (2006 Aug). East Indian sandalwood and alpha-santalol odor increase physiological and self-rated arousal in humans. Planta Med, 72(9), 792-800.

Hiramatsu N, Xiufen W, Takechi R, Itoh Y, Mamo J, Pal S (2004). "Antimutagenicity of Japanese traditional herbs, gennoshoko, yomogi, senburi and iwa-tobacco," Biofactors. 22(1-4):123-5.

Hitokoto H, Morozumi S, Wauke T, Sakai S, Kurata H (1980 Apr). "Inhibitory effects of spices on growth and toxin production of toxigenic fungi," Appl Environ Microbiol. 39(4):818-22.

Hölzle E (1992 Sep). "Pigmented lesions as a sign of photodamage," Br J Dermatol. 17(Suppl 41):48-50.

Hongratanaworakit T (2009 Feb). "Relaxing effect of rose oil on humans," Nat Prod Commun. 4(2):291-6.

Hongratanaworakit T, Buchbauer G (2004 Jul). "Evaluation of the harmonizing effect of ylang-ylang oil on humans after inhalation," Planta Med. 70(7):632-6.

Hongratanaworakit T, Buchbauer G (2006 Sep). "Relaxing effect of ylang ylang oil on humans after transdermal absorption," Phytother Res. 20(9):758-63.

Hongratanaworakit, T., Heuberger, E., & Buchbauer, G. (2004 Jan). Evaluation of the effects of East Indian sandalwood oil and alpha-santalol on humans after transdermal absorption. Planta Med, 70(1), 3-7.

Hosseini, M., Ghasemzadeh Rahbardar, M., Sadeghnia, H. R., & Rakhshandeh, H. (2011 Oct). Effects of different extracts of Rosa damascena on pentylenetetrazol-induced seizures in mice. Zhong Xi Yi Jie He Xue Bao, 9(10), 1118-1124.

Hosseini, M., Jafarianheris, T., Seddighi, N., Parvaneh, M., Ghorbani, A., Sadeghnia, H. R., & Rakhshandeh, H. (2012 Dec). Effects of different extracts of Eugenia caryophyllata on pentylenetetrazole-induced seizures in mice. Zhong Xi Yi Jie He Xue Bao, 10(12), 1476-1481.

Hosseinzadeh H., Karimi, G. R., & Ameri, M. (2002 Dec). Effects of Anethum graveolens L. seed extracts on experimental gastric irritation models in mice. BMC Pharmacol, 2, 1-5.

Modern Essentials Usage Guide

Hostanska K, Daum G, Saller R (2002 Sep-Oct). "Cytostatic and apoptosis-inducing activity of boswellic acids toward malignant cell lines in vitro," Anticancer Res. 22(5):2853-62.

Howard J., Hyman A.A. (2003) Dynamics and mechanics of the microtubule plus end. Nature. 422: 753-758.

Hoya Y, Matsumura I, Fujita T, Yanaga K. (2008 Nov-Dec). "The use of nonpharmacological interventions to reduce anxiety in patients undergoing gastroscopy in a setting with an optimal soothing environment," Gastroenterol Nurs. 31(6):395-9.

Huang, C. S., Yin, M. C., & Chiu, L. C. (2011 Sep). Antihyperglycemic and antioxidative potential of Psidium guajava fruit in streptozotocin-induced diabetic rats. Food Chem Toxicol, 49(9), 2189-2195.

Huang L, Abuhamdah S, Howes MJ, Dixon CL, Elliot MS, Ballard C, Holmes C, Burns A, Perry EK, Francis PT, Lees G, Chazot PL (2008 Nov). "Pharmacological profile of essential oils derived from Lavandula angustifolia and Melissa officinalis with anti-agitation properties: focus on ligand-gated channels," J Pharm Pharmacol. 60(11):1515-22.

Huang MT, Badmaev V, Ding Y, Liu Y, Xie JG, Ho CT (2000). "Anti-tumor and anti-carcinogenic activities of triterpenoid, beta-boswellic acid," Biofactors. 13(1-4):225-30.

Hudaib, M., Speroni, E., Di Pietra, A. M., & Cavrini, V. (2002 Jul). GC/MS evaluation of thyme (Thymus vulgaris L.) oil composition and variations during the vegetative cycle. J Pharm Biomed Anal, 29(4), 691-700.

Hunan Yi Ke Da Xue Xue Bao (1999). "Experimental study on induction of apoptosis of leukemic cells by Boswellia carterii Birdw extractive," Hunan Yi Ke Da Xue Xue Bao. 24(1):23-5.

Hudson, J., Kuo, M., & Vimalanathan, S. (2011 Dec). The antimicrobial properties of cedar leaf (Thuja plicata) oil; a safe and efficient decontamination agent for buildings. Int J Environ Res Public Health, 8(12), 4477-4487.

Hussein G, Miyashiro H, Nakamura N, Hattori M, Kakiuchi N, Shimotohno K (2000 Nov). "Inhibitory effects of sudanese medicinal plant extracts on hepatitis C virus (HCV) protease," Phytother Res. 14(7):510-6.

Hyldgaard, M., Mygind, T., & Meyer, R. L. (2012 Feb). Essential oils in food preservation: mode of action, synergies, and interactions with food matrix components. Frontiers in Microbiology, 3, 1-24.

Idaomar M, El-Hamss R, Bakkali F, Mezzoug N, Zhiri A, Baudoux D, Muñoz-Serrano A, Liemans V, Alonso-Moraga A (2002 Jan 15). "Genotoxicity and antig-enotoxicity of some essential oils evaluated by wing spot test of Drosophila melanogaster," Mutat Res. 13(1-2):61-8.

Iamsaard, S., Prabsattroo, T., Sukhorum, W., Muchimapura, S., Srisaard, P., Uabundit, N., . . . Wattanathorn, J. (2013 Mar). Anethum graveolens Linn. (dill) extract enhances the mounting frequency and level of testicular tyrosine protein phosphorylation in rats. J Zhejiang Univ Sci B, 14(3), 247-252.

Imai H, Osawa K, Yasuda H, Hamashima H, Arai T, Sasatsu M (2001). "Inhibition by the essential oils of peppermint and spearmint of the growth of pathogenic bacteria," Microbios. 106(Suppl 1):31-9.

Imokawa G (2009 Jul). "A possible mechanism underlying the ceramide deficiency in atopic dermatitis: expression of a deacylase enzyme that cleaves the N-acyl linkage of sphingomyelin and glucosylceramide," J Dermatol Sci. 55(1):1-9.

Inouye S, Nishiyama Y, Uchida K, Hasumi Y, Yamaguchi H, Abe S (2006 Dec). "The vapor activity of oregano, perilla, tea tree, lavender, clove, and geranium oils against a Trichophyton mentagrophytes in a closed box," J Infect Chemother. 12(6):349-54.

Inouye S, Takizawa T, Yamaguchi H (2001 May). "Antibacterial activity of essential oils and their major constituents against respiratory tract pathogens by gaseous contact," J Antimicrob Chemother. 47(5):565-73.

Inouye S, Yamaguchi H, Takizawa T (2001 Dec). "Screening of the antibacterial effects of a variety of essential oils on respiratory tract pathogens, using a modified dilution assay method," J Infect Chemother. 7(4):251-4.

Iori A, Grazioli D, Gentile E, Marano G, Salvatore G (2005 Apr 20). "Acaricidal properties of the essential oil of Melaleuca alternifolia Cheel (tea tree oil) against nymphs of Ixodes ricinus," Vet Parasitol. 129(1-2):173-6.

Ishida T, Mizushina Y, Yagi S, Irino Y, Nishiumi S, Miki I, Kondo Y, Mizuno S, Yoshida H, Azuma T, Yoshida M (2012). "Inhibitory effects of glycyrrhetinic Acid on DNA polymerase and inflammatory activities," Evid Based Complement Alternat Med. 2012:650514.

Itai T, Amayasu H, Kuribayashi M, Kawamura N, Okada M, Momose A, Tateyama T, Narumi K, Uematsu W, Kaneko S (2000 Aug). "Psychological effects of aromatherapy on chronic hemodialysis patients," Psychiatry Clin Neurosci. 54(4):393-7.

Itai T, Amayasu H, Kuribayashi M, Kawamura N, Okada M, Momose A, Tateyama T, Narumi K, Uematsu W, Kaneko S (2000 Aug). "Psychological effects of aromatherapy on chronic hemodialysis patients," Psychiatry Clin Neurosci. 54(4):393-7.

Iwata, J., LeDoux, J. E., Meeley, M. P., Arneric, S., & Reis, D. J. (1986 Sep). Intrinsic neurons in the amygdaloid field projected to by the medial geniculate body mediate emotional responses conditioned to acoustic stimuli. Brain Res, 383(1-2), 195-214.

Jafarzadeh, M., Arman, S., & Pour, F. F. (2013 Aug). Effect of aromatherapy with orange essential oil on salivary cortisol and pulse rate in children during dental treatment: A randomized controlled clinical trial. Adv Biomed Res, 2, 1-10.

Jager, W., Buchbauer, G., Jirovetz, L., & Fritzer, M. (1992). Percutaneous absorption of lavender oil from a massage oil. J Soc Cosmet Chem, 43(1), 49-54.

Jager, W., Nasel, B., Nasel, C., Binder, R., Stimpfl, T., Vycudilik, W., & Buchbauer, G. (1996 Aug). Pharmacokinetic studies of the fragrance compound 1,8-cineol in humans during inhalation. Chem Senses, 21(4), 477-480.

Jamal A, Javed K, Aslam M, Jafri MA (2006 Jan 16). "Gastroprotective effect of cardamom, Elettaria cardamomum Maton. fruits in rats," J Ethnopharmacol. 103(2):149-53.

Janahmadi M, Niazi F, Danyali S, Kamalinejad M (2006 Mar 8). "Effects of the fruit essential oil of Cuminum cyminum Linn. (Apiaceae) on pentylenetetrazol-induced epileptiform activity in F1 neurones of Helix aspersa," J Ethnopharmacol. 104(1-2):278-82.

Jang M, Cai L, Udeani GO, Slowing KV, Thomas CF, Beecher CW, Fong HH, Farnsworth NR, Kinghorn AD, Mehta RG, Moon RC, Pezzuto JM (1997 Jan 10). "Cancer chemopreventive activity of resveratrol, a natural product derived from grapes," Science. 275 (5297):218-20.

Jefferies H., Coster J., Khalil A., Bot J., McCauley R.D., Hall J.C. (2003) Glutathione. ANZ Journal of Surgery. 73: 517-522.

Jeon, S., Bose, S., Hur, J., Jun, K., Kim, Y. K., Cho, K. S., & Koo, B. S. (2011 Sep). A modified formulation of Chinese traditional medicine improves memory impairment and reduces Abeta level in the Tg-APPswe/PS1dE9 mouse model of Alzheimer's disease. J Ethnopharmacol, 137(1), 783-789.

Jimenez A, Santos A, Alonso G, Vazquez D (1976 Mar 17). "Inhibitors of protein synthesis in eukarytic cells. Comparative effects of some amaryllidaceae alkaloids," Biochim Biophys Acta. 425(3):342-8.

Jing, L., Zhang, Y., Fan, S., Gu, M., Guan, Y., Lu, X., . . . Zhou, Z. (2013 Sep). Preventive and ameliorating effects of citrus D-limonene on dyslipidemia and hyperglycemia in mice with high-fat diet-induced obesity. Eur J Pharmacol, 715(1-3), 46-55.

Jing Y, Nakajo S, Xia L, Nakaya K, Fang Q, Waxman S, Han R (1999 Jan). "Boswellic acid acetate induces differentiation and apoptosis in leukemia cell lines," Leuk Res. 23(1):43-50.

Jing Y, Xia L, Han R (1992 Mar). "Growth inhibition and differentiation of promyelocytic cells (HL-60) induced by BC-4, an active principle from Boswellia carterii Birdw," Chin Med Sci J. 7(1):12-5.

Johnson, L. R., Ghishan,F.K., Kaunitz, J.D., Merchant, J., Said, H.M., & Wood, J. (Eds.). (2012 Jul). Physiology of the gastrointestinal tract (5th ed.). London: Elsevier.

Johnson, M., Pace, R. D., Dawkins, N. L., & Willian, K. R. (2013 Nov). Diets containing traditional and novel green leafy vegetables improve liver fatty acid profiles of spontaneously hypertensive rats. Lipids Health Dis, 12, 168.

Johny AK, Baskaran SA, Charles AS, Amalaradjou MA, Darre MJ, Khan MI, Hoagland TA, Schreiber DT, Donoghue AM, Donoghue DJ, Venkitarayanan K. (2009 Apr). "Prophylactic supplementation of caprylic acid in feed reduces Salmonella enteritidis colonization in commercial broiler chicks," J. Food Prot. 72(4):722-7.

Juergens U.R., Dethlefsen U., Steinkamp G., Gillissen A., Repges R., Vetter H. (2003) Anti-inflammatory activity of 1.8-cineol (eucalyptol) in bronchial asthma: a double-blind placebo-controlled trial. Respiratory Medicine. 97: 250-256.

Juergens UR, Stöber M, Schmidt-Schilling L, Kleuver T, Vetter H (1998 Sep 17). "Anti-inflammatory effects of euclyptol (1.8-cineole) in bronchial asthma: inhibition of arachidonic acid metabolism in human blood monocytes ex vivo," Eur J Med Res. 3(9):407-12.

Juergens UR, Stöber M, Vetter H (1998 Dec 16). "The anti-inflammatory activity of L-menthol compared to mint oil in human monocytes in vitro: a novel perspective for its therapeutic use in inflammatory diseases," Eur J Med Res. 3(12):539-45.

Juglal S, Govinden R, Odhav B (2002 Apr). "Spice oils for the control of co-occurring mycotoxin-producing fungi," J Food Prot. 65(4):683-7.

Jun, H. J., Lee, J. H., Jia, Y., Hoang, M. H., Byun, H., Kim, K. H., & Lee, S. J. (2012 Mar). Melissa officinalis essential oil reduces plasma triglycerides in human apolipoprotein E2 transgenic mice by inhibiting sterol regulatory element-binding protein-1c-dependent fatty acid synthesis. J Nutr, 142(3), 432-440.

Jung K, Kim IH, Han D (2004). "Effect of medicinal plant extracts on forced swimming capacity in mice," J Ethnopharmacol. 93:75-81.

Jung SH, Kang KD, Ju D, Fawcen RJ, Safa R, Kamalden TA, Osborne NN (2008 Sep). "The flavanoid baicalin counteracts ischemic and oxidative insults to retinal cells and lipid peroxidation to brain membranes," Neurochem Int.

Jung, Y. H., Kwon, S. H., Hong, S. I., Lee, S. O., Kim, S. Y., Lee, S. Y., & Jang, C. G. (2012 Dec). 5-HT(1A) receptor binding in the dorsal raphe nucleus is implicated in the anxiolytic-like effects of Cinnamomum cassia. Pharmacol Biochem Behav, 103(2), 367-372.

Kabuto, H., Tada, M., & Kohno, M. (2007 Mar). Eugenol [2-methoxy-4-(2-propenyl)phenol] prevents 6-hydroxydopamine-induced dopamine depression and lipid peroxidation inductivity in mouse striatum. Biol Pharm Bull, 30(3), 423-427.

Kadekaro AL, Kanto H, Kavanagh R, Abdel-Malek ZA (2003 Jun). "Significance of the melanocortin 1 receptor in regulating human melanocyte pigmentation, proliferation, and survival," Ann N Y Acad Sci. 994:359-65.

Kadohisa, M. (2013 Oct). Effects of odor on emotion, with implications. Front Syst Neurosci, 7, 1-6.

Kambara T, Zhou Y, Kawashima Y, Kishida N, Mizutani K, Ikeda T, Kamayama K (2003). "A New Dermatological Availability of the Flavonoid Fraction from Licorice Roots—Effect on Acne," J Soc Cosmet Chem Jpn. 37(3)179-85.

Kamiyama, M., & Shibamoto, T. (2012 Jun). Flavonoids with potent antioxidant activity found in young green barley leaves. J Agric Food Chem, 60(25), 6260-6267.

Kane FM, Brodie EE, Coull A, Coyne L, Howd A, Milne A, Niven CC, Robbins R (2004 Oct 28-Nov 10). "The analgesic effect of odour and music upon dressing change," Br J Nurs. 13(19):S4-12.

Kanehara S, Ohtani T, Uede K, Furukawa F (2007 Dec). "Clinical effects of undershirts coated with borage oil on children with atopic dermatitis: a double-blind, placebo-controlled clinical trial," J Dermatol. 34(12):811-5.

Katdare M, Singhal H, Newmark H, Osborne MP, Telang NT (1997 Jan 1). "Prevention of mammary preneoplastic transformation by naturally-occurring tumor inhibitors," Cancer Lett. 111(1-2):141-7.

Kato K., Cox A.D., Hisaka M.M., Graham S.M., Buss J.E., Der C.J. (1992) Isoprenoid addition to Ras protein is the critical modification for its membrane associa-tion and transforming activity. Proc. Natl. Sci. USA. 89: 6403-6407.

Kato T, Hancock RL, Mohammadpour H, McGregor B, Manalo P, Khaiboullina S, Hall MR, Pardini L, Pardini RS (2002 Dec). "Influence of omega-3 fatty acids on the growth of human colon carcinoma in nude mice," Cancer Lett. 187(1-2):169-77.

Kaur M, Agarwal C, Singh RP, Guan X, Dwivedi C, Agarwal R (2005 Feb). "Skin cancer chemopreventive agent, {alpha}-santalol, induces apoptotic death of human epidermoid carcinoma A431 cells via caspase activation together with dissipation of mitochondrial membrane potential and cytochrome c release," Carcinogenesis. 26(2):369-80.

Kee Y, Lin RC, Hsu SC, Scheller RH (1995 May). "Distinct domains of syntaxin are required for synaptic vesicle fusion complex formation and dissociation," Neuron. 14(5):991-8.

Kéita SM, Vincent C, Schmit J, Arnason JT, Bélanger A (2001 Oct). "Efficacy of essential oil of Ocimum basilicum L. and O. gratissimum L. applied as an insecticidal fumigant and powder to control Callosobruchus maculatus (Fab.)," J Stored Prod Res. 37(4):339-349.

Kennedy DO, Little W, Haskell CF, Scholey AB (2006 Feb). "Anxiolytic effects of a combination of Melissa officinalis and Valeriana officinalis during laboratory induced stress," Phytother Res. 20(2):96-102.

Keogh A, Fenton S, Leslie C, Aboyoun C, Macdonald P, Zhao YC, Bailey M, Rosenfeldt F (2003). "Randomised double-blind, placebo-controlled trial of coenzyme Q₁₀ therapy in class II and III systolic heart failure," Heart Lung Circ. 12(3):135-41.

Khallouki F, Younos C, Soulimani R, Oster T, Charrouf Z, Spiegelhalder B, Bartsch H, Owen RW (2003 Feb). "Consumption of argan oil (Morocco) with its unique profile of fatty acids, tocopherols, squalene, sterols and phenolic compounds should confer valuable cancer chemopreventive effects," Eur J Cancer Prev. 12(1):67-75.

Khan AU, Gilani AH (2009 Dec 10). "Antispasmodic and bronchodilator activities of Artemisia vulgaris are mediated through dual blockade of muscarinic receptors and calcium influx," J Ethnopharmacol. 126(3):480-6.

Khatibi A, Haghparast A, Shams J, Dianati E, Komaki A, Kamalinejad M (2008 Dec 19). "Effects of the fruit essential oil of Cuminum cyminum L. on the acquisition and expression of morphine-induced conditioned place preference in mice," Neurosci Lett. 448(1):94-8.

Kheirkhah A, Casas V, Li W, Raju VK, Tseng SC (2007 May). "Corneal manifestations of ocular demodex infestation," Am J Ophthalmol. 143(5):743-749.

Kiecolt-Glaser JK, Graham JE, Malarkey WB, Porter K, Lemeshow S, Glaser R (2008 Apr). "Olfactory influences on mood and autonomic, endocrine, and immune function," Psychoneuroendocrinology. 33(3):328-39.

Kim, H. J., Yang, H. M., Kim, D. H., Kim, H. G., Jang, W. C., & Lee, Y. R. (2003 Jun). Effects of ylang-ylang essential oil on the relaxation of rat bladder muscle in vitro and white rabbit bladder in vivo. J Korean Med Sci, 18(3), 409-414.

Kim HM, Cho SH (1999 Feb). "Lavender oil inhibits immediate-type allergic reaction in mice and rats," J Pharm Pharmacol. 51(2):221-6.

Kim, I. H., Kim, C., Seong, K., Hur, M. H., Lim, H. M., & Lee, M. S. (2012 Dec). Essential oil inhalation on blood pressure and salivary cortisol levels in prehyper-tensive and hypertensive subjects. Evid Based Complement Alternat Med, 2012, 1-9.

Kim MA, Sakong JK, Kim EJ, Kim EH, Kim EH (2005 Feb). "Effect of aromatherapy massage for the relief of constipation in the elderly," Taehan Kanho Hakhoe Chi. 35(1):56-64.

Kim MJ, Nam ES, Paik SI (2005 Feb). "The effects of aromatherapy on pain, depression, and life satisfaction of arthritis patients," Taehan Kanho Hakhoe Chi. 35(1):186-94.

Kim, T. H., Kim, H. J., Lee, S. H., & Kim, S. Y. (2012 Jun). Potent inhibitory effect of Foeniculum vulgare Miller extract on osteoclast differentiation and ovariectomy-induced bone loss. Int J Mol Med, 29(6), 1053-1059.

Kite SM, Thaler EJ, Anderson K, Young T, Young J, Wood J, Howells N, Bradburn J (1998 May). "Development of an aromatherapy service at a Cancer Centre," Palliat Med. 12(3):171-80.

Kline RM, Kline JJ, Di Palma J, Barbero GJ (2001 Jan). "Enteric-coated, pH-dependent peppermint oil capsules for the treatment of irritable bowel syndrome in children," J Pediatr. 138(1):125-8.

Klug W.S., Cummings M.R., Spencer C., Palladino M.A. Concepts of Genetics. San Francisco: Pearson Custom Publishing, 2009.

Kobayashi Y, Takahashi R, Ogino F (2005 Oct 3). "Antipruritic effect of the single oral administration of German chamomile flower extract and its combined effect with antiallergic agents in ddY mice," J Ethnopharmacol. 101(1-3):308-12.

Modern Essentials Usage Guide

Kocevski, D., Du, M., Kan, J., Jing, C., Lacanin, I., & Pavlovic, H. (2013 May). Antifungal effect of Allium tuberosum, Cinnamomum cassia, and Pogostemon cablin essential oils and their components against population of Aspergillus species. J Food Sci, 78(5), M731-737.

Koh KJ, Pearce AL, Marshman G, Finlay-Jones JJ, Hart PH (2002 Dec). "Tea tree oil reduces histamine-induced skin inflammation," Br J Dermatol. 147(6):1212-7.

Kohlert, C., van Rensen, I., Marz, R., Schindler, G., Graefe, E. U., & Veit, M. (2000 Aug). Bioavailability and pharmacokinetics of natural volatile terpenes in animals and humans. Planta Med, 66(6), 495-505.

Komiya M, Takeuchi T, Harada E (2006 Sep 25). "Lemon oil vapor causes an anti-stress effect via modulating the 5-HT and DA activities in mice," Behav Brain Res. 172(2):240-9.

Komori T, Fujiwara R, Tanida M, Nomura J (1995 Dec). "Potential antidepressant effects of lemon odor in rats," Eur Neuropsychopharmacol. 5(4):477-80.

Komori T, Fujiwara R, Tanida M, Nomura J, Yokoyama MM (1995 May-Jun). "Effects of citrus fragrance on immune function and depressive states," Neuroimmunomodulation. 2(3):174-80.

Koo HN, Hong SH, Kim CY, Ahn JW, Lee YG, Kim JJ, Lyu YS, Kim HM (2002 Jun). "Inhibitory effect of apoptosis in human astrocytes CCF-STTG1 cells by lemon oil," Pharmacol Res. 45(6):469-73.

Koo HN, Jeong HJ, Kim CH, Park ST, Lee SJ, Seong KK, Lee SK, Lyu YS, Kim HM (2001 Dec). "Inhibition of heat shock-induced apoptosis by peppermint oil in astrocytes," J Mol Neurosci. 17(3):391-6.

Kooncumchoo P, Sharma S, Porter J, Govitrapong P, Ebadi M (2006). "Coenzyme Q(10) provides neuroprotection in iron-induced apoptosis in dopaminergic neurons," J Mol Neurosci. 28(2):125-41.

Kosalec I, Pepeljnjak S, Kustrak D. (2005 Dec). "Antifungal activity of fluid extract and essential oil from anise fruits (Pimpinella anisum L, Apiaceae)," Acta Pharm. 55(4):377-85.

Koutroumanidou, E., Kimbaris, A., Kortsaris, A., Bezirtzoglou, E., Polissiou, M., Charalabopoulos, K., & Pagonopoulou, O. (2013 Aug). Increased seizure latency and decreased severity of pentylenetetrazol-induced seizures in mice after essential oil administration. Epilepsy Res Treat, 2013.

Krishnakumar A, Abraham PM, Paul J, Paulose CS (2009 Sep 15). "Down-regulation of cerebellar 5-HT(2C) receptors in pilocarpine-induced epilepsy in rats: therapeutic role of Bacopa monnieri extract," J Neurol Sci. 284(1-2):124-8.

Krishnakumar A, Nandhu MS, Paulose CS (2009 Oct). "Upregulation of 5-HT2C receptors in hippocampus of pilocarpine-induced epileptic rats: antagonism by Bacopa monnieri," Epilepsy Behav. 16(2):225-30.

Kuettner A, Pieper A, Koch J, Enzmann F, Schroeder S (2005 Feb 28). "Influence of coenzyme Q(10) and cerivastatin on the flow-mediated vasodilation of the brachial artery: results of the ENDOTACT study," Int J Cardiol. 98(3):413-9.

Kumar A, Malik F, Bhushan S, Sethi VK, Shahi AK, Kaur J, Taneja SC, Qazi GN, Singh J (2008 Feb 15). "An essential oil and its major constituent isointermedeol induce apoptosis by increased expression of mitochondrial cytochrome c and apical death receptors in human leukaemia HL-60 cells," Chem Biol Interact. 171(3):332-47.

Kumar P, Kumar A (2003 Jun). "Possible neuroprotective effect of Withania somnifera root extract against 3-nitropropionic acid-induced behavioral, biochemical, and mitochondrial dysfunction in an animal model of Huntington's disease," J Med Food. 12(3):591-600.

Kumaran AM, D'Souza P, Agarwal A, Bokkolla RM, Balasubramaniam M (2003 Sep). "Geraniol, the putative anthelmintic principle of Cymbopogon martinii," Phytother Res. 17(8):957.

Kumari, S., & Dutta, A. (2013 Jul). Protective effect of Eleteria cardamomum (L.) Maton against Pan masala induced damage in lung of male Swiss mice. Asian Pac J Trop Med, 6(7), 525-531.

Kuo YM, Hayflick SJ, Gitschier J (2007 Jun). "Deprivation of pantothenic acid elicits a movement disorder and azoospermia in a mouse model of pantothenate kinase-associated neurodegeneration," J Inherit Metab Dis. 30(3):310-7.

Kuwahata, H., Komatsu, T., Katsuyama, S., Corasaniti, M. T., Bagetta, G., Sakurada, S., . . . Takahama, K. (2013 Feb). Peripherally injected linalool and bergamot essential oil attenuate mechanical allodynia via inhibiting spinal ERK phosphorylation. Pharmacol Biochem Behav, 103(4), 735-741.

Kwieciński J, Eick S, Wójcik K (2009 Apr). "Effects of tea tree (Melaleuca alternifolia) oil on Staphylococcus aureus in biofilms and stationary growth phase," Int J Antimicrob Agents. 33(4):343-7.

Lachowicz, K., Jones, G., Briggs, D., Bienvenu, F., Wan, J., Wilcock, A., & Coventry, M. (1998). The synergistic preservative effects of the essential oils of sweet basil (Ocimum basilicum L.) against acid-tolerant food microflora. Letters in Applied Microbiology, 26(3), 209-214.

Lagouge M et al. (2006 Dec 15). "Resveratrol improves mitochondrial function and protects against metabolic disease by activating SIRT1 and PGC-1alpha," Cell. 127(6):1109-22.

Lahlou S, Figueiredo AF, Magalhães PJ, Leal-Cardoso JH (2002 Dec). "Cardiovascular effects of 1,8-cineole, a terpenoid oxide present in many plant essential oils, in normotensive rats," Can J Physiol Pharmacol. 80(12):1125-31.

Lahlou S., Interaminense L.F.L., Magalhaes P.J.C., Leal-Cardoso J.H., Duarte G.P. (2004) Cardiovascular Effects of Eugenol, a Phenolic Compound Present in Many Plant Essential Oils, in Normotensive Rats. Journal of Cardiovascular Pharmacology. 43: 250-257.

Lambert R.J.W., Skandamis P.N., Coote P.J., Nychas G-J.E. (2001) A study of the minimun inhibitory concentration and mode of action of oregano essential oil, thymol and carvacrol. Journal of Applied Microbiology. 91: 453-462.

Lampronti I, Saab AM, Gambari R (2006 Oct). "Antiproliferative activity of essential oils derived from plants belonging to the Magnoliophyta division," Int J Oncol. 29(4):989-95.

Langeveld, W. T., Veldhuizen, E. J., & Burt, S. A. (2014 Feb). Synergy between essential oil components and antibiotics: a review. Crit Rev Microbiol, 40(1), 76-94.

Lantry LE, Zhang Z, Gao F, Crist KA, Wang Y, Kelloff GJ, Lubet RA, You M (1997). "Chemopreventive effect of perillyl alcohol on 4-(methylnitrosamino)-1-(3-pyridyl)-1-butanone induced tumorigenesis in (C3H/HeJ X A/J)F1 mouse lung," J Cell Biochem Suppl. 27:20-5.

Larder B.A., Kemp S.D., Harrigan P.R. (1995) Potential Mechanism for Sustained Antiretroviral Efficacy of AZT-3TC Combination Therapy. Science. 269: 696-699.

Laurent TC, Laurent UB, Frazer JR (1995 May). "Functions of hyaluronan," Ann Rheum Dis. 54(5):429-32.

Lawrence, H. A., & Palombo, E. A. (2009 Dec). Activity of essential oils against Bacillus subtilis spores. J Microbiol Biotechnol, 19(12), 1590-1595.

LeDoux, J. (2003). The emotional brain, fear, and the amygdala. Cellular and molecular neurobiology, 23(4-5), 727-738.

LeDoux, J. E., Iwata, J., Cicchetti, P., & Reis, D. J. (1988 Jul). Different projections of the central amygdaloid nucleus mediate autonomic and behavioral correlates of conditioned fear. J Neurosci, 8(7), 2517-2529.

Ledoux, J. E., Romanski, L., & Xagoraris, A. (1989 Jul). Indelibility of subcortical emotional memories. J Cogn Neurosci, 1(3), 238-243.

Lee, H. S. (2002 Dec). Inhibitory activity of Cinnamomum cassia bark-derived component against rat lens aldose reductase. J Pharm Pharm Sci, 5(3), 226-230.

Lee HS (2005 Apr 6). "Cuminaldehyde: Aldose Reductase and alpha-Glucosidase Inhibitor Derived from Cuminum cyminum L. Seeds," J Agric Food Chem. 53(7):2446-50.

Lee, H. S., & Ahn, Y. J. (1998 Jan). Growth-Inhibiting Effects of Cinnamomum cassia Bark-Derived Materials on Human Intestinal Bacteria. J Agric Food Chem, 46(1), 8-12.

Lee IS, Lee GJ (2006 Feb). "Effects of lavender aromatherapy on insomnia and depression in women college students," Taehan Kanho Hakhoe Chi. 36(1):136-43.

Lee SK, Zhang W, Sanderson BJ (2008 Aug). "Selective growth inhibition of human leukemia and human lymphoblastoid cells by resveratrol via cell cycle arrest and apoptosis induction," J Agric Food Chem. 56(16):7572-7.

Lee SU, Shim KS, Ryu SY, Min YK, Kim SH (2009 Feb). "Machilin A isolated from Myristica fragrans stimulates osteoblast differentiation," Planta Med. 75(2):152-7.

Lee, T., Lee, S., Ho Kim, K., Oh, K. B., Shin, J., & Mar, W. (2013 Sep). Effects of magnolialide isolated from the leaves of Laurus nobilis L. (Lauraceae) on immuno-globulin E-mediated type I hypersensitivity in vitro. J Ethnopharmacol, 149(2), 550-556.

Leffa, D. D., da Silva, J., Daumann, F., Dajori, A. L., Longaretti, L. M., Damiani, A. P., . . . de Andrade, V. M. (2013 Dec). Corrective effects of acerola (Malpighia emarginata DC.) juice intake on biochemical and genotoxical parameters in mice fed on a high-fat diet. Mutat Res.

Legault J, Dahl W, Debiton E, Pichette A, Madelmont JC (2003 May). "Antitumor activity of balsam fir oil: production of reactive oxygen species induced by alpha-humulene as possible mechanism of action," Planta Med. 69(5):402-7.

Legault J, Pichette A (2007 Dec). "Potentiating effect of beta-caryophyllene on anticancer activity of alpha-humulene, isocaryophyllene and paclitaxel," J Pharm Pharmacol. 59(12):1643-7.

Lehrer J, Eckersberger C, Walla P, Pötsch G, Deecke L (2000 Oct 1-15). "Ambient odor of orange in a dental office reduces anxiety and improves mood in female patients," Physiol Behav. 71(1-2):83-6.

Lehrer J, Marwinski G, Lehr S, Johren P, Deecke L. (2005 Sep 15). "Ambient odors of orange and lavender reduce anxiety and improve mood in a dental office," Physiol Behav. 86(1-2):92-5.

Letawe C, Boone M, Piérard GE (1998 Mar). "Digital image analysis of the effect of topically applied linoleic acid on acne microcomedones," Clin Exp Dermatol. 23(2):56-8.

Leung LH (1995 Jun). "Pantothenic acid deficiency as the pathogenesis of acne vulgaris," Med Hypotheses. 44(6):490-2.

Lewith GT, Godfrey AD, Prescott P (2005 Aug). "A single-blinded, randomized pilot study evaluating the aroma of Lavandula augustifolia as a treatment for mild insomnia," J Altern Complement Med. 11(4):631-7.

Li SP, Li P, Dont TT, Tsim KW (2001). "Anti-oxidation activity of different types of natural Cordyceps sinensis and cultured Cordyceps mycelia," Phytomedicine. 8:207-12.

Li QQ, Lee RX, Liang H, Zhong Y (2013 Jan). "Anticancer activity of beta-elemene and its synthetic analogs in human malignant brain tumor cells," Anticancer Res. 33(1):65-76.

Li QQ, Wang G, Huang F, Li JM, Cuff CF, Reed E. (2013 Mar). "Sensitization of lung cancer cells to cisplatin by beta-elemene is mediated through blockade of cell cycle progression: antitumor efficacies of beta-elemene and its synthetic analogs," Med Oncol. 30(1):488.

Li QQ, Wang G, Liang H, Li JM, Huang F, Agarwal PK, Zhong Y, Reed E (2013). "Beta element promotes cisplatin-induced cell death in human bladder cancer and other carcinomas," Anticancer Res. 33(4):1421-8.

Li, R., Liang, T., Xu, L., Li, Y., Zhang, S., & Duan, X. (2013 Jan). Protective effect of cinnamon polyphenols against STZ-diabetic mice fed high-sugar, high-fat diet and its underlying mechanism. Food Chem Toxicol, 51, 419-425.

Li, Y. P., Yuan, S. F., Cai, G. H., Wang, H., Wang, L., Yu, L., . . . Yun, J. (2014 May). Patchouli Alcohol Dampens Lipopolysaccharide Induced Mastitis in Mice. Inflammation.

Li, X., Duan, S., Chu, C., Xu, J., Zeng, G., Lam, A. K., . . . Jiang, L. (2013 Aug). Melaleuca alternifolia concentrate inhibits in vitro entry of influenza virus into host cells. Molecules, 18(8), 9550-9566.

Liapi C, Anifandis G, Chinou I, Kourounakis AP, Theodosopoulos S, Galanopoulou P (2007 Oct). "Antinociceptive properties of 1,8-Cineole and beta-pinene, from the essential oil of Eucalyptus camaldulensis leaves, in rodents," Planta Med. 73(12):1247-54.

Lima CF, Azevedo MF, Araujo R, Fernandes-Ferreira M, Pereira-Wilson C (2006 Aug). "Metformin-like effect of Salvia officinalis (common sage): is it useful in diabetes prevention?," Br J Nutr. 96(2):326-33.

Lima DF, Brandao MS, Moura JB, Leitao JM Carvalho FA, Miura LM, Leite JR, Sousa DP, Almeida FR (2012 Feb). "Antinociceptive activity of the monoterpene a-phellandrene in rodents: possible mechanisms of action," J Pharm Pharmacol. 64(2):283-92.

Lin PW, Chan WC, Ng BF, Lam LC (2007 May). "Efficacy of aromatherapy (Lavandula angustifolia) as an intervention for agitated behaviours in Chinese older persons with dementia: a cross-over randomized trial," Int J Geriatr Psychiatry. 22(5):405-10.

Lin SC, Chung TC, Lin CC, Ueng TH, Lin YH, Lin SY, Wang I.Y (2000). "Hepatoprotective effects of Arctium lappa on carbon tetrachloride- and acetaminophen-induced liver damage," Am J Chin Med. 28(2):163-73.

Linck V.M., da Silva A.L., Figueiro M., Piato A.L., Herrmann A.P., Birck F.D., Moreno P.R.H., Elisabetsky E. (2009) Inhaled linalool-induced sedation in mice. Phytomedicine. 16: 303-307.

Lipovac M, Chedraui P, Gruenhut C, Gocan A, Stammler M, Imhof M (2010 Mar). "Improvement of postmenopausal depressive and anxiety symptoms after treatment with isoflavones derived from red clover extracts," Maturitas. 65(3):258-61.

Lis-Balchin M, Hart S (1999 Sep). "Studies on the mode of action of the essential oil of lavender (Lavandula angustifolia P. Miller)," Phytother Res. 13(6):540-2.

Lis-Balchin M, Hart S, Wan Hang Lo B (2002 Aug). "Jasmine absolute (Jasminum grandiflora L.) and its mode of action on guinea-pig ileum in vitro," Phytother Res. 16(5):437-9.

Liu, C. T., Raghu, R., Lin, S. H., Wang, S. Y., Kuo, C. H., Tseng, Y. J., & Sheen, L. Y. (2013 Nov). Metabolomics of ginger essential oil against alcoholic fatty liver in mice. J Agric Food Chem, 61(46), 11231-11240.

Liu J, Head E, Gharib AM, Yuan W, Ingersoll RT, Hagen TM, Cotman CW, Ames BN (2002 Feb). "Memory loss in old rats is associated with brain mitochondrial decay and RNA/DNA oxidation: partial reversal by feeding acetyl-L-carnitine and/or R-alpha -lipoic acid," Proc Natl Acad Sci U S A. 99(4):2356-61.

Liu J, Killilea DW, Ames BN (2002 Feb 19). "Age-associated mitochondrial oxidative decay: improvement of carnitine acetyltransferase substrate-binding affinity and activity in brain by feeding old rats acetyl-L- carnitine and/or R-alpha-lipoic acid," Proc Natl Acad Sci U S A. 99(4):1876-81.

Liu JH, Chen GH, Yeh HZ, Huang CK, Poon SK (1997 Dec). "Enteric-coated peppermint-oil capsules in the treatment of irritable bowel syndrome: a prospective, randomized trial," J Gastroenterol. 32(6):765-8.

Liu JJ, Nilsson A, Oredsson S, Badmaev V, Duan RD (2002 Oct). "Keto- and acetyl-keto-boswellic acids inhibit proliferation and induce apoptosis in Hep G2 cells via a caspase-8 dependent pathway," Int J Mol Med. 10(4):501-5.

Liu JJ, Nilsson A, Oredsson S, Badmaev V, Zhao WZ, Duan RD (2002 Dec). "Boswellic acids trigger apoptosis via a pathway dependent on caspase-8 activation but independent on Fas/Fas ligand interaction in colon cancer HT-29 cells," Carcinogenesis. 23(12):2087-93.

Lobo, V., Patil, A., Phatak, A., & Chandra, N. (2010 Jul). Free radicals, antioxidants and functional foods: Impact on human health. Pharmacogn Rev, 4(8), 118-126.

Loew O. (1900) A New Enzyme of General Occurrence in Organisms. Science. 11: 701-702.

Lohidasan S, Paradkar AR, Mahadik KR (2009 Nov). "Nootropic activity of lipid-based extract of Bacopa monniera Linn. compared with traditional preparation and extracts," J Pharm Pharmacol. 61(11):1537-44.

Loizzo MR, Tundis R, Menichini F, Saab AM, Statti GA, Menichini F (2007 Sep-Oct). "Cytotoxic activity of essential oils from labiatae and lauraceae families against in vitro human tumor models," Anticancer Res. 27(5A):3293-9.

Long J, Gao F, Tong L, Cotman CW, Ames BN, Liu J (2009 Apr). "Mitochondrial decay in the brains of old rats: ameliorating effect of alpha-lipoic acid and acetyl-L-carnitine," Neurochem Res. 34(4):755-63.

Longley D.B. Harkin D.P., Johnston P.G. (2003) 5-Fluorouracil: Mechanisms of Action and Clinical Strategies. Nature Reviews. 3: 330-338.

Loughlin R, Gilmore BF, McCarron PA, Tunney MM (2008 Apr). "Comparison of the cidal activity of tea tree oil and terpinen-4-ol against clinical bacterial skin isolates and human fibroblast cells.," Lett Appl Microbiol. 46(4):428-33.

Lu LJ, Cree M, Josyula S, Nagamani M, Grady JJ, Anderson KE (2000 Mar 1). "Increased urinary excretion of 2-hydroxyestrone but not 16alpha-hydroxyestrone in premenopausal women during a soya diet containing isoflavones," Cancer Res. 60(5):1299-305.

Lu M, Battinelli L, Daniele C, Melchioni C, Salvatore G, Mazzanti G (2002 Mar). "Muscle relaxing activity of Hyssopus officinalis essential oil on isolated intestinal preparations," Planta Med. 68(3):213-6.

Lu M, Xia L, Hua H, Jing Y (2008 Feb 15). "Acetyl-keto-beta-boswellic acid induces apoptosis through a death receptor 5-mediated pathway in prostate cancer cells," Cancer Res. 68(4):1180-6.

Lu, T., Sheng, H., Wu, J., Cheng, Y., Zhu, J., & Chen, Y. (2012 Jun). Cinnamon extract improves fasting blood glucose and glycosylated hemoglobin level in Chinese patients with type 2 diabetes. Nutr Res, 32(6), 408-412.

Lu XQ, Tang FD, Wang Y, Zhao T, Bian RL (2004 Feb). "Effect of Eucalyptus globulus oil on lipopolysaccharide-induced chronic bronchitis and mucin hypersecretion in rats," Zhongguo Zhong Yao Za Zhi. 29(2):168-71.

Lucas M, Asselin G, Mérette C, Poulin MJ, Dodin S (2009 Feb). "Ethyl-eicosapentaenoic acid for the treatment of psychological distress and depressive symptoms in middle-aged women: a double-blind, placebo-controlled, randomized clinical trial," Am J Clin Nutr. 89(2):641-51.

Maatta-Riihinen KR, Kahkonen MP, Torronen AR, Heinonen IM (2005 Nov 2). "Catechins and procyanidins in berries of vaccinium species and their antioxidant activity," J Agric Food Chem. 53(22):8485-91.

Mabrok HB, Klopfleisch R, Ghanem KZ, Clavel T, Blaut M, Loh G (2012 Jan). "Lignan transformation by gut bacteria lowers tumor burden in a gnotobiotic rat model of breast cancer," Carcinogenesis. 33(1):203-8.

Machado, D. G., Cunha, M. P., Neis, V. B., Balen, G. O., Colla, A., Bettio, L. E., . . . Rodrigues, A. L. (2013 Jan). Antidepressant-like effects of fractions, essential oil, carnosol and betulinic acid isolated from Rosmarinus officinalis L. Food Chem, 136(2), 999-1005.

Maddocks-Jennings W, Wilkinson JM, Cavanagh HM, Shillington D (2009 Apr). "Evaluating the effects of the essential oils Leptospermum scoparium (manuka) and Kunzea ericoides (kanuka) on radiotherapy induced mucositis: a randomized, placebo controlled feasibility study," Eur J Oncol Nurs. 13(2):87-93.

Mahesh A, Jeyachandran R, Cindrella L, Thangadurai D, Veerapur VP, Muralidhara Rao D (2010 Jun). "Hepatocurative potential of sesquiterpene lactones of Taraxacum officinale on carbon tetrachloride induced liver toxicity in mice," Acta Biol Hung. 61(2):175-90.

Maickel, R. P., & Snodgrass, W. R. (1973 Oct). Physicochemical factors in maternal-fetal distribution of drugs. Toxicology and Applied Pharmacology, 26(2), 218-230.

Malaguarnera M, Cammalleri L, Gargante MP, Vacante M, Colonna V, Motta M (2007 Dec). "L-Carnitine treatment reduces severity of physical and mental fatigue and increases cognitive functions in centenarians: a randomized and controlled clinical trial," Am J Clin Nutr. 86(6):1738-44.

Mandel S, Stoner GD (1990 Jan). "Inhibition of N-nitrosobenzylmethylamine-induced esophageal tumorigenesis in rats by ellagic acid," Carcinogenisis. 11(1):55-61.

Manohar V, Ingram C, Gray J, Talpur NA, Echard BW, Bagchi D, Preuss HG (2001 Dec). "Antifungal activities of origanum oil against Candida albicans," Mol Cell Biochem. 228(1-2):111-7.

Maquart FX, Siméon A, Pasco S, Monboisse JC (1999). "[Regulation of cell activity by the extracellular matrix: the concept of matrikines]," J Soc Biol. 193(4-5):423-8.

Marder M, Viola H, Wasowski C, Fernández S, Medina JH, Paladini AC (2003 Jun). "6-methylapigenin and hesperidin: new valeriana flavonoids with activity on the CNS," Pharmacol Biochem Behav. 75(3):537-45.

Margetts, L., & Sawyer, R. (2007). Transdermal drug delivery: principles and opioid therapy. Continuing Education in Anaesthesia, Critical Care & Pain, 7(5), 171-176.

Marinangeli CP, Jones PJ (2012 Aug). "Pulse grain consumption and obesity: effects on energy expenditure, substrate oxidation, body composition, fat deposition and satiety," Br J Nutr. 108 Suppl 1:246-51.

Marounek M, Skrivanova E, Rada V, (2003). "Susceptibility of Escherichia coli to C2-C18 fatty acids," Folia Microbiol (Praha). 48(6):731-5.

Maruyama N, Sekimoto Y, Ishibashi H, Inouye S, Oshima H, Yamaguchi H, Abe S (2005 Feb 10). "Suppression of neutrophil accumulation in mice by cutaneous application of geranium essential oil," J Inflamm (Lond). 2(1):1.

Masango, P. (2005). Cleaner production of essential oils by steam distillation. Journal of Cleaner Production, 13(8), 833-839.

Masukawa Y., Narita H., Sato H., Naoe A., Kondo N., Sugai Y., Oba T., Homma R., Ishikawa J., Takagi Y., Kitahara T. (2009) Comprehensive quantification of ceramide species in human stratum corneum. Journal of Lipid Research. 50: 1708-1719.

May B, Kuntz HD, Kieser M, Köhler S (1996 Dec). "Efficacy of a fixed peppermint oil/caraway oil combination in non-ulcer dyspepsia," Arzneimittelforschung. 46(12):1149-53.

McCord J.M., Fridovich I. (1969) Superoxide Dismutase: an enzymic function for erytrocuprein (hemocuprein). The Journal of Biological Chemistry. 244: 6049-6055.

Meamarbashi, A., & Rajabi, A. (2013 Mar). The effects of peppermint on exercise performance. J Int Soc Sports Nutr, 10(1), 15.

Meier B, Berger D, Hoberg E, Sticher O, Schaffner W, (2000). "Pharmacological Activities of Vitex agnus-castus Extracts in Vitro," Phytomedicine. 7(5):373-81.

Meier , L., Stange, R., Michalsen, A., & Uehleke, B. (2012 May). Clay jojoba oil facial mask for lesioned skin and mild acne--results of a prospective, observational pilot study. Forsch Komplementmed, 19(2), 75-79.

Meiller, T. F., Silva, A., Ferreira, S. M., Jabra-Rizk, M. A., Kelley, J. I., & DePaola, L. G. (2005 Apr). Efficacy of Listerine Antiseptic in reducing viral contamination of saliva. J Clin Periodontol, 32(4), 341-346.

Meldrum B.S. (1994) The role of glutamate in epilepsy and other CNS disorders. Neurology. 44: S14-S23.

Meldrum B.S., Akbar M.T., Chapman A.G. (1999) Glutamate receptors and transporters in genetic and acquired models of epilepsy. Epilepsy Research. 36: 189-204.

Melo, F. H., Venancio, E. T., de Sousa, D. P., de Franca Fonteles, M. M., de Vasconcelos, S. M., Viana, G. S., & de Sousa, F. C. (2010 Aug). Anxiolytic-like effect of Carvacrol (5-isopropyl-2-methylphenol) in mice: involvement with GABAergic transmission. Fundam Clin Pharmacol, 24(4), 437-443.

Melov S., Ravenscroft J., Malik S., Gill M.S., Walker D.W., Clayton P.E., Wallace D.C., Malfroy B., Doctrow S.R., Lithgow G.J. (2000) Extension of Life-Span with Superoxide Dismutase/Catalase Mimetics. Science. 289: 1567-1569.

Mercier B., Prost J., Prost M. (2009) The Essential Oil of Turpentine and Its Major Volatile Fraction (α- and β-Pinenes): A Review. International Journal of Occupational Medicine and Environmental Health. 22: 331-342.

Miguel, M. G. (2010 Dec). Antioxidant and anti-inflammatory activities of essential oils: a short review. Molecules, 15(12), 9252-9287.

Mills JJ, Chari RS, Boyer IJ, Gould MN, Jirtle RL (1995 Mar 1). "Induction of apoptosis in liver tumors by the monoterpene perillyl alcohol," Cancer Res. 55(5):979-83.

Mimica-Dukić N, Bozin B, Soković M, Mihajlović B, Matavulj M (2003 May). "Antimicrobial and antioxidant activities of three Mentha species essential oils," Planta Med. 69(5):413-9.

Minaiyan, M., Ghannadi, A. R., Afsharipour, M., & Mahzouni, P. (2011 Jan). Effects of extract and essential oil of Rosmarinus officinalis L. on TNBS-induced colitis in rats. Res Pharm Sci, 6(1), 13-21.

Miocinovic R et al. (2005 Jan). "In vivo and in vitro effect of baicalin on human prostate cancer cells," Int J Oncol. 26(1):241-6.

Mishra, A., Bhatti, R., Singh, A., & Singh Ishar, M. P. (2010 Mar). Ameliorative effect of the cinnamon oil from Cinnamomum zeylanicum upon early stage diabetic nephropathy. Planta Med, 76(5), 412-417.

Misharina TA, Bulakova EB, Fatkullina LD, Terinina MB, Krikunova NI, Vorob'eva AK, Erokhin VN, Goloshchapov AN (2011 Nov–Dec). "Changes in fatty acid composition in the brain and liver in aging mice of high cancer risk AKR strain and effect of savory essential oil administration on leukemic process," biomed Khim. 57(6):604-14.

Mkolo MN, Magano SR (2007 Sep). "Repellent effects of the essential oil of Lavendula angustifolia against adults of Hyalomma marginatum rufipes," J S Afr Vet Assoc. 78(3):149-52.

Mohsenzadeh M (2007 Oct 15). "Evaluation of antibacterial activity of selected Iranian essential oils against Staphylococcus aureus and Escherichia coli in nutrient broth medium," Pak J Biol Sci. 10(20):3693-7.

Mondello F, De Bernardis F, Girolamo A, Cassone A, Salvatore G (2006 Nov 3). "In vivo activity of terpinen-4-ol, the main bioactive component of Melaleuca alternifolia Cheel (tea tree) oil against azole-susceptible and -resistant human pathogenic Candida species," BMC Infect Dis. 6:158.

Monfalouti HE, Guillaume D, Denhez C, Charrouf Z (2010 Dec). "Therapeutic potential of argan oil: a review," J Pharm Pharmacol. 62(12):1669-75.

Monsefi, M., Zahmati, M., Masoudi, M., & Javidnia, K. (2011 Dec). Effects of Anethum graveolens L. on fertility in male rats. Eur J Contracept Reprod Health Care, 16(6), 488-497.

Moon HJ, Park KS, Ku MJ, Lee MS, Jeong SH, Imbs TI, Zvyagintseva TN, Ermakova SP, Lee YH (2009 Oct). "Effect of Costaria costata fucoidan on expression of matrix metalloproteinase-1 promoter, mRNA, and protein," J Nat Prod. 72(10):1731-4.

Moon T, Wilkinson JM, Cavanagh HM (2006 Nov). "Antiparasitic activity of two Lavandula essential oils against Giardia duodenalis, Trichomonas vaginalis and Hexamita inflata," Parasitol Res. 99(6):722-8.

Moore LE, Brennan P, Karami S, Hung RJ, Hsu C, Boffetta P, Toro J, Zaridze D, Janout V, Bencko V, Navratilova M, Szeszenia-Dabrowska N, Mates D, Mukeria A, Holcatova I, Welch R, Chanock S, Rothman N, Chow WH (2007 Sep). "Glutathione S-transferase polymorphisms, cruciferous vegetable intake and cancer risk in the Central and Eastern European Kidney Cancer Study," Carcinogenesis. 28(9):1960-4.

Moreno S, Scheyer T, Romano CS, Vojnov AA (2006 Feb). "Antioxidant and antimicrobial activities of rosemary extracts linked to their polyphenol composition," Free Radic Res. 40(2):223-31.

Moretti MD, Sanna-Passino G, Demontis S, Bazzoni E (2002). "Essential oil formulations useful as a new tool for insect pest control," AAPS PharmSciTech. 3(2):E13.

Mori TA, Bao DQ, Burke V, Puddey IB, Beilin LJ (1999 Aug). "Docosahexaenoic acid but not eicosapentaenoic acid lowers ambulatory blood pressure and heart rate in humans," Hypertension. 34(2):253-60.

Morinobu A et al. (2008 Jul). "-Epigallocatechin-3-gallate suppresses osteoclast differentiation and ameliorates experimental arthritis in mice," Arthritis Rheum. 58(7):2012-8.

Morris MC, Sacks F, Rosner B (1993 Aug). "Does fish oil lower blood pressure? A meta-analysis of controlled trials," Circulation. 88(2):523-33.

Morse M.A., Stoner G.D. (1993) Cancer chemoprevention: principles and prospects. Carcinogenesis. 14: 1737-1746.

Mosaffa F, Behravan J, Karimi G, Iranshahi M (2006 Feb). "Antigenotoxic effects of Satureja hortensis L. on rat lymphocytes exposed to oxidative stress," Arch Pharm Res. 29(2):159-64.

Moss M, Cook J, Wesnes K, Duckett P (2003 Jan). "Aromas of rosemary and lavender essential oils differentially affect cognition and mood in healthy adults," Int J Neurosci. 113(1):15-38.

Moss M, Hewitt S, Moss L, Wesnes K (2008 Jan). "Modulation of cognitive performance and mood by aromas of peppermint and ylang-ylang," Int J Neurosci. 118(1):59-77.

Motomura N, Sakurai A, Yotsuya Y (2001 Dec). "Reduction of mental stress with lavender odorant," Percept Mot Skills. 93(3):713-8.

Moussaieff A, Rimmerman N, Bregman T, Straiker A, Felder CC, Shoham S, Kashman Y, Huang SM, Lee H, Shohami E, Mackie K, Caterina MJ, Walker JM, Fride E, Mechoulam R (2008 Aug). "Incensole acetate, an incense component, elicits psychoactivity by activating TRPV3 channels in the brain," FASEB J. 22(8):3024-34.

Moussaieff A, Shein NA, Tsenter J, Grigoriadis S, Simeonidou C, Alexandrovich AG, Trembovler V, Ben-Neriah Y, Schmitz ML, Fiebich BL, Munoz E, Mechoulam R, Shohami E (2008 Jul). "Incensole acetate: a novel neuroprotective agent isolated from Boswellia carterii," J Cereb Blood Flow Metab. 28(7):1341-52.

Moustafa. A. H., Ali, E. M., Moselhy, S. S., Tousson, E., & El-Said, K. S. (2012 Oct). Effect of coriander on thioacetamide-induced hepatotoxicity in rats. Toxicol Ind Health, 1-10.

Moy KA, Yuan JM, Chung FL, Wang XL, Van Den Berg D, Wang R, Gao YT, Yu MC (2009 Dec 1). "Isothiocyanates, glutathione S-transferase M1 and T1 polymorphisms and gastric cancer risk: a prospective study of men in Shanghai, China," Int J Cancer. 125(11):2652-9.

Mugnaini, L., Nardoni, S., Pinto, L., Pistelli, L., Leonardi, M., Pisseri, F., & Mancianti, F. (2012 Jun). In vitro and in vivo antifungal activity of some essential oils against feline isolates of Microsporum canis. J Mycol Med, 22(2), 179-184.

Muhlbauer, R. C., Lozano, A., Palacio, S., Reinli, A., & Felix, R. (2003 Apr). Common herbs, essential oils, and monoterpenes potently modulate bone metabolism. Bone, 32(4), 372-380.

Mukherjee P.K., Chandra J., Kuhn D.M., Ghannoum M.A. (2003) Mechanism of Fluconazole Resistance in Candida albicansBiofilms: Phase-Specific Role of Efflux Pumps and Membrane Sterols. Infection and Immunity. 71: 4333-4340.

Mumcuoglu KY, Magdassi S, Miller J, Ben-Ishai F, Zentner G, Helbin V, Friger M, Kahana F, Ingber A (2004 Dec). "Repellency of citronella for head lice: double-blind randomized trial of efficacy and safety," Isr Med Assoc J. 6(12):756-9.

Munzel T., Feil R., Mulsch A., Lohmann S.M., Hofmann F., Walter U. (2003) Physiology and Pathophysiology of Vascular Signaling Controlled by Cyclic Guanosine 3',5' –Cyclic Monophospate—Dependent Protein Kinase. Circulation. 108: 2172-2183.

Na HJ, Koo HN, Lee GG, Yoo SJ, Park JH, Lyu YS, Kim HM (2001 Dec). "Juniper oil inhibits the heat shock-induced apoptosis via preventing the caspase-3 activation in human astrocytes CCF-STTG1 cells," Clin Chim Acta. 314(1-2):215-20.

Nagashyana N, Sankarankutt P, Nampoothiri MRV, Moahan P, Mohan Kumar P (2000). "Association of L-dopa with recovery following Ayurvedic medication in Parkinson's disease," J Neurol Sci. 176:1121-7.

Naguib YM (2000 Apr). "Antioxidant activities of astaxanthin and related carotenoids," J Agric Food Chem. 48(4):1150-4.

Nair B (2001). "Final report on the safety assessment of Mentha Piperita (Peppermint) Oil, Mentha Piperita (Peppermint) Leaf Extract, Mentha Piperita (Peppermint) Leaf, and Mentha Piperita (Peppermint) Leaf Water," Int J Toxicol. 20(Suppl 3):61-73..

Nair MK, Joy J, Vasudevan P, Hinckley L, Hoagland TA, Venkitanarayanan KS (2009 Mar 30). "Antibacterial effect of caprylic acid and monocaprylin on major bacterial mastitis pathogens," Vet Microbiol. 135(3-4):358-62.

Nair, V., Singh, S., & Gupta, Y. K. (2012 Mar). Evaluation of disease modifying activity of Coriandrum sativum in experimental models. Indian J Med Res, 135, 240-245.

Nanthakomon T, Pongrojpaw D (2006 Oct). "The efficacy of ginger in prevention of postoperative nausea and vomiting after major gynecologic surgery," J Med Assoc Thai. 89(4):S130-6.

Nardoni, S., Mugnaini, L., Pistelli, L., Leonardi, M., Sanna, V., Perrucci, S., . . . Mancianti, F. (2014 Apr). Clinical and mycological evaluation of an herbal antifungal formulation in canine Malassezia dermatitis. J Mycol Med.

Narishetty S.T.K., Panchagnula R. (2004) Transdermal delivey of zidovudine: effect of terpenes and their mechanism of action. Journal of Controlled Release. 95: 367-379.

Narishetty S.T.K., Panchagnula R. (2005) Effects of L-menthol and 1,8-cineole on phase behavior and molecular organization of SC lipids and skin permeation of zidovudine. Journal of Controlled Release. 102: 59-70.

Nasel C, Nasel B, Samec P, Schindler E, Buchbauer G (1994 Aug). "Functional imaging of effects of fragrances on the human brain after prolonged inhalation," Chem Senses. 19(4):359-64.

Naseri, M., Mojab, F., Khodadoost, M., Kamalinejad, M., Davati, A., Choopani, R., . . . Emtiazy, M. (2012 Nov). The Study of Anti-Inflammatory Activity of Oil-Based Dill (Anethum graveolens L.) Extract Used Topically in Formalin-Induced Inflammation Male Rat Paw. Iran J Pharm Res, 11(4), 1169-1174.

Navarra, M., Ursino, M. R., Ferlazzo, N., Russo, M., Schumacher, U., & Valentiner, U. (2014 Jun). Effect of Citrus bergamia juice on human neuroblastoma cells in vitro and in metastatic xenograft models. Fitoterapia, 95, 83-92.

Modern Essentials Usage Guide

Navarro SL, Chang JL, Peterson S, Chen C, King IB, Schwarz Y, Li SS, Li L, Potter JD, Lampe JW (2009 Nov). "Modulation of human serum glutathione S-transferase A1/2 concentration by cruciferous vegetables in a controlled feeding study is influenced by GSTM1 and GSTT1 genotypes," Cancer Epidemiol Biomarkers Prev. 18(11):2974-8.

Navarro SL, Peterson S, Chen C, Makar KW, Schwarz Y, King IB, Li SS, Li L, Kestin M, Lampe JW. (2009 Apr). "Cruciferous vegetable feeding alters UGT1A1 activity: diet- and genotype-dependent changes in serum bilirubin in a controlled feeding trial," Cancer Prev Res (Phila Pa). 2(4):345-52.

Nielsen FH, Hunt CD, Mullen LM, Hunt JR (1987 Nov). "Effect of dietary boron on mineral, estrogen, and testosterone metabolism in postmenopausal women," FASEB J. 1(5):394-7.

Nikolaevski VV, Kononova NS, Pertsovski AI, Shinkarchuk IF (1990 Sep-Oct). "Effect of essential oils on the course of experimental atherosclerosis," Patol Fiziol Eksp Ter. (5):52-3.

Ninomiya K, Matsuda H, Shimoda H, Nishida N, Kasajima N, Yoshino T, Morikawa T, Yoshikawa M (2004 Apr 19). "Carnosic acid, a new class of lipid absorption inhibitor from sage," Bioorg Med Chem Lett. 14(8):1943-6.

Nishio M, Kawmata H, Fujita K, Ishizaki T, Hayman R, Idemi T (2004). "A new enamel restoring agent for use after PMTC," Journal of Dental Research 83(1920):SpclIssueA.

Noori, S., Hassan, Z. M., & Salehian, O. (2013 Mar). Sclareol reduces CD4+ CD25+ FoxP3+ Treg cells in a breast cancer model in vivo. Iran J Immunol, 10(1), 10-21.

Norazmir, M. N., Jr., & Ayub, M. Y. (2010 Apr). Beneficial lipid-lowering effects of pink guava puree in high fat diet induced-obese rats. Malays J Nutr, 16(1), 171-185.

Nostro A, Bisignano G, Angela Cannatelli M, Crisafi G, Paola Germanò M, Alonzo V (2001 Jun). "Effects of Helichrysum italicum extract on growth and enzymatic activity of Staphylococcus aureus," Int J Antimicrob Agents. 17(6):517-20.

Nostro A, Blanco AR, Cannatelli MA, Enea V, Flamini G, Morelli I, Sudano Roccaro A, Alonzo V (2004 Jan 30). "Susceptibility of methicillin-resistant staphylococci to oregano essential oil, carvacrol and thymol," FEMS Microbiol Lett. 230(2):191-5.

Nostro A, Cannatelli MA, Marino A, Picerno I, Pizzimenti FC, Scoglio ME, Spataro P (2003 Jan). "Evaluation of antiherpesvirus-1 and genotoxic activities of Helichrysum italicum extract," New Microbiol. 26(1):125-8.

Nothlings U, Murphy SP, Wilkens LR, Henderson BE, Kolonel LN (2007 Oct). "Flavonols and pancreatic cancer risk: the multiethnic cohort study," Am J Epidemiol. 166(8):924-31.

Nyadjeu, P., Nguelefack-Mbuyo, E. P., Atsamo, A. D., Nguelefack, T. B., Dongmo, A. B., & Kamanyi, A. (2013 Feb). Acute and chronic antihypertensive effects of Cinnamomum zeylanicum stem bark methanol extract in L-NAME-induced hypertensive rats. BMC Complement Altern Med, 13, 1-10.

Oboh, G., Olasehinde, T. A., & Ademosun, A. O. (2014 Mar). Essential oil from lemon peels inhibit key enzymes linked to neurodegenerative conditions and pro-oxidant induced lipid peroxidation. J Oleo Sci, 63(4), 373-381.

Ogeturk, M., Kose, E., Sarsilmaz, M., Akpinar, B., Kus, I., & Meydan, S. (2010 Oct). Effects of lemon essential oil aroma on the learning behaviors of rats. Neurosciences (Riyadh), 15(4), 292-293.

Ohno T, Kita M, Yamaoka Y, Imamura S, Yamamoto T, Mitsufuji S, Kodama T, Kashima K, Imanishi J (2003 Jun). "Antimicrobial activity of essential oils against Helicobacter pylori," Helicobacter. 8(3):207-15.

Okugawa, H., Ueda, R., Matsumoto, K., Kawanishi, K., & Kato, K. (2000 Oct). Effects of sesquiterpenoids from Oriental incenses on acetic acid-induced writhing and D2 and 5-HT2A receptors in rat brain. Phytomedicine, 7(5), 417-422.

Olajide OA, Ajayi FF, Ekhelar AI, Awe SO, Makinde JM, Alada AR (1999 Jun). "Biological effects of Myristica fragrans (nutmeg) extract," Phytother Res. 13(4):344-5.

Olapour, A., Behaeen, K., Akhondzadeh, R., Soltani, F., Al Sadat Razavi, F., & Bekhradi, R. (2013 Nov). The Effect of Inhalation of Aromatherapy Blend containing Lavender Essential Oil on Cesarean Postoperative Pain. Anesth Pain Med, 3(1), 203-207.

Onawunmi GO, Yisak WA, Ogunlana EO (1984 Dec). "Antibacterial constituents in the essential oil of Cymbopogon citratus (DC.) Stapf.," J Ethnopharmacol. 12(3):279-86.

Onocha, P., Oloyede, G., & Afolabi, Q. (2011). Chemical composition, cytotoxicity and antioxidant activity of essential oils of Acalypha hispida flowers. Inter J Pharm, 7(1), 144-148.

Opalchenova G, Obreshkova D (2003 Jul). "Comparative studies on the activity of basil—an essential oil from Ocimum basilicum L.--against multidrug resistant clinical isolates of the genera Staphylococcus, Enterococcus and Pseudomonas by using different test methods," J Microbiol Methods. 54(1):105-10.

Orafidiya LO, Agbani EO, Abereoje OA, Awe T, Abudu A, Fakoya FA (2003 Oct). "An investigation into the wound-healing properties of essential oil of Ocimum gratissimum linn," J Wound Care. 12(9):331-4.

Osher Y, Bersudsky Y, Belmaker RH (2005 Jun). "Omega-3 eicosapentaenoic acid in bipolar depression: report of a small open-label study," J Clin Psychiatry. 66(6):726-9.

Ostad SN, Soodi M, Shariffzadeh M, Khorshidi N, Marzban H (2001 Aug). "The effect of fennel essential oil on uterine contraction as a model for dysmenorrhea, pharmacology and toxicology study," J Ethnopharmacol. 76(3):299-304.

Ou, M. C., Hsu, T. F., Lai, A. C., Lin, Y. T., & Lin, C. C. (2012 May). Pain relief assessment by aromatic essential oil massage on outpatients with primary dysmenorrhea: a randomized, double-blind clinical trial. J Obstet Gynaecol Res, 38(5), 817-822.

Paliwal S, J Sundaram and S Mitragotri (2005). "Induction of cancer-specific cytotoxicity towards human prostate and skin cells using quercetin and ultrasound," British Journal of Cancer. 92:499-502.

Palozza P, Krinsky NI (1992 Sep). "Astaxanthin and canthaxanthin are potent antioxidants in a membrane model," Arch Biochem Biophys. 297(2):291-5.

Pandey, A., Bigoniya, P., Raj, V., & Patel, K. K. (2011 Jul). Pharmacological screening of Coriandrum sativum Linn. for hepatoprotective activity. J Pharm Bioallied Sci, 3(3), 435-441.

Paoletti P., Neyton J. (2007) NMDA receptor subunits: functions and pharmacology. Current Opinion in Pharmacology. 7: 39-47.

Pardridge, W. M. (2003 Mar). Blood-brain barrier drug targeting: the future of brain drug development. Mol Interv, 3(2).

Pardridge, W. M. (2009 Sep). Alzheimer's disease drug development and the problem of the blood-brain barrier. Alzheimers Dement, 5(5), 427-432.

Park, G., Kim, H. G., Kim, Y. O., Park, S. H., Kim, S. Y., & Oh, M. S. (2012 Feb). Coriandrum sativum L. protects human keratinocytes from oxidative stress by regulating oxidative defense systems. Skin Pharmacol Physiol, 25(2), 93-99.

Park, H. J., Kim, S. K., Kang, W. S., Woo, J. M., & Kim, J. W. (2014 Feb). Effects of essential oil from Chamaecyparis obtusa on cytokine genes in the hippocampus of maternal separation rats. Can J Physiol Pharmacol, 92(2), 95-101.

Park SY, Kim HS, Cho EK, Kwon BY, Phark S, Hwang KW, Sul D (2008 Aug). "Curcumin protected PC12 cells against beta-amyloid-induced toxicity through the inhibition of oxidative damage and tau hyperphosphorylation," Food Chem Toxicol. 46(8):2881-7.

Pause, B. M., Raack, N., Sojka, B., Goder, R., Aldenhoff, J. B., & Ferstl, R. (2003 Mar). Convergent and divergent effects of odors and emotions in depression. Psychophysiology, 40(2), 209-225.

Pavela R (2005 Dec). "Insecticidal activity of some essential oils against larvae of Spodoptera littoralis," Fitoterapia. 76(7-8):691-6.

Pavela R (2008 Feb). "Insecticidal properties of several essential oils on the house fly (Musca domestica L.)," Phytother Res. 22(2):274-8.

Peana AT, D'Aquila PS, Panin F, Serra G, Pippia P, Moretti MD (2002 Dec). "Anti-inflammatory activity of linalool and linalyl acetate constituents of essential oils," Phytomedicine. 9(8):721-6.

Peana A.T., D'Aquila P.S., Chessa M. L., Moretti M.D.L., Serra G., Pippia P. (2003) (-)-Linalool produces antinociception in two experimental models of pain. European Journal of Pharmacology. 460: 37-41.

Pearce AL, Finlay-Jones JJ, Hart PH (2005 Jan). "Reduction of nickel-induced contact hypersensitivity reactions by topical tea tree oil in humans," Inflamm Res. 54(1):22-30.

Pemberton E, Turpin PG (2008 Mar-Apr). "The effect of essential oils on work-related stress in intensive care unit nurses," Holist Nurs Pract. 22(2):97-102.

Penalvo JL, Lopez-Romero P (2012 Feb 29). "Urinary enterolignan concentrations are positively associated with serum HDL cholesterol and negatively associated with serum triglycerides in U.S. adults," J Nutr. [Epub ahead of print].

Peng SM, Koo M, Yu ZR (2009 Jan). "Effects of music and essential oil inhalation on cardiac autonomic balance in healthy individuals," J Altern Complement Med. 15(1):53-7.

Pengelly, A. (2004). The Constituents of Medicinal Plants (2nd ed.). Singapore: Allen and Unwin.

Perry N, Perry E (2006). "Aromatherapy in the management of psychiatric disorders: clinical and neuropharmacological perspectives," CNS Drugs. 20(4):257-80.

Peters G.J., Backus H.H.J., Freemantle S., van Triest B., Codacci-Pisanelli G., van der Wilt C.L., Smid K., Lunec J., Calvert A.H., Marsh S., McLeod H.L., Bloemena E., Meijer S., Jansen G., van Groeningen C.J., Pinedo H.M. (2002) Induction of thymidylate synthase as a 5-fluorouracil resistance mechanism. Biochimica et Biophysica Acta. 1587: 194-205.

Pevsner J, Hsu SC, Braun JE, Calakos N, Ting AE, Bennett MK, Scheller RH (1994 Aug). "Specificity and regulation of a synaptic vesicle docking complex," Neuron. 13(2):353-61.

Philippe M, Garson JC, Gilard P, Hocquaux M, Hussler G, Leroy F, Mahieu C, Semeria D, Vanlerberghe G (1994 Aug). "Synthesis of 2-N-oleoylamino-octadec-ane-1,3-diol: a new ceramide highly effective for the treatment of skin and hair," Int J Cosmet Sci. 17(4):133-46.

Piazza GA, Ritter JL, Baracka CA (1995 Jan). "Lysophosphatidic acid induction of transforming growth factors alpha and beta: modulation of proliferation and differentiation in cultured human keratinocytes and mouse skin," Exp Cell Res. 216(1):51-64.

Pichette A, Larouche PL, Lebrun M, Legault J (2006 May). "Composition and antibacterial activity of Abies balsamea essential oil," Phytother Res. 20(5):371-3.

Pietruck F, Busch S, Virchow S, Brockmeyer N, Siffert W (1997 Jan). "Signalling properties of lysophosphatidic acid in primary human skin fibroblasts: role of pertussis toxin-sensitive GTP-binding proteins," Naunyn Schmiedebergs Arch Pharmacol. 355(1):1-7.

Pina-Vaz C, Gonçalves Rodrigues A, Pinto E, Costa-de-Oliveira S, Tavares C, Salgueiro L, Cavaleiro C, Gonçalves MJ, Martinez-de-Oliveira J (2004 Jan). "Antifungal activity of Thymus oils and their major compounds," J Eur Acad Dermatol Venereol. 18(1):73-8.

Ping H, Zhang G, Ren G (2010 Aug-Sep). "Antidiabetic effects of cinnamon oil in diabetic KK-Ay mice," Food Chem Toxicol. 48(8-9):2344-9.

Pistone G, Marino A, Leotta C, Dell'Arte S, Finocchiaro G, Malaguarnera M (2003). "Levocarnitine administration in elderly subjects with rapid muscle fatigue: effect on body composition, lipid profile and fatigue," Drugs Aging. 20(10):761-7.

Pouvreau L, Gruppen H, Piersma SR, van den Broek LA, van Koningsveld GA, Voragen AG (2001 Jun). "Relative abundance and inhibitory distribution of protease inhibitors in potato juice from cv. Elkana," J Agric Food Chem. 49(6):2864-74.

Preuss HG, Echard B, Enig M, Brook I, Elliott TB (2005 Apr). "Minimum inhibitory concentrations of herbal essential oils and monolaurin for gram-positive and gram-negative bacteria," Mol Cell Biochem. 272(1-2):29-34.

Puatanachokchai R, Kishida H, Denda A, Murata N, Konishi Y, Vinitketkumnuen U, Nakae D (2002 Sep 8). "Inhibitory effects of lemon grass (Cymbopogon citratus, Stapf) extract on the early phase of hepatocarcinogenesis after initiation with diethylnitrosamine in male Fischer 344 rats," Cancer Lett. 183(1):9-15.

Qiu Y, Du GH, Qu ZW, Zhang JT (1995). "Protective effects of ginsenoside on the learning and memory impairment induced by transient cerebral ischemia-reperfusion in mice," Chin Pharmacol Bull. 11:299-302.

Qureshi A.A., Mangels W.R., Din A.A., Elson C.E. (1988) Inhibition of Hepatic Mevalonate Biosynthesis by the Monoterpene, d-Limonene. J. Agric. Food Chem. 36: 1220-1224.

Ragho R., Postlethwaite AE, Keski-Oja J, Moses HL., Kang AH (1987 Apr). "Transforming growth factor-beta increases steady state levels of type I procollagen and fibronectin messenger RNAs posttranscriptionally in cultured human dermal fibroblasts," J Clin Invest. 79(4):1285-8.

Rahman MM, Ichiyanagi T, Komiyama T, Sato S, Konishi T (2008 Aug). "Effects of anthocyanins on psychological stress-induced oxidative stress and neurotransmitter status," J Agric Food Chem. 56(16):7545-50.

Ra Kovi, A., Milanovi, I., Pavlovi, N. A., Ebovi, T., Vukmirovi, S. A., & Mikov, M. (2014 Jul). Antioxidant activity of rosemary (Rosmarinus officinalis L.) essential oil and its hepatoprotective potential. BMC Complement Altern Med, 14(1), 1-20.

Raman A, Weir U, Bloomfield SF (1995 Oct). "Antimicrobial effects of tea-tree oil and its major components on Staphylococcus aureus, Staph. epidermidis and Propionibacterium acnes," Lett Appl Microbiol. 21(4):242-5.

Ramezani, R., Moghimi, A., Rakhshandeh, H., Ejtehadi, H., & Kheirabadi, M. (2008 Mar). The effect of Rosa damascena essential oil on the amygdala electrical kindling seizures in rat. Pak J Biol Sci, 11(5), 746-751.

Ranzato, E., Martinotti, S., & Burlando, B. (2011 Mar). Wound healing properties of jojoba liquid wax: an in vitro study. J Ethnopharmacol, 134(2), 443-449.

Rao S., Krauss N.E., Heerding J.M., Swindell C.S., Ringel I., Orr G.A., Horwitz S.B. (1994) 3'-(p-Azidobenzamido)taxol Photolabels the N-terminal 31 AminoAcids of β-Tubulin. The Journal of Biological Chemistry. 269: 3132-3134.

Rao S., Orr G.A., Chaudhary A.G., Kingston D.G.I., Horwitz S.B. (1995) Characterization of the Taxol Binding Site on the Microtubule. The Journal of Biological Chemistry. 270: 20235-20238.

Rasooli I, Fakoor MH, Yadegarinia D, Gachkar L, Allameh A, Rezaei MB (2008 Feb 29). "Antimycotoxigenic characteristics of Rosmarinus officinalis and Trachyspermum copticum L. essential oils," Int J Food Microbiol. 122(1-2):135-9.

Rasooli I, Shayegh S, Taghizadeh M, Astaneh SD (2008 Sep). "Phytotherapeutic prevention of dental biofilm formation," Phytother Res. 22(9):1162-7.

Rathi, B., Bodhankar, S., Mohan, V., & Thakurdesai, P. (2013 Jun). Ameliorative Effects of a Polyphenolic Fraction of Cinnamomum zeylanicum L. Bark in Animal Models of Inflammation and Arthritis. Sci Pharm, 81(2), 567-589.

Reddy AC, Lokesh BR (1994). "Studies on anti-inflammatory activity of spice principles and dietary n-3 polyunsaturated fatty acids on carrageenan-induced inflammation in rats," Ann Nutr Metab. 38(6):349-58.

Reddy BS, Wang CX, Samaha H, Lubet R, Steele VE, Kelloff GJ, Rao CV (1997 Feb 1). "Chemoprevention of colon carcinogenesis by dietary perillyl alcohol," Cancer Res. 57(3):420-5.

Rees WD, Evans BK, Rhodes J (1979 Oct 6). "Treating irritable bowel syndrome with peppermint oil," Br Med J. 2(6194):835-6.

Reeve, V. E., Allanson, M., Arun, S. J., Domanski, D., & Painter, N. (2010 Apr). Mice drinking goji berry juice (Lycium barbarum) are protected from UV radiation-induced skin damage via antioxidant pathways. Photochem Photobiol Sci, 9(4), 601-607. Reichling J, Fitzi J, Hellmann K, Wegener T, Bucher S, Saller R (2004 Oct). "Topical tea tree oil effective in canine localised pruritic dermatitis--a multi centre randomised double-blind controlled clinical trial in the veterinary practice," Dtsch Tierarztl Wochenschr. 111(10):408-14.

Reichling J, Koch C, Stahl-Biskup E, Sojka C, Schnitzler P (2005 Dec). "Virucidal activity of a beta-triketone-rich essential oil of Leptospermum scoparium (manuka oil) against HSV-1 and HSV-2 in cell culture," Planta Med. 71(12):1123-7.

Renimel I, Andre P (Inventors) (1995). "Method for treatment of allergic disorders and cosmetic compositions using cucurbitine," USPTO 5714164.

Rhee SG (2006 Jun). "Cell signaling. H2O2, a necessary evil for cell signaling," Science. 312(5782):1882-3.

Rigano L, Dell'Acqua G, Leporatti R (2000). "Benefits of Trimethylglycine (Betaine) in Personal-Care Formulations," Cosm Toil. 115(12):47-54.

Ritschel, W. A., Brady, M. E., & Tan, H. S. (1979 Mar). First-pass effect of coumarin in man. Int J Clin Pharmacol Biopharm, 17(3), 99-103.

Modern Essentials Usage Guide

Rivero-Cruz B, Rojas MA, Rodríguez-Sotres R, Cerda-García-Rojas CM, Mata R (2005 Apr). "Smooth muscle relaxant action of benzyl benzoates and salicylic acid derivatives from Brickellia veronicaefolia on isolated guinea-pig ileum," Planta Med. 71(4):320-5.

Romero-Jiménez M, Campos-Sánchez J, Analla M, Muñoz-Serrano A, Alonso-Moraga A (2005 Aug 1). "Genotoxicity and anti-genotoxicity of some traditional medicinal herbs," Mutat Res. 585(1-2):147-55.

Rosa A, Deiana M, Atzeri A, Corona G, Incani A, Melis MP, Appendino G, Dessì MA (2007 Jan 30). "Evaluation of the antioxidant and cytotoxic activity of arzanol, a prenylated alpha-pyrone-phloroglucinol etherodimer from Helichrysum italicum subsp.microphyllum," Chem Biol Interact. 165(2):117-26.

Rose JE, Behm FM (1994 Feb). "Inhalation of vapor from black pepper extract reduces smoking withdrawal symptoms," Drug Alcohol Depend. 34(3):225-9.

Rowinsky E.K., Donehower R.C. (1995) Paclitaxel (Taxol). The New England Journal of Medicine. 332: 1004-1014.

Roy S, Khanna S, Krishnaraju AV, Subbaraju GV, Yasmin T, Bagchi D, Sen CK (2006 Mar-Apr). "Regulation of vascular responses to inflammation: inducible matrix metalloproteinase-3 expression in human microvascular endothelial cells is sensitive to antiinflammatory Boswellia," Antioxid Redox Signal. 8(3-4):653-60.

Roy S, Khanna S, Shah H, Rink C, Phillips C, Preuss H, Subbaraju GV, Trimurtulu G, Krishnaraju AV, Bagchi M, Bagchi D, Sen CK (2005 Apr). "Human genome screen to identify the genetic basis of the anti-inflammatory effects of Boswellia in microvascular endothelial cells," DNA Cell Biol. 24(4):244-55.

Roy S, Khanna S, Alessio HM, Vider J, Bagchi D, Bagchi M, Sen CK (2002 Sep). "Anti-angiogenic property of edible berries," Free Radic Res. 36(9):1023-31.

Rozza, A. L., Moraes Tde, M., Kushima, H., Tanimoto, A., Marques, M. O., Bauab, T. M., . . . Pellizzon, C. H. (2011 Jan). Gastroprotective mechanisms of Citrus lemon (Rutaceae) essential oil and its majority compounds limonene and beta-pinene: involvement of heat-shock protein-70, vasoactive intestinal peptide, glutathione, sulfhydryl compounds, nitric oxide and prostaglandin E(2). Chem Biol Interact, 189(1-2), 82-89.

Ruthig DJ, Meckling-Gill KA (1999 Oct). "Both (n-3) and (n-6) fatty acids stimulate wound healing in the rat intestinal epithelial cell line, IEC-6," J Nutr. 129(10):1791-8.

Sabzghabaee AM, Davoodi N, Ebadian B, Aslani A, Ghannadi A (2012 Mar). "Clinical evaluation of the essential oil of "Satureja hortensis" for the treatment of denture stomatitis," Dent Res J (isfahan). 9(2):198-202.

Sadraei, H., Asghari, G., & Emami, S. (2013 Jan). Inhibitory effect of Rosa damascena Mill flower essential oil, geraniol and citronellol on rat ileum contraction. Res Pharm Sci, 8(1), 17-23.

Sadraei H, Asghari GR, Hajhashemi V, Kolagar A, Ebrahimi M. (2001 Sep). "Spasmolytic activity of essential oil and various extracts of Ferula gummosa Boiss. on ileum contractions," Phytomedicine. 8(5):370-6.

Saeed SA, Gilani AH (1994 May). "Antithrombotic activity of clove oil," J Pak Med Assoc. 44(5):112-5.

Saeedi M, Morteza, Semnani K, Ghoreishi MR (2003 Sep). "The treatment of atopic dermatitis with licorice gel," J Dermatolog Treat. 14(3):153-7.

Saerens KM, Zhang J, Saey L, Van Bogaert IN, Soetaert W (2011 Apr). "Cloning and functional characterization of the UDP-glucosyltransferase UgtB1 involved in sophorolipid production by Candida bombicola and creation of a glucolipid-producing yeast strain," Yeast. 28(4):279-92.

Safayhi H, Sabieraj J, Sailer ER, Ammon HP (1994 Oct). "Chamazulene: an antioxidant-type inhibitor of leukotriene B4 formation," Planta Med. 60(5):410-3.

Saha SS, Ghosh M (2009 Jul 18). "Comparative study of antioxidant activity of alpha-eleostearic acid and punicic acid against oxidative stress generated by sodium arsenite," Food Chem Toxicol. [Epub ahead of print].

Said T, Dutot M, Martin C, Beaudeux JL, Boucher C, Enee E, Baudouin C, Warnet JM, Rat P (2007 Mar). "Cytoprotective effect against UV-induced DNA damage and oxidative stress: role of new biological UV filter," Eur J Pharm Sci. 30(3-4):203-10.

Saikia, D., Parveen, S., Gupta, V. K., & Luqman, S. (2012 Dec). Anti-tuberculosis activity of Indian grass KHUS (Vetiveria zizanioides L. Nash). Complement Ther Med, 20(6), 434-436.

Saiyudthong, S., & Marsden, C. A. (2011 Jun). Acute effects of bergamot oil on anxiety-related behaviour and corticosterone level in rats. Phytother Res, 25(6), 858-862.

Salmalian, H., Saghebi, R., Moghadamnia, A. A., Bijani, A., Faramarzi, M., Nasiri Amiri, F., . . . Bekhradi, R. (2014 Apr). Comparative effect of thymus vulgaris and ibuprofen on primary dysmenorrhea: A triple-blind clinical study. Caspian J Intern Med, 5(2), 82-88.

Samarth RM (2007 Nov). "Protection against radiation induced hematopoietic damage in bone marrow of Swiss albino mice by Mentha piperita (Linn)," J Radiat Res (Tokyo). 48(6):523-8.

Samarth RM, Goyal PK, Kumar A (2004 Jul). "Protection of swiss albino mice against whole-body gamma irradiation by Mentha piperita (Linn).," Phytother Res. 18(7):546-50.

Samarth RM, Kumar A (2003 Jun). "Radioprotection of Swiss albino mice by plant extract Mentha piperita (Linn.)," J Radiat Res (Tokyo). 44(2):101-9.

Samarth RM, Panwar M, Kumar M, Kumar A (2006 May). "Radioprotective influence of Mentha piperita (Linn) against gamma irradiation in mice: Antioxidant and radical scavenging activity," Int J Radiat Biol. 82(5):331-7.

Samarth RM, Samarth M (2009 Apr). "Protection against radiation-induced testicular damage in Swiss albino mice by Mentha piperita (Linn.)," Basic Clin Pharmacol Toxicol. 104(4):329-34.

Samman S, Naghii MR, Lyons Wall PM, Verus AP (1998 Winter). "The nutritional and metabolic effects of boron in humans and animals," Biol Trace Elem Res. 66(1-3):227-35.

Sanguinetti, M., Posteraro, B., Romano, L., Battaglia, F., Lopizzo, T., De Carolis, E., & Fadda, G. (2007 Feb). In vitro activity of Citrus bergamia (bergamot) oil against clinical isolates of dermatophytes. J Antimicrob Chemother, 59(2), 305-308.

Santamaria, M., Jr., Petermann, K. D., Vedovello, S. A., Degan, V., Lucato, A., & Franzini, C. M. (2014 Feb). Antimicrobial effect of Melaleuca alternifolia dental gel in orthodontic patients. Am J Orthod Dentofacial Orthop, 145(2), 198-202.

Santos AO, Ueda-Nakamura T, Dias Filho BP, Veiga Junior VF, Pinto AC, Nakamura CV (2008 May). "Antimicrobial activity of Brazilian copaiba oils obtained from different species of the Copaifera genus," Mem Inst Oswaldo Cruz. 103(3):277-81.

Santos AO, Ueda-Nakamura T, Dias Filho BP, Veiga Junior VF, Pinto AC, Nakamura CV (2008 Nov 20). "Effect of Brazilian copaiba oils on Leishmania amazonensis," J Ethnopharmacol. 120(2):204-8.

Santos FA, Rao VS (2000 Jun). "Anti-inflammatory and antinociceptive effects of 1,8-cineole a terpenoid oxide present in many plant essential oils," Phytother Res. 14(4):240-4.

Sarahroodi, S., Esmaeili, S., Mikaili, P., Hemmati, Z., & Saberi, Y. (2012 Apr). The effects of green Ocimum basilicum hydroalcoholic extract on retention and retrieval of memory in mice. Anc Sci Life, 31(4), 185-189.

Sasannejad, P., Saeedi, M., Shoeibi, A., Gorji, A., Abbasi, M., & Foroughipour, M. (2012 Apr). Lavender essential oil in the treatment of migraine headache: a placebo-controlled clinical trial. Eur Neurol, 67(5), 288-291.

Satchell AC, Saurajen A, Bell C, Barnetson RS (2002 Aug). "Treatment of interdigital tinea pedis with 25% and 50% tea tree oil solution: a randomized, placebo-controlled, blinded study," Australas J Dermatol. 43(3):175-8.

Satou, T., Takahashi, M., Kasuya, H., Murakami, S., Hayashi, S., Sadamoto, K., & Koike, K. (2013 Feb). Organ accumulation in mice after inhalation of single or mixed essential oil compounds. Phytother Res, 27(2), 306-311.

Savelev SU, Okello EJ, Perry EK (2004 Apr). "Butyryl- and acetyl-cholinesterase inhibitory activities in essential oils of Salvia species and their constituents," Phytother Res. 18(4):315-24.

Savino F, Cresi F, Castagno E, Silvestro L, Oggero R (2005 Apr). "A randomized double-blind placebo-controlled trial of a standardized extract of Matricariae recutita, Foeniculum vulgare and Melissa officinalis (ColiMil) in the treatment of breastfed colicky infants," Phytother Res. 19(4):335-40.

Sayyah M, Nadjafnia L, Kamalinejad M (2004 Oct). "Anticonvulsant activity and chemical composition of Artemisia dracunculus L. essential oil," J Ethnopharmacol. 94(2-3):283-7.

Sayyah M, Saroukhani G, Peirovi A, Kamalinejad M (2003 Aug). "Analgesic and anti-inflammatory activity of the leaf essential oil of Laurus nobilis Linn," Phytother Res. 17(7):733-6.

Sayyah M, Valizadeh J, Kamalinejad M (2002 Apr). "Anticonvulsant activity of the leaf essential oil of Laurus nobilis against pentylenetetrazole- and maximal electroshock-induced seizures," Phytomedicine. 9(3):212-6.

Scalbert A, Johnson IT, and Saltmarsh M (2005 Jan). "Polyphenols: antioxidants and beyond," Presented at the 1st International Conference on Polyphenols and Health, Vichy, France. Am J Clin Nut. 81(1):215S-7S.

Schecter A., Birnbaum L., Ryan J.J., Constable J.D. (2006) Dioxins: An overview. Environmental Research. 101: 419-428.

Scheinfeld NS, Mones J (2005 May). "Granular parakeratosis: pathologic and clinical correlation of 18 cases of granular parakeratosis," J Am Acad Dermatol. 52(5):863-7.

Schellack, G. (2011). Series on nursing pharmacology and medicine management part 3: drug dosage forms and the routes of drug administration. Profession Nurse Today, 15(6), 10-15.

Schlachterman A et al. (2008 Mar). "Combined resveratrol, quercetin, and catechin treatment reduces breast tumor growth in a nude mouse model," Transl Oncol. 1(1):19-27.

Schmitt, S., Schaefer, U. F., Doebler, L., & Reichling, J. (2009 Oct). Cooperative interaction of monoterpenes and phenylpropanoids on the in vitro human skin permeation of complex composed essential oils. Planta Med, 75(13), 1381-1385.

Schnitzler P, Schön K, Reichling J (2001 Apr). "Antiviral activity of Australian tea tree oil and eucalyptus oil against herpes simplex virus in cell culture," Pharmazie. 56(4):343-7.

Schnitzler P, Schuhmacher A, Astani A, Reichling J (2008 Sep). "Melissa officinalis oil affects infectivity of enveloped herpesviruses," Phytomedicine. 15(9):734-40.

Schreckinger, M. E., Lotton, J., Lila, M. A., & de Mejia, E. G. (2010 Apr). Berries from South America: a comprehensive review on chemistry, health potential, and commercialization. J Med Food, 13(2), 233-246.

Schroter A., Kessner D., Kiselev M.A., Haub T., Dante S., Neubert R.H.H. (2009) Basic Nanostructure of Stratum Corneum Lipid Matrices Based on Ceramides [EOS] and [AP]: A Neutron Diffraction Study. Biophysical Journal. 97: 1104-1114.

Schuhmacher A, Reichling J, Schnitzler P (2003). "Virucidal effect of peppermint oil on the enveloped viruses herpes simplex virus type 1 and type 2 in vitro," Phytomedicine. 10(6-7):504-10.

Selim, S. A., Adam, M. E., Hassan, S. M., & Albalawi, A. R. (2014). Chemical composition, antimicrobial and antibiofilm activity of the essential oil and methanol extract of the Mediterranean cypress (Cupressus sempervirens L.). BMC Complement Altern Med, 14(1), 1-8.

Sell, C. (Ed.). (2006). The Chemistry of Fragrances From Perfumer to Consumer (2nd ed.). Dorchester, UK: The Royal Society of Chemistry.

Senapati S, Banerjee S, Gangopadhyay DN (2008 Sep-Oct). "Evening primrose oil is effective in atopic dermatitis: a randomized placebo-controlled trial," Indian J Dermatol Venereol Leprol. 74(5):447-52.

Senni K, Gueniche F, Foucault-Bertaud A, Igondjo-Tchen S, Fioretti F, Colliec-Jouault S, Durand P, Guezennec J, Godeau G, Letourneur D (2006 Jan 1). "Fucoidan a sulfated polysaccharide from brown algae is a potent modulator of connective tissue proteolysis," Arch Biochem Biophys. 445(1):56-64.

Seol, G. H., Shim, H. S., Kim, P. J., Moon, H. K., Lee, K. H., Shim, I., . . . Min, S. S. (2010 Jul). Antidepressant-like effect of Salvia sclarea is explained by modulation of dopamine activities in rats. J Ethnopharmacol, 130(1), 187-190.

Serafino, A., Sinibaldi Vallebona, P., Andreola, F., Zonfrillo, M., Mercuri, L., Federici, M., . . . Pierimarchi, P. (2008 Apr). Stimulatory effect of eucalyptus essential oil on innate cell-mediated immune response. BMC Immunol, 9, 17.

Shaikh IA, Brown I, Schofield AC, Wahle KW, Heys SD (2008 Nov). "Docosahexaenoic acid enhances the efficacy of docetaxel in prostate cancer cells by modulation of apoptosis: the role of genes associated with the NF-kappaB pathway," Prostate. 68(15):1635-46.

Shaltiel-Karyo, R., Davidi, D., Frenkel-Pinter, M., Ovadia, M., Segal, D., & Gazit, E. (2012 Oct). Differential inhibition of alpha-synuclein oligomeric and fibrillar assembly in parkinson's disease model by cinnamon extract. Biochim Biophys Acta, 1820(10), 1628-1635.

Shankar GM, Li S, Mehta TH, Garcia-Munoz A, Shepardson NE, Smith I, Brett FM, Farrell MA, Rowan MJ, Lemere CA, Regan CM, Walsh DM, Sabatini BL, Selkoe DJ (2008 Jun 22). "Amyloid-protein dimers isolated directly from Alzheimer's brains impair synaptic plasticity and memory," Nat Med. 14(8):837-42.

Shankar S, Ganapathy S, Hingorani SR, Srivastava RK (2008 Jan). "EGCG inhibits growth, invasion, angiogenesis and metastasis of pancreatic cancer," Front Biosci. 13:440-52.

Shapiro S., Guggenheim B. (1995) The action of thymol on oral bacteria. Oral Microbiology and Immunology. 10: 241-246.

Shapiro S, Meier A, Guggenheim B (1994 Aug). "The antimicrobial activity of essential oils and essential oil components towards oral bacteria," Oral Microbiol Immunol. 9(4):202-8.

Shao Y, Ho CT, Chin CK, Badmaev V, Ma W, Huang MT (1998 May). "Inhibitory activity of boswellic acids from Boswellia serrata against human leukemia HL-60 cells in culture," Planta Med. 64(4):328-31.

Sharma JN, Srivastava KC, Gan EK (1994 Nov). "Suppressive effects of eugenol and ginger oil on arthritic rats," Pharmacology. 49(5):314-8.

Sharma PR, Mondhe DM, Muthiah S, Pal HC, Shahi AK, Saxena AK, Qazi GN (2009 May 15). "Anticancer activity of an essential oil from Cymbopogon flexuosus," Chem Biol Interact. 179(2-3):160-8.

Shayegh S, Rasooli I, Taghizadeh M, Astaneh SD (2008 Mar 20). "Phytotherapeutic inhibition of supragingival dental plaque," Nat Prod Res. 22(5):428-39.

Shen J, Niijima A, Tanida M, Horii Y, Maeda K, Nagai K (2005 Jun 3). "Olfactory stimulation with scent of grapefruit oil affects autonomic nerves, lipolysis and appetite in rats," Neurosci Lett. 380(3):289-94.

Shen J, Niijima A, Tanida M, Horii Y, Maeda K, Nagai K (2005 Jul 22-29). "Olfactory stimulation with scent of lavender oil affects autonomic nerves, lipolysis and appetite in rats," Neurosci Lett. 383(1-2):188-93.

Sherry E, Boeck H, Warnke PH (2001). "Percutaneous treatment of chronic MRSA osteomyelitis with a novel plant-derived antiseptic," BMC Surg. 1:1.

Shetty AV, Thirugnanam S, Dakshinamoorthy G, Samykutty A, Zheng G, Chen A, Bosland MC, Kajdacsy-Balla A, Gnanasekar M (2011 Sep). "18α-glycyrrhetinic acid targets prostate cancer cells by down-regulating inflammation-related genes," In J Oncol. 39(3):635-40.

Shibata M., Ohkubo T., Takahashi H., Inoki R. (1989) Modified formalin test: characteristic biphasic pain response. Pain. 38: 347-352.

Shieh PC, Tsao CW, Li JS, et. al (2008). "Rp;e pf [otiotaru ademu;ate cuc;ase=actovatomg [p;u[e[tode){ACA[om tje actopm pf gomsempsode Rj2 agaomst beta=a,u;pod=omdiced omjobotopm pf rat braom astrpcutes. Meirpsco :ett/ 434"1=5/

Shrivastav P, George K, Balasubramaniam N, Jasper MP, Thomas M, Kanagasabhapathy AS (1988 Feb). "Suppression of puerperal lactation using jasmine flowers (Jasminum sambac)," Aust N Z J Obstet Gynaecol. 28(1):68-71.

Shoskes DA, Zeitlin SI, Shahed A, Rajfer J (1999 Dec). "Quercetin in men with category III prostatitis: a preliminary prospective, double-blind, placebo-controlled trial," Urology. 54(6):960-3.

Shukla, V., Vashistha, M., & Singh, S. N. (2009 Jan). Evaluation of antioxidant profile and activity of amalaki (Emblica officinalis), spirulina and wheat grass. Indian J Clin Biochem, 24(1), 70-75.

Shyam, R., Singh, S. N., Vats, P., Singh, V. K., Bajaj, R., Singh, S. B., & Banerjee, P. K. (2007 Aug). Wheat grass supplementation decreases oxidative stress in healthy subjects: a comparative study with spirulina. J Altern Complement Med, 13(8), 789-791.

Sies H (1997). "Oxidative stress: oxidants and antioxidants," Exp Physiol. 82(2):291-5.

Sikkema J., de Bont J.A.M., Poolman B. (1995) Mechanisms of Membrane Toxicity of Hydrocarbons. Microbiological Reviews. 59: 201-222.

Appendix

Modern Essentials Usage Guide

Sikora, E., & Bodziarczyk, I. (2012). Composition and antioxidant activity of kale (Brassica oleracea L. var. acephala) raw and cooked. Acta Sci Pol Technol Aliment, 11(3), 239-248.

Silva Brum L.F., Emanuelli T., Souza D.O., Elisabetsky E. (2001) Effects of Linalool on Glutamate Release and Uptake in Mouse Cortical Synaptosomes. Neurochemical Research. 26: 191-194

Silva Brum L.F., Elisabetsky E., Souza D. (2001) Effects of Linalool on [3H] MK801 and [3H] Muscimol Binding in Mouse Cortical Membranes. Phytotherapy Research. 15: 422-425.

Silva J, Abebe W, Sousa SM, Duarte VG, Machado MI, Matos FJ (2003 Dec). "Analgesic and anti-inflammatory effects of essential oils of Eucalyptus," J Ethnopharmacol. 89(2-3):277-83.

Siméon A, Monier F, Emonard H, Gillery P, Birembaut P, Hornebeck W, Maquart FX (1999 Jun). "Expression and activation of matrix metalloproteinases in wounds: modulation by the tripeptide-copper complex glycyl-L-histidyl-L-lysine-Cu2+," J Invest Dermatol. 112(3):957-64.

Singh, D., Rao, S. M., & Tripathi, A. K. (1984 May). Cedarwood oil as a potential insecticidal agent against mosquitoes. Naturwissenschaften, 71(5), 265-266.

Singh HB, Srivastava M, Singh AB, Srivastava AK (1995 Dec). "Cinnamon bark oil, a potent fungitoxicant against fungi causing respiratory tract mycoses," Allergy. 50(12):995-9.

Singh N, Bhalla M, deJager P, Gilca M (2011). "An overview on ashwagandha: a rasayana (rejuvenator) of ayurveda," Afr J Tradit Complement Altern Med. 8(s):208-13.

Singh RH, Udupa KN (1993). "Clinical and experimental studies on rasayana drugs and rasayana therapy," Special Research Monograph, Central Council for Research in Ayurveda and Siddha (CCRAS), Ministry of Health and Family Welfare, New Delhi.

Singletary K, MacDonald C, Wallig M (1996 Jun 24). "Inhibition by rosemary and carnosol of 7,12-dimethylbenz[a]anthracene (DMBA)-induced rat mammary tumorigenesis and in vivo DMBA-DNA adduct formation," Cancer Lett. 104(1):43-8.

Siu KM, Mak DH, CHiu PY, Poon MK, Du Y, Ko KM "2004). "Pharmacological basis of "Yin-nourishing" and "Yang-invigorating" actions of Cordyceps, a Chinese tonifying herb," Life Sci. 76:385-95.

Siurin SA (1997). "Effects of essential oil on lipid peroxidation and lipid metabolism in patients with chronic bronchitis," Klin Med (Mosk). 75(10):43-5.

Skocibusić M, Bezić N (2004 Dec). "Phytochemical analysis and in vitro antimicrobial activity of two Satureja species essential oils," Phytother Res. 18(12):967-70.

Skold M., Borje A., Matura M., Karlberg A-T. (2002) Studies on the autoxidation and sensitizing capacity of the fragrance chemical linalool, identifying a linalool hydroperoxide. Contact Dermatitis. 46: 267-272.

Skrivanova E, Savka OG, Marounek M (2004). "In vitro effect of C2-C18 fatty acids on Salmonellas," Folia Microbiol (Praha). 49(2):199-202.

Slamenova D, Kuboskova K, Horvathova E, Robichova S. (2002 Mar 28). "Rosemary-stimulated reduction of DNA strand breaks and FPG-sensitive sites in mammalian cells treated with H2O2 or visible light-excited Methylene Blue," Cancer Lett. 177(2):145-53.

Slima, A. B., Ali, M. B., Barkallah, M., Traore, A. I., Boudawara, T., Allouche, N., & Gdoura, R. (2013 Mar). Antioxidant properties of Pelargonium graveolens L'Her essential oil on the reproductive damage induced by deltamethrin in mice as compared to alpha-tocopherol. Lipids Health Dis, 12(1), 30.

Smith DG, Standing L, de Man A (1992 Apr). "Verbal memory elicited by ambient odor," Percept Mot Skills. 74(2):339-43.

Smith-Palmer A, Stewart J, Fyfe L (2004 Oct). "Influence of subinhibitory concentrations of plant essential oils on the production of enterotoxins A and B and alpha-toxin by Staphylococcus aureus," J Med Microbiol. 53(Pt 10):1023-7.

Soares SF, Borges LM, de Sousa Braga R, Ferreira LL, Louly CC, Tresvenzol LM, de Paula JR, Ferri PH (2009 Oct 7). "Repellent activity of plant-derived compounds against Amblyomma cajennense (Acari: Ixodidae) nymphs," Vet Parasitol. Epub ahead of print.

Sorentino S., Landmesser U. (2005) Nonlipid-lowering Effects of Statins. Current Treatment Options to Cardiovascular Medicine. 7: 459-466.

Sriram N, Kalayarasan S, Sudhandiran G (2008 Jul). "Enhancement of antioxidant defense system by epigallocatechin-3-gallate during bleomycin induced experimental Pulmonary Fibrosis," Biol Pharm Bull. 31(7):1306-11.

Stanzl K, Zastrow L, Röding J, Artmann C (1996 Jun). "The effectiveness of molecular oxygen in cosmetic formulations," Int J Cosmet Sci. 18(3):137-50.

Steiner M, Priel I, Giat J, Levy J, Sharoni Y, Danilenko M (2001). "Carnosic acid inhibits proliferation and augments differentiation of human leukemic cells induced by 1,25-dihydroxyvitamin D3 and retinoic acid," Nutr Cancer. 41(1-2):135-44.

Strati A, Papoutsi Z, Lianidou E, Moutsatsou P (2009 Sep). "Effect of ellagic acid on the expression of human telomerase reverse transcriptase (hTERT) alpha+Beta+ transcript in estrogen receptor-positive MCF-7 breast cancer cells," Clin Biochem. 42(13-14):1358-62.

Stratton S.P., Alberts D.S., Einspahr J.G. (2010) A Phase 2a Study of Topical Perillyl Alcohol Cream for Chemoprevention of Skin Cancer. Cancer Prevention Research. 3: 160-169.

Stratton S.P., Saboda K.L., Myrdal P.B., Gupta A., McKenzie N.E., Brooks C., Salasche S.J., Warneke J.A., Ranger-Moore J., Bozzo P.D., Blanchard J., Einspahr J.G. (2008) Phase 1 Study of Topical Perillyl Alcohol Cream for Chemoprevention of Skin Cancer. Nutrition and Cancer. 60: 325-330.

Su KP, Huang SY, Chiu TH, Huang KC, Huang CL, Chang HC, Pariante CM (2008 Apr). "Omega-3 fatty acids for major depressive disorder during pregnancy: results from a randomized, double-blind, placebo-controlled trial," J Clin Psychiatry. 69(4):644-51.

Subash Babu P, Prabuseenivasan S, Ignacimuthu S. (2007 Jan). "Cinnamaldehyde--a potential antidiabetic agent," Phytomedicine.14(1):15-22.

Südhof TC (1995 Jun 22). "The synaptic vesicle cycle: a cascade of protein-protein interactions," Nature. 375(6533):645-53.

Suneetha, W. J., & Krishnakantha, T. P. (2005 May). Cardamom extract as inhibitor of human platelet aggregation. Phytother Res, 19(5), 437-440.

Tabanca, N., Wang, M., Avonto, C., Chittiboyina, A. G., Parcher, J. F., Carroll, J. F., . . . Khan, I. A. (2013 May). Bioactivity-guided investigation of geranium essential oils as natural tick repellents. J Agric Food Chem, 61(17), 4101-4107.

Taherian, A. A., Vafaei, A. A., & Ameri, J. (2012 Apr). Opiate System Mediate the Antinociceptive Effects of Coriandrum sativum in Mice. Iran J Pharm Res, 11(2), 679-688.

Takahashi, N., Yao, L., Kim, M., Sasako, H., Aoyagi, M., Shono, J., . . . Kawada, T. (2013 Jul). Dill seed extract improves abnormalities in lipid metabolism through peroxisome proliferator-activated receptor-alpha (PPAR-alpha) activation in diabetic obese mice. Mol Nutr Food Res, 57(7), 1295-1299.

Takaki I, Bersani-Amado LE, Vendruscolo A, Sartoretto SM, Diniz SP, Bersani-Amado CA, Cuman RK (2008 Dec). "Anti-inflammatory and antinociceptive effects of Rosmarinus officinalis L. essential oil in experimental animal models," J Med Food. 11(4):741-6.

Takarada K, Kimizuka R, Takahashi N, Honma K, Okuda K, Kato T (2004 Feb). "A comparison of the antibacterial efficacies of essential oils against oral pathogens," Oral Microbiol Immunol. 19(1):61-4.

Tan P, Zhong W, Cai W (2000 Sep). "Clinical study on treatment of 40 cases of malignant brain tumor by elemene emulsion injection," Zhongguo Zhong Xi Yi Jie He Za Zhi. 20(9):645-8.

Tang J, Wingerchuk DM, Crum BA, Rubin DI, Demaerschalk BM (2007 May). "Alpha-lipoic acid may improve symptomatic diabetic polyneuropathy," Neurologist. 12(3):164-7.

Tanida M, Niijima A, Shen J, Nakamura T, Nagai K (2005 Oct 5). "Olfactory stimulation with scent of essential oil of grapefruit affects autonomic neurotransmission and blood pressure," Brain Res. 1058(1-2):44-55.

Tanida M, Niijima A, Shen J, Nakamura T, Nagai K (2006 May 1). "Olfactory stimulation with scent of lavender oil affects autonomic neurotransmission and blood pressure in rats," Neurosci Lett. 398(1-2):155-60.

Tantaoui-Elaraki A, Beraoud L (1994). "Inhibition of growth and aflatoxin production in Aspergillus parasiticus by essential oils of selected plant materials," J Environ Pathol Toxicol Oncol. 13(1):67-72.

Tao L, Zhou L, Zheng L, Yao M (2006 Jul). "Elemene displays anti-cancer ability on laryngeal cancer cells in vitro and in vivo," Cancer Chemother Pharmacol. 58(1):24-34.

Tare V, Deshpande S, Sharma RN (2004 Oct). "Susceptibility of two different strains of Aedes aegypti (Diptera: Culicidae) to plant oils," J Econ Entomol. 97(5):1734-6.

Tavares AC, Gonçalves MJ, Cavaleiro C, Cruz MT, Lopes MC, Canhoto J, Salgueiro LR (2008 Sep 2). "Essential oil of Daucus carota subsp. halophilus: composition, antifungal activity and cytotoxicity," J Ethnopharmacol. 119(1):129-34.

Tayarani-Najaran, Z., Talasaz-Firoozi, E., Nasiri, R., Jalali, N., & Hassanzadeh, M. (2013 Jan). Antiemetic activity of volatile oil from Mentha spicata and Mentha x piperita in chemotherapy-induced nausea and vomiting. Ecancermedicalscience, 7, 1-6.

Terzi V, Morcia C, Faccioli P, Vale G, Tacconi G, Malnati M (2007 Jun). "In vitro antifungal activity of the tea tree (Melaleuca alternifolia) essential oil and its major components against plant pathogens," Lett Appl Microbiol. 44(6):613-8.

Thavara U, Tawatsin A, Bhakdeenuan P, Wongsinkongman P, Boonruad T, Bansiddhi J, Chavalittumrong P, Komalamisra N, Siriyasatien P, Mulla MS (2007 Jul). "Repellent activity of essential oils against cockroaches (Dictyoptera: Blattidae, Blattellidae, and Blaberidae) in Thailand," Southeast Asian J Trop Med Public Health. 38(4):663-73.

Thompson, J. D., Chalchat, J. C., Michet, A., Linhart, Y. B., & Ehlers, B. (2003). Qualitative and quantitative variation in monoterpene co-occurrence and composition in the essential oil of Thymus vulgaris chemotypes. Journal of Chemical Ecology, 29(4), 873.

Thukham-Mee, W., & Wattanathorn, J. (2012). Evaluation of Safety and Protective Effect of Combined Extract of Cissampelos pareira and Anethum graveolens (PM52) against Age-Related Cognitive Impairment. Evid Based Complement Alternat Med, 2012, 1-10.

Tiano L, Belardinelli R, Carnevali P, Principi F, Seddaiu G, Littarru GP (2007 Sep). "Effect of coenzyme Q10 administration on endothelial function and extracellular superoxide dismutase in patients with ischaemic heart disease: a double-blind, randomized controlled study," Eur Heart J. 28(18):2249-55.

Tildesley NT, Kennedy DO, Perry EK, Ballard CG, Wesnes KA, Scholey AB (2005 Jan 17). "Positive modulation of mood and cognitive performance following administration of acute doses of Salvia lavandulaefolia essential oil to healthy young volunteers," Physiol Behav. 83(5):699-709.

Tipton DA, Hamman NR, Dabbous MKh (2006 Mar). "Effect of myrrh oil on IL-1beta stimulation of NF-kappaB activation and PGE(2) production in human gingival fibroblasts and epithelial cells," Toxicol In Vitro. 20(2):248-55.

Tipton DA, Lyle B, Babich H, Dabbous MKh (2003 Jun). "In vitro cytotoxic and anti-inflammatory effects of myrrh oil on human gingival fibroblasts and epithelial cells," Toxicol In Vitro. 17(3):301-10.

Tisserand, R. & Young, R. (2014). Essential oil safety a guide for health care professionals (2nd ed.). China: Churchill Livingstone Elsevier.

Tognolini M, Ballabeni V, Bertoni S, Bruni R, Impicciatore M, Barocelli E (2007 Sep). "Protective effect of Foeniculum vulgare essential oil and anethole in an experimental model of thrombosis," Pharmacol Res. 56(3):254-60.

Tortora G.J., Funke B.R., Case C.L. Microbiology: An Introduction. 9th ed. San Francisco: Pearson Benjamin Cummings, 2007.

Traka M, Gasper AV, Melchini A, Bacon JR, Needs PW, Frost V, Chantry A, Jones AM, Ortori CA, Barrett DA, Ball RY, Mills RD, Mithen RF (2008 Jul 2). "Broccoli consumption interacts with GSTM1 to perturb oncogenic signalling pathways in the prostate," PLoS One. 3(7):e2568.

Tran KT, Griffith L, Wells A (2004 May-Jun). "palmitoyl-glycyl-histidyl-lysine," Wound Repair Regen. 12(3):262-8.

Trautmann M, Peskar BM, Peskar BA (1991 Aug 16). "Aspirin-like drugs, ethanol-induced rat gastric injury and mucosal eicosanoid release," Eur J Pharmacol. 201(1):53-8.

Trigg JK (1996 Jun). "Evaluation of a eucalyptus-based repellent against Anopheles spp. in Tanzania," J Am Mosq Control Assoc. 12(2 Pt 1):243-6.

Tripathi, P., Tripathi, R., Patel, R. K., & Pancholi, S. S. (2013 Jan). Investigation of antimutagenic potential of Foeniculum vulgare essential oil on cyclophosphamide induced genotoxicity and oxidative stress in mice. Drug Chem Toxicol, 36(1), 35-41.

Trongtokit Y, Rongsriyam Y, Komalamisra N, Apiwathnasorn C (2005 Apr). "Comparative repellency of 38 essential oils against mosquito bites," Phytother Res. 19(4):303-9.

Trovato, A., Taviano, M. F., Pergolizzi, S., Campolo, L., De Pasquale, R., & Miceli, N. (2010 Apr). Citrus bergamia Risso & Poiteau juice protects against renal injury of diet-induced hypercholesterolemia in rats. Phytother Res, 24(4), 514-519.

Truan JS, Chen JM, Thompson LU (2012). "Comparative effects of sesame seed lignan and flaxseed lignan in reducing the growth of human breast tumors (MCF-7) at high levels of circulating estrogen in athymic mice," Nutr Cancer. 64(1):65-71.

Tsiri, D., Graikou, K., Poblocka-Olech, L., Krauze-Baranowska, M., Spyropoulos, C., & Chinou, I. (2009 Nov). Chemosystematic value of the essential oil composition of Thuja species cultivated in Poland-antimicrobial activity. Molecules, 14(11), 4707-4715.

Tso MOM, Lam TT (1994 Oct 27). "Method of retarding and ameliorating central nervous system and eye damage," University of Illinois: USPatent #5527533.

Tumen, I., Suntar, I., Eller, F. J., Keles, H., & Akkol, E. K. (2013 Jan). Topical wound-healing effects and phytochemical composition of heartwood essential oils of Juniperus virginiana L., Juniperus occidentalis Hook., and Juniperus ashei J. Buchholz. J Med Food, 16(1), 48-55.

Turley, S.M. (2009). Understanding pharmacology for health professionals (4th ed.). Prentice Hall.

Turrens J.F. (2003) Mitochondrial formation of reactive oxygen species. Journal of Physiology.552: 335-344.

Tuzcu M, Sahin N, Karatepe M, Cikim G, Kilinc U, Sahin K (2008 Sep). "Epigallocatechin-3-gallate supplementation can improve antioxidant status in stressed quail," Br Poult Sci. 49(5):643-8.

Tyagi, A., & Malik, A. (2010). Antimicrobial action of essential oil vapours and negative air ions against Pseudomonas fluorescens. Int J Food Microbiol, 143(3), 205-210.

Tyagi, A. K., & Malik, A. (2012). Bactericidal action of lemon grass oil vapors and negative air ions. Innovative Food Science & Emerging Technologies, 13(0), 169-177.

Ueno-Iio, T., Shibakura, M., Yokota, K., Aoe, M., Hyoda, T., Shinohata, R., . . . Kataoka, M. (2014 Jun). Lavender essential oil inhalation suppresses allergic airway inflammation and mucous cell hyperplasia in a murine model of asthma. Life Sci.

Ulusoy S, Boşgelmez-Tinaz G, Seçilmiş-Canbay H (2009 Nov). "Tocopherol, carotene, phenolic contents and antibacterial properties of rose essential oil, hydrosol and absolute," Curr Microbiol. 59(5):554-8.

Umezu T (2000 Jun). "Behavioral effects of plant-derived essential oils in the geller type conflict test in mice," Jpn J Pharmacol. 83(2):150-3.

Umezu T (1999 Sep). "Anticonflict effects of plant-derived essential oils," Pharmacol Biochem Behav. 64(1):35-40.

Umezu T, Ito H, Nagano K, Yamakoshi M, Oouchi H, Sakaniwa M, Morita M (2002 Nov 22). "Anticonflict effects of rose oil and identification of its active constituents," Life Sci. 72(1):91-102.

Uribe S., Ramírez J., Pena A. (1985) Effects of β-Pinene on Yeast Membrane Functions. Journal of Bacteriology. 161: 1195-1200.

Urso, M. L., & Clarkson, P. M. (2003). Oxidative stress, exercise, and antioxidant supplementation. Toxicology, 189(1), 41-54.

Vallianou, I., Peroulis, N., Pantazis, P., & Hadzopoulou-Cladaras, M. (2011 Nov). Camphene, a plant-derived monoterpene, reduces plasma cholesterol and triglycerides in hyperlipidemic rats independently of HMG-CoA reductase activity. PLoS ONE, 6(11), e20516.

van Poppel G, Verhoeven DT, Verhagen H, Goldbohm RA (1999). "Brassica vegetables and cancer prevention. Epidemiology and mechanisms," Adv Exp Med Biol. 472:159-68.

van Tol RW, Swarts HJ, van der Linden A, Visser JH (2007 May). "Repellence of the red bud borer Resseliella oculiperda from grafted apple trees by impregnation of rubber budding strips with essential oils," Pest Manag Sci. 63(5):483-90.

Varga J, Jimenez SA (1986 Jul 31). "Stimulation of normal human fibroblast collagen production and processing by transforming growth factor-beta," Biochem Biophys Res Commun. 138(2):974-80.

Vazquez JA, Arganoza MT, Boikov D, Akins RA, Vaishampayan JK (2000 Jun). "In vitro susceptibilities of Candida and Aspergillus species to Melaleuca alternafolia (tea tree) oil," Rev Iberoam Micol. 17(2):60-3.

Modern Essentials Usage Guide

Velaga, M. K., Yallapragada, P. R., Williams, D., Rajanna, S., & Bettaiya, R. (2014 Jun). Hydroalcoholic Seed Extract of Coriandrum sativum (Coriander) Alleviates Lead-Induced Oxidative Stress in Different Regions of Rat Brain. Biol Trace Elem Res, 159(1-3), 351-363.

Venegas C, Cabrera-Vique C, Garcia-Corzo L, Escames G, Acuna-Castroviejo D, Lopez LC (2011 Nov). "Determination of coenzyme Q10, coenzyme Q9, and melatonin contents in virgin argan oils: comparison with other edible vegetable oils," J Agric Food Chem. 59(22):12102-8.

Veratti E, Rossi T, Giudice S, Benassi L, Bertazzoni G, Morini D, Azzoni P, Bruni E, Giannnetti A, MaqnoniC. (2011 Jun). "18beta-glycyrrhetinic acid and glabridin prevent oxidative DNA fragmentation in UVB-irradiated human keratinocyte cultures," Anticancer Res. 31(6):2209-15.

Verma, S. K., Jain, V., & Katewa, S. S. (2009 Dec). Blood pressure lowering, fibrinolysis enhancing and antioxidant activities of cardamom (Elettaria cardamomum). Indian J Biochem Biophys, 46(6), 503-506.

Vertuani S, Angusti A, Manfredini S (2004). "The antioxidants and pro-antioxidants network: an overview," Curr Pharm Des. 10(14):1677–94.

Vigo E, Cepeda A, Gualillo O, Perez-Fernandez R (2005 Mar). "In-vitro anti-inflammatory activity of Pinus sylvestris and Plantago lanceolata extracts: effect on inducible NOS, COX-1, COX-2 and their products in J774A.1 murine macrophages," J Pharm Pharmacol. 57(3):383-91.

Vigo E, Cepeda A, Gualillo O, Perez-Fernandez R (2004 Feb). "In-vitro anti-inflammatory effect of Eucalyptus globulus and Thymus vulgaris: nitric oxide inhibition in J774A.1 murine macrophages," J Pharm Pharmacol. 56(2):257-63.

Vigushin DM, Poon GK, Boddy A, English J, Halbert GW, Pagonis C, Jarman M, Coombes RC (1998). "Phase I and pharmacokinetic study of D-limonene in patients with advanced cancer. Cancer Research Campaign Phase I/II Clinical Trials Committee," Cancer Chemother Pharmacol. 42(2):111-7.

Vujosević M, Blagojević J (2004). "Antimutagenic effects of extracts from sage (Salvia officinalis) in mammalian system in vivo," Acta Vet Hung. 52(4):439-43.

Vuković-Gačić B, Nikcević S, Berić-Bjedov T, Knezević-Vukcević J, Simić D (2006 Oct). "Antimutagenic effect of essential oil of sage (Salvia officinalis L.) and its monoterpenes against UV-induced mutations in Escherichia coli and Saccharomyces cerevisiae," Food Chem Toxicol. 44(10):1730-8.

Vutyavanich T, Kraisarin T, Ruangsri R (2001 Apr). "Ginger for nausea and vomiting in pregnancy: randomized, double-masked, placebo-controlled trial," Obstet Gynecol. 97(4):577-82.

Walker AF, Bundy R, Hicks SM, Middleton RW (2002 Dec). "Bromelain reduces mild acute knee pain and improves well-being in a dose-dependent fashion in an open study of otherwise healthy adults," Phytomedicine. 9(8):681-6.

Walker TB, Smith J, Herrera M, Lebegue B, Pinchak A, Fischer J (2010 Oct). "The influence of 8 weeks of whey-protein and leucine supplementation on physical and cognitive performance," Int J Sport Nutr Exerc Metab. 20(5):409-17.

Wallerius S, Rosmond R, Ljung T, Holm G, Björntorp P (2003 Jul). "Rise in morning saliva cortisol is associated with abdominal obesity in men: a preliminary report," J Endocrinol Invest. 26(7):616-9. Walter BM, Bilkei G (2004 Mar 15). "Immunostimulatory effect of dietary oregano etheric oils on lymphocytes from growth-retarded, low-weight growing-finishing pigs and productivity," Tijdschr Diergeneeskd. 129(6):178-81.

Wang, K., & Su, C. Y. (2000 Oct). Pharmacokinetics and disposition of beta-elemene in rats. Yao Xue Xue Bao, 35(10), 725-728.

Wang, L., Li, W. G., Huang, C., Zhu, M. X., Xu, T. L., Wu, D. Z., & Li, Y. (2012 Nov). Subunit-specific inhibition of glycine receptors by curcumol. J Pharmacol Exp Ther, 343(2), 371-379.

Wang, W., Zu, Y., Fu, Y., Reichling, J., Suschke, U., Nokemper, S., & Zhang, Y. (2009 Feb). In vitro antioxidant, antimicrobial and anti-herpes simplex virus type 1 activity of Phellodendron amurense Rupr. from China. Am J Chin Med, 37(1), 195-203.

Warskulat U, Brookmann S, Felsner I, Brenden H, Grether-Beck S, Haussinger D (2008 Dec). "Ultraviolet A induces transport of compatible organic osmolytes in human derman fibroblasts," Exp Dermatol. 17(12):1031-6.

Warskulat U, Reinen A, Grether-Beck S, Krutmann J, Haussinger D (2004Sep). "The osmolyte strategy of normal human keratinocyts in maintaining cell homeostasis," J Invest Dermatol. 123(3):516-21.

Watanabe, S., Hara, K., Ohta, K., Iino, H., Miyajima, M., Matsuda, A., . . . Matsushima, E. (2013 Jan). Aroma helps to preserve information processing resources of the brain in healthy subjects but not in temporal lobe epilepsy. Seizure, 22(1), 59-63.

Weaver CM, Martin BR, Jackson GS, McCabe GP, Nolan JR, McCabe LD, Barnes S, Reinwald S, Boris ME, Peacock M (2009 Oct). "Antiresorptive effects of phytoestrogen supplements compared with estradiol or risedronate in postmenopausal women using (41)Ca methodology," J Clin Endocrinol Metab. 94(10):3798-805.

Weaver R.F. Molecular Biology. 4th ed. New York: McGraw Hill, 2008.

Wee, JJ, Park, KM, Chug A (2011). "Biological Activities of Ginseng and Its Application to Human Health," *Herbal Medicine: Biomolecular and Clinical Aspects*. 2nd ed.

Wei A, Shibamoto T (2007). "Antioxidant activities of essential oil mixtures toward skin lipid squalene oxidized by UV irradiation," Cutan Ocul Toxicol. 26(3):227-33.

Wiig, H., & Swartz, M. A. (2012). Interstitial fluid and lymph formation and transport: physiological regulation and roles in inflammation and cancer. Physiological Reviews, 92(3), 1005-1060.

Wilkinson JM, Hipwell M, Ryan T, Cavanagh HM (2003 Jan 1). "Bioactivity of Backhousia citriodora: antibacterial and antifungal activity," J Agric Food Chem. 51(1):76-81.

Wilkinson S, Aldridge J, Salmon I, Cain E, Wilson B (1999 Sep). "An evaluation of aromatherapy massage in palliative care," Palliat Med. 13(5):409-17.

Wilkinson, S. M., Love, S. B., Westcombe, A. M., Gambles, M. A., Burgess, C. C., Cargill, A., . . . Ramirez, A. J. (2007 Feb). Effectiveness of aromatherapy massage in the management of anxiety and depression in patients with cancer: a multicenter randomized controlled trial. Journal of Clinical Oncology, 25(5), 532-539.

Williamson EM, Priestley CM, Burgess IF (2007 Dec). "An investigation and comparison of the bioactivity of selected essential oils on human lice and house dust mites," Fitoterapia. 78(7-8):521-5.

Winkler-Stuck K, Wiedemann FR, Wallesch CW, Kunz WS (2004 May 15). "Effect of coenzyme Q10 on the mitochondrial function of skin fibroblasts from Parkinson patients," J Neurol Sci. 220(1-2):41-8.

Woodruff J (2002 Mar). "Improving Hair Strength," Cosm Toil. :33-5.

Xia L, Chen D, Han R, Fang Q, Waxman S, Jing Y (2005 Mar). "Boswellic acid acetate induces apoptosis through caspase-mediated pathways in myeloid leukemia cells," Mol Cancer Ther. 4(3):381-8.

Xiao D, Powolny AA, Barbi de Moura M, Kelley EE, Bommareddy A, Kim SH, Hahm ER, Normolle D, Van Houten B, Singh SV (2010 Jun 22). "Phenethyl isothiocyanate inhibits oxidative phosphorylation to trigger reactive oxygen species-mediated death of human prostate cancer cells," J Biol Chem Epub ahead of print. Epub ahead of print.

Xiufen W, Hiramatsu N, Matsubara M (2004). "The antioxidative activity of traditional Japanese herbs," Biofactors. 21(1-4):281-4.

Xu, J., Guo, Y., Zhao, P., Xie, C., Jin, D. Q., Hou, W., & Zhang, T. (2011 Dec). Neuroprotective cadinane sesquiterpenes from the resinous exudates of Commiphora myrrha. Fitoterapia, 82(8), 1198-1201.

Xu J., Zhou F., Ji B-P., Pei R-S., Xu N. (2008) The antibacterial mechanism of carvacrol and thymol against Escherichia coli. Letters in Applied Microbiology. 47: 174-179.

Xu X, Duncan AM, Merz BE, Kurzer MS (1998 Dec). "Effects of soy isoflavones on estrogen and phytoestrogen metabolism in premenopausal women," Cancer Epidemiol Biomarkers Prev. 7(12):1101-8.

Xu X, Duncan AM, Wangen KE, Kurzer MS (2000 Aug). "Soy consumption alters endogenous estrogen metabolism in postmenopausal women," Cancer Epidemiol biomarkers Prev. 9(8):781-6.

Yamada, K., Mimaki, Y., & Sashida, Y. (2005 Feb). Effects of inhaling the vapor of Lavandula burnatii super-derived essential oil and linalool on plasma adrenocorticotropic hormone (ACTH), catecholamine and gonadotropin levels in experimental menopausal female rats. Biol Pharm Bull, 28(2), 378-379.

Yan, H., Sun, X., Sun, S., Wang, S., Zhang, J., Wang, R., . . . Kang, W. (2011 Jun). Anti-ultraviolet radiation effects of Coptis chinensis and Phellodendron amurense glycans by immunomodulating and inhibiting oxidative injury. Int J Biol Macromol, 48(5), 720-725.

Yang F. et al. (2005 Feb 18). "Curcumin inhibits formation of amyloid beta oligomers and fibrils, binds plaques, and reduces amyloid in vivo," J Biol Chem. 280(7):5892-901.

Yang GY, Wang W (1994 Sep). "Clinical studies on the treatment of coronary heart disease with Valeriana officinalis var latifolia," Zhongguo Zhong Xi Yi Jie He Za Zhi. 14(9):540-2.

Yang L, Hao J, Zhang J (2009). "Ginsenoside Rg3 promotes beta-amyloid peptide degradation by enhancing gene expression of neprilysin," J Pharm Pharmacol. 61:375-80.

Yang SA, Jeon SK, Lee EJ, Im NK, Jhee KH, Lee SP, Lee IS (2009 May). "Radical Scavenging Activity of the Essential Oil of Silver Fir (Abies alba)," J Clin Biochem Nutr. 44(3):253-9.

Yap, P. S., Krishnan, T., Yiap, B. C., Hu, C. P., Chan, K. G., & Lim, S. H. (2014 May). Membrane disruption and anti-quorum sensing effects of synergistic interaction between Lavandula angustifolia (lavender oil) in combination with antibiotic against plasmid-conferred multi-drug-resistant Escherichia coli. J Appl Microbiol, 116(5), 1119-1128.

Yavari Kia, P., Safajou, F., Shahnazi, M., & Nazemiyeh, H. (2014 Mar). The effect of lemon inhalation aromatherapy on nausea and vomiting of pregnancy: a double-blinded, randomized, controlled clinical trial. Iran Red Crescent Med J, 16(3).

Yazdanparast R, Shahriyari L (2008 Jan). "Comparative effects of Artemisia dracunculus, Satureja hortensis and Origanum majorana on inhibition of blood platelet adhesion, aggregation and secretion," Vascul Pharmacol. 48:1):32-7.

Yip YB, Tam AC. (2008 Jun). "An experimental study on the effectiveness of massage with aromatic ginger and orange essential oil for moderate-to-severe knee pain among the elderly in Hong Kong," Complement Ther Med. 16(3):131-8.

Yoo, C. B., Han, K. T., Cho, K. S., Ha, J., Park, H. J., Nam, J. H., . . . Lee, K. T. (2005 Jul). Eugenol isolated from the essential oil of Eugenia caryophyllata induces a reactive oxygen species-mediated apoptosis in HL-60 human promyelocytic leukemia cells. Cancer Lett, 225(1), 41-52.

Youdim KA, Deans SG (1999 Sep 8). "Dietary supplementation of thyme (Thymus vulgaris L.) essential oil during the lifetime of the rat: its effects on the antioxidant status in liver, kidney and heart tissues," Mech Ageing Dev. 109(3):163-75.

Youdim KA, Deans SG (2000 Jan). "Effect of thyme oil and thymol dietary supplementation on the antioxidant status and fatty acid composition of the ageing rat brain," Br J Nutr. 83(1):87-93.

Youn L.J., Yoon J.W., Hovde C.J. (2010) A Brief Overview of Escherichia coli O157:H7 and Its Plasmid O157. Journal of Microbiology and Biotechnology. 20: 1-10.

Younis F, Mirelman D, Rabinkov A, Rosenthal T (2010 Jun). "S-allyl-mercapto-captopril: a novel compound in the treatment of Cohen-Rosenthal diabetic hypertensive rats," J Clin Hypertens (Greenwich) 12(6):451-5.

Yu B.P. (1994) Cellular Defenses Against Damage From Reactive Oxygen Species. Physiological Reviews. 74: 139-162.

Yu YM, Chang WC, Wu CH, Chiang SY (2005 Nov). "Reduction of oxidative stress and apoptosis in hyperlipidemic rabbits by ellagic acid," J Nutr Biochem. 16(11):675-81.

Yu Z, Wang R, Xu L, Xie S, Dong J, Jing Y (2011 Jan 25). "β-Elemene piperazine derivatives induce apoptosis in human leukemia cells through downregulation of c-FLIP and generation of ROS," PLos One 6(1)e15843.

Yuan HQ, Kong F, Wang XL, Young CY, Hu XY, Lou HX (2008 Jun 1). "Inhibitory effect of acetyl-11-keto-beta-boswellic acid on androgen receptor by interference of Sp1 binding activity in prostate cancer cells," Biochem Pharmacol. 75(11):2112-21.

Yuan YV, Walsh NA (2006 Jul). "Antioxidant and antiproliferative activities of extracts from a variety of edible seaweeds," Food Chem Toxicol. 44(7):1144-50.

Yüce, A., Turk, G., Ceribasi, S., Guvenc, M., Ciftci, M., Sonmez, M., . . . Aksakal, M. (2014 Apr). Effectiveness of cinnamon (Cinnamomum zeylanicum) bark oil in the prevention of carbon tetrachloride-induced damages on the male reproductive system. Andrologia, 46(3), 263-272.

Yun, J. (2014 Jan). Limonene inhibits methamphetamine-induced locomotor activity via regulation of 5-HT neuronal function and dopamine release. Phytomedicine. Retrieved from http://dx.doi.org/10.1016/j.phymed.2013.12.004

Zembron-Lacny A, Szyszka K, Szygula Z (2007 Dec). "Effect of cysteine derivatives administration in healthy men exposed to intense resistance exercise by evaluation of pro-antioxidant ratio," J Physiol Sci. 57(6):343-8.

Zha C., Brown G.B., Brouillette W.J. (2004) Synthesis and Structure-Activity Relationship Studies for Hydantoins and Analogues as Voltage-Gasted Sodium Channel Ligands. Journal of Medicinal Chemistry. 47: 6519-6528.

Zhang, J., Kang, M. J., Kim, M. J., Kim, M. E., Song, J. H., Lee, Y. M., & Kim, J. I. (2008 Jan). Pancreatic lipase inhibitory activity of taraxacum officinale in vitro and in vivo. Nutr Res Pract, 2(4), 200-203.

Zhang, R., Wang, B., Zhao, H., Wei, C., Yuan, G., & Guo, R. (2009). Tissue distribution of curcumol in rats after intravenous injection of zedoary turmeric oil fat emulsion. Asian Journal of Pharmacodynamics and Pharmacokinetics, 1608, 51-57.

Zhang W, Wang X, Liu Y, Tian H, Flickinger B, Empie MW, Sun SZ (2008 Jun). "Dietary flaxseed lignan extract lowers plasma cholesterol and glucose concentrations in hypercholesterolaemic subjects," Br J Nutr. 99(6):1301-9.

Zhang X, Zhang Y, Li Y (2013 Aug). "Beta element decreases cell invasion by upregulating E-cadherin expression in MCF-7 human breast cancer cells," Oncol Rep. 30(2):745-50.

Zhang Z, Li Y, Zhang Y, Song J, Wang Q, Zheng L, Liu D. (2013). "Beta-element blocks epithelial mesenchymal transition in human breast cancer cell line MCF-7 through Smad3-mediated down-regulation of nuclear transcription factors," PLoS One 8(3):e58719.

Zhang, Z., Liu, X., Zhang, X., Liu, J., Hao, Y., Yang, X., & Wang, Y. (2011 May). Comparative evaluation of the antioxidant effects of the natural vitamin C analog 2-O-beta-D-glucopyranosyl-L-ascorbic acid isolated from Goji berry fruit. Arch Pharm Res, 34(5), 801-810.

Zhao W, Entschladen F, Liu H, Niggemann B, Fang Q, Zaenker KS, Han R (2003). "Boswellic acid acetate induces differentiation and apoptosis in highly metastatic melanoma and fibrosarcoma cells," Cancer Detect Prev. 27(1):67-75.

Zheng GQ, Kenney PM, Lam LK. (1992 Aug). "Anethofuran, carvone, and limonene: potential cancer chemopreventive agents from dill weed oil and caraway oil," Planta Med. 58(4):338-41.

Zheng GQ, Kenney PM, Zhang J, Lam LK (1993). "Chemoprevention of benzo[a]pyrene-induced forestomach cancer in mice by natural phthalides from celery seed oil," Nutr Cancer. 19(1):77-86.

Zhou BR, Luo D, Wei FD, Chen XE, Gao J (2008 Jul). "Baicalin protects human fibroblasts against ultraviolet B-induced cyclobutane pyrimidine dimers formation," Arch Dermatol Res. 300(6):331-4.

Zhou, J., Tang F., Bian R. (2004) Effect of α-pinene on nuclear translocation of NF-ϰB in THP-1 cells. Acta Pharmacol Sin. 25: 480-484.

Zhou J, Zhou S, Tang J, Zhang K, Guang L, Huang Y, Xu Y, Ying Y, Zhang L, Li D (2009 Mar 15). "Protective effect of berberine on beta cells in streptozotocin-and high-carbohydrate/high-fat diet-induced diabetic rats," Eur J Pharmacol. 606(1-3):262-8.

Zhou, X. M., Zhao, Y., He, C. C., & Li, J. X. (2012 Feb). Preventive effects of Citrus reticulata essential oil on bleomycin-induced pulmonary fibrosis in rats and the mechanism. Zhong Xi Yi Jie He Xue Bao, 10(2), 200-209.

Zhu BC, Henderson G, Chen F, Fei H, Laine RA (2001 Aug). "Evaluation of vetiver oil and seven insect-active essential oils against the Formosan subterranean termite," J Chem Ecol. 27(8):1617-25.

Zhu BC, Henderson G, Yu Y, Laine RA (2003 Jul 30). "Toxicity and repellency of patchouli oil and patchouli alcohol against Formosan subterranean termites Coptotermes formosanus Shiraki (Isoptera: Rhinotermitidae)," J Agric Food Chem. 51(16):4585-8

Zhu JS, Halpern GM, Jones K (1998). "The scientific rediscovery of a precious ancient Chinese herbal regimen: Cordyceps sinensis. Part I," J Altern Complement Med. 4:289-303.

Ziegler D, Ametov A, Barinov A, Dyck PJ, Gurieva I, Low PA, Munzel U, Yakhno N, Raz I, Novosadova M, Maus J, Samigullin R (2006 Nov). "Oral treatment with alpha-lipoic acid improves symptomatic diabetic polyneuropathy: the SYDNEY 2 trial," Diabetes Care. 29(11):2365-70.
Ziegler G, Ploch M, Miettinen-Baumann A, Collet W (2002 Nov 25). "Efficacy and tolerability of valerian extract LI 156 compared with oxazepam in the treatment of non-organic insomnia--a randomized, double-blind, comparative clinical study," Eur J Med Res. 7(11):480-6.
Zore G.B., Thakre A.D., Jadhav S., Karuppayil S.M. (2011) Terpenoids inhibit Candida albicans growth by affecting membrane integrity and arrest of cell cycle. Phytomedicine. doi: 10.1016/j.phymed.2011.03.008.
Zou B, Li QQ, Zhao J, Li JM, Cuff CF, Reed E (2013 Mar). "Beta-Elemene and taxanes synergistically induce cytotoxicity and inhibit proliferation in ovarian cancer and other tumor cells," Anticancer Res. 33(3):929-40.

Bibliography

Balch, M.D., James, and Phyllis Balch, C.N.C. *Prescription for Nutritional Healing.* Garden City Park, NY: Avery Publishing Group, 1990.
Başer, Kemal Hüsnü Can & Gerhard Buchbauer. *Handbook of Essential Oils: Science, Technology, and Applications.* Florida: CRC Press, 2010. Print.
Becker, M.D., Robert O. *The Body Electric.* New York, NY: Wm. Morrow, 1985.
Brown T.L., LeMay H.E., Bursten B.E. *Chemistry: The Central Science. 10th ed.* Upper Saddle River: Pearson Prentice Hall, 2006.
Burroughs, Stanley. *Healing for the Age of Enlightenment.* Auburn, CA: Burroughs Books, 1993.
Burton Goldberg Group, The. *Alternative Medicine: The Definitive Guide.* Fife, WA: Future Medicine Publishing, Inc., 1994.
Can Baser, K Husnu, Buchbauer, Gerhard. Handbood of Essential Oils: Science Technology, and Applications. Boca Raton, FL: Taylor & Francis Group, 2010.
Carter, Howard. *The Tomb of Tutankhamen.* Washington, D.C.: National Geographic Society, 2003. Print.
Cowan M.K., Talaro K.P. *Microbiology: A Systems Approach. 2nd ed.* New York: McGraw Hill, 2009.
Fischer-Rizzi, Suzanne. *Complete Aromatherapy Handbook.* New York, NY: Sterling Publishing, 1990.
Gattefosse, Rene-Maurice. *Gattefosse's Aromatherapy.* Essex, England: The C.W. Daniel Company Ltd., 1937 English translation.
Gawronski, Donald. *Medical Choices.* Lincoln, Nebraska: Authors Choice Press, 2002. Print.
Guyton A.C., Hall J.E. *Textbook of Medical Physiology. 10th ed.* Philadelphia: W.B. Saunders Company, 2000.
Green, Mindy. *Natural Perfumes: Simple Aromatherapy Recipes.* Loveland CO: Interweave Press Inc., 1999.
Hill, David K. *Frankincense.* Spanish Fork, UT: AromaTools, 2010.
Integrated Aromatic Medicine. Proceedings from the First International Symposium, Grasse, France. Essential Science Publishing, March 2000.
Lis-Balchin, Maria. *Aromatherapy Science: A Guide for Healthcare Professionals.* London, UK: Pharmaceutical Press, 2006.
Keville, Kathi. "A History of Fragrance." Healthy.net. 1995. Web. 9 Aug. 2012.
Lawless, Julia. *The Encyclopaedia of Essential Oils.* Rockport, MA: Element, Inc., 1992.
Maury, Marguerite. *Marguerite Maury's Guide to Aromatherapy.* C.W. Daniel, 1989.
Pénoël, M.D., Daniel and Pierre Franchomme. L'aromatherapie exactement. Limoges, France: Jollois, 1990.
Petrovska, Biljana Bauer. "Historical Review of Medicinal Plants' Usage." *Pharmacognosy Reviews* 2012 (6:11): 1–5. Print. Print.
Porter, Stephen. *The Great Plague.* Stroud, Gloucestershire: Amberly Publishing, 2009. Print.
Price, Shirley, and Len Price. *Aromatherapy for Health Professionals.* New York, NY: Churchill Livingstone Inc., 1995.
Price, Shirley, and Penny Price Parr. *Aromatherapy for Babies and Children.* San Francisco, CA: Thorsons, 1996.
Rose, Jeanne. *375 Essential Oils and Hydrosols.* Berkeley, CA: North Atlantic Books, 1999.
Rose, Jeanne. *The Aromatherapy Book: Applications and Inhalations.* Berkeley, CA: North Atlantic Books, 1992.
Ryman, Danièle. *Aromatherapy: The Complete Guide to Plant & Flower Essences for Health and Beauty.* New York: Bantam Books, 1993.
Sheppard-Hanger, Sylla. *The Aromatherapy Practitioner Reference Manual.* Tampa, FL: Atlantic Institute of Aromatherapy, Twelfth Printing February 2000.

Tisserand, Maggie. *Aromatherapy for Women: a Practical Guide to Essential Oils for Health and Beauty.* Rochester, VT: Healing Arts Press, 1996.
Tisserand, Robert. *Aromatherapy: to Heal and Tend the Body.* Wilmot, WI: Lotus Press, 1988.
Tisserand, Robert. *The Art of Aromatherapy.* Rochester, VT: Healing Arts Press, 1977.
Tisserand, Robert, and Tony Balacs. *Essential Oil Safety: A Guide for Health Care Professionals.* New York, NY: Churchill Livingstone, 1995.
Tortora G.J., Funke B.R., Case C.L. *Microbiology: An Introduction. 9th ed.* San Francisco: Pearson Benjamin Cummings, 2007.
Valnet, M.D., Jean. *The Practice of Aromatherapy: a Classic Compendium of Plant Medicines and their Healing Properties.* Rochester, VT: Healing Arts Press, 1980.
Valnet, Jean. *The Practice of Aromatherapy.* Rochester Vermont: Healing Arts Press, 1982. Print.
Watson, Franzesca. *Aromatherapy Blends & Remedies.* San Francisco, CA: Thorsons, 1995.
Weaver R.F. *Molecular Biology. 4th ed.* New York: McGraw Hill, 2008.
Wilson, Roberta. *Aromatherapy for Vibrant Health and Beauty: a practical A-to-Z reference to aromatherapy treatments for health, skin, and hair problems.* Honesdale, PA: Paragon Press, 1995.
Worwood, Valerie Ann. *The Complete Book of Essential Oils & Aromatherapy.* San Rafael, CA: New World Library, 1991.

Index

INDEX

Modern Essentials Usage Guide

Essential Oils & Blends *Quick Usage Chart* – Part 1

Single Oil Name	Topical			Aromatic			Internal			Common Uses (see the Single Oils chapter for additional uses)
	Adult	Child/Sensitive	Pregnancy	Adult	Child	Pregnancy	Adult	Child (6+)	Pregnancy	
Arborvitae	●	●	●	●	●	●	✕	✕	✕	Antibacterial, Antifungal, Calming, Repellent
Basil	●	●	●	●	●	●	●	●	✕	Autism, Bronchitis, Earache, Cramps/Spasms, Bug Bites, Wounds
Bergamot**	●	●	●	●	●	●	●	●	●	Brain Injury, Colic, Depression, Respiratory Infection, Stress
Birch	●	●	✕	●	●	✕	✕	✕	✕	Muscle Aches, Pain
Black Pepper	●	●	●	●	●	●	●	●	●	Addictions, Cooking, Circulation
Cardamom	●	●	●	●	●	●	●	●	●	Coughs, Inflammation, Muscle Aches, Nausea, Respiratory Ailments
Cassia	●	●	✕	●	●	●	●	●	✕	Antibacterial, Antiviral, Disinfectant, Warming
Cedarwood	●	●	●	●	●	●	✕	✕	✕	Calming, Tension, Tuberculosis, Urinary Infection, Yoga
Cilantro	●	●	●	●	●	●	●	●	●	Anxiety, Cooking
Cinnamon	●	●	✕	●	●	●	●	●	✕	Antibacterial, Antifungal, Diabetes, Mold, Respiratory Infection, Warming
Clary Sage	●	●	●	●	●	●	●	●	●	Cholesterol, Cramps, Hot Flashes, PMS, Respiratory Infection
Clove	●	●	●	●	●	●	●	●	●	Antifungal, Antioxidant, Antiviral, Corns, Hypothyroidism, Toothache
Coriander	●	●	●	●	●	●	●	●	●	Cartilage Injury, Muscle Aches, Muscle Development, Whiplash
Cypress	●	●	●	●	●	●	✕	✕	✕	Aneurysm, Carpal Tunnel, Concussion, Muscle Fatigue, Pain, Stroke
Dill	●	●	●	●	●	●	●	●	●	Cholesterol, Cooking, Flavoring
Eucalyptus	●	●	●	●	●	●	✕	✕	✕	Inflammation, Neuralgia, Pain, Respiratory Issues, Shingles
Fennel	●	●	●	●	●	●	●	●	●	Blood Clots, Bruises, Digestive Support, Skin, Wrinkles
Frankincense	●	●	●	●	●	●	●	●	●	Arthritis, Inflammation, Mental Fatigue, Respiratory Issues, Skin, Warts
Geranium	●	●	●	●	●	●	●	●	●	Air Purification, Bleeding, Diabetes, Dry Skin, Vertigo, Wrinkles
Ginger*	●	●	●	●	●	●	●	●	●	Digestive Issues, Morning Sickness, Nausea, Rheumatic Fever
Grapefruit	●	●	●	●	●	●	●	●	●	Anorexia, Appetite Suppressant, Cellulite, Hangover
Helichrysum	●	●	●	●	●	●	●	●	●	Antiviral, Bleeding, Cholesterol, Earache, Herpes, Sciatica, Wounds
Juniper Berry	●	●	●	●	●	●	●	●	●	Acne, Alcoholism, Dermatitis/Eczema, Kidney Stones, Tinnitus
Lavender	●	●	●	●	●	●	●	●	●	Allergies, Boils, Burns, Calming, Itching, Pain, Skin, Sleep, Wrinkles
Lemon*	●	●	●	●	●	●	●	●	●	Anxiety, Cleansing, Depression, Disinfectant, Grease, Heartburn, Stress
Lemongrass	●	●	●	●	●	●	●	●	●	Air Purification, Cholesterol, Cramps, Joint Injuries, Tissue Repair
Lime*	●	●	●	●	●	●	●	●	●	Bacterial Infections, Fever, Gum/Grease Removal, Skin
Marjoram	●	●	●	●	●	●	●	●	●	Arthritis, Cramps, Muscle Ache/Spasm, Neuralgia, Whiplash
Melaleuca	●	●	●	●	●	●	●	●	●	Acne, Antifungal, Boils, Cold Sores, Disinfectant, Sore Throat, Wounds
Melissa	●	●	●	●	●	●	●	●	●	Antiviral, Calming, Cold Sores, Viral Infection
Myrrh	●	●	●	●	●	●	●	●	●	Allergies (Skin), Gum Disease, Infection, Skin Wounds/Problems
Orange*	●	●	●	●	●	●	●	●	●	Anxiety, Digestion, Fear, Insomnia, Menopause, Nervousness, Uplifting
Oregano	●	●	●	●	●	●	●	●	●	Antifungal, Candida, Muscle Aches, Parasites, MRSA, Warts
Patchouli	●	●	●	●	●	●	●	●	●	Diuretic, Fever, Mosquito Repellent, Termite Repellent
Peppermint	●	●	●	●	●	●	●	●	●	Alertness, Allergies, Cooling, Headache, Indigestion, Nausea, Sinusitis

Essential Oils & Blends *Quick Usage Chart*—Part 2

Single Oil Name	Topical Adult	Child/Sensitive	Pregnancy	Aromatic Adult	Child	Pregnancy	Internal Adult	Child (6+)	Pregnancy	Common Uses (see the Single Oils chapter for additional uses)
Roman Chamomile	●	●	●	●	●	●	●	●	●	Allergies, Diaper Rash, Dry Skin, Insomnia, Neuritis, Shock, Stings
Rose	●	●	●	●	●	●	●	●	●	Aphrodisiac, Poison Ivy/Oak, Scarring (Prevention)
Rosemary	●	●	×	●	●	×	●	●	×	Antioxidant, Arthritis, Diabetes, Flu, Headache, Memory, Sinusitis
Sandalwood	●	●	●	●	●	●	●	●	●	Back Pain, Clarity, Laryngitis, Meditation, Rashes, Sunscreen, Yoga
Spearmint	●	●	●	●	●	●	●	●	●	Cooking, Indigestion
Thyme	●	●	×	●	●	×	●	●	×	Antibacterial, Antifungal, Colds, Dermatitis, Respiratory Infections
Vetiver	●	●	●	●	●	●	●	●	●	ADD/ADHD, Balance, Termite Repellent, Vitiligo
White Fir	●	●	●	●	●	●	●	●	●	Cleansing, Bronchitis, Bursitis, Energizing, Muscle Fatigue/Pain
Wintergreen	●	●	×	●	●	×	×	×	×	Arthritic Pain, Bone Pain, Dandruff, Joint Pain/Inflammation,
Ylang Ylang	●	●	●	●	●	●	●	●	●	Calming, Crying, High Blood Pressure, Hyperpnea, Relaxing, Stress

Oil Blend Name	Topical Adult	Child/Sensitive	Pregnancy	Aromatic Adult	Child	Pregnancy	Internal Adult	Child (6+)	Pregnancy	Common Uses (see the Oil Blends chapter for additional uses)
Anti-aging Blend	●	●	●	×	×	×	×	×	×	Aging, Chapped/Cracked Skin, Dry Skin, Revitalizing, Wrinkles
Calming Blend	●	●	●	●	●	×	×	×	×	ADD/ADHD, Anxiety, Calming, Insomnia, Sedative, Stress, Tension
Cleansing Blend	●	●	●	●	●	×	×	×	×	Air Pollution, Allergies, Boils, Deodorizing, Infection, Mildew, Stings
Cellular Complex	●	●	●	●	●	●	●	●	●	Aging, Antioxidant, Atherosclerosis, Cancer, Cellular Vitality, Tumors
Detoxification Blend*	●	●	●	●	●	●	●	●	●	Cleansing, Endocrine Support, Hormonal Balance, Tissue Support
Digestive Blend	●	●	●	●	●	●	●	●	●	Bloating, Cramps, Gastritis, Heartburn, Nausea, Parasites, Sinusitis
Focus Blend	●	●	●	●	●	●	×	×	×	ADD/ADHD, Anxiety, Concentration, Focus, Hyperactive, Stress
Grounding Blend	●	●	●	●	●	●	×	×	×	Anxiety, Back Pain, Balance, Depression, Energy, Mood Swings, Seizure
Headache Tension Blend	●	●	●	●	●	●	×	×	×	Headaches, Migraines, Muscle Tension, Tension Headaches
Invigorating Blend*	●	●	●	●	●	●	×	×	×	Calming, Depression, Eating Disorders, Mastitis, Sedative
Joyful Blend*	●	●	●	●	●	●	×	×	×	Anxiety, Depression, Energizing, Grief/Sorrow, Stress, Uplifting
Massage Blend	●	●	●	×	×	×	×	×	×	Anxiety, Muscle Aches/Pain, Muscular Dystrophy, Relaxation, Tension
Metabolic Blend	●	●	●	●	●	●	●	●	●	Appetite Suppressant, Cellulite, Obesity, Weight Loss
Protective Blend	●	●	●	●	●	●	●	●	●	Air Pollution, Antibacterial, Antifungal, Antiviral, Cleansing, Disinfecting
Respiratory Blend	●	●	●	●	●	●	×	×	×	Antiviral, Asthma, Congestion, Cough, Influenza, Pneumonia, Sinusitis
Repellent Blend	●	●	●	●	●	●	×	×	×	Bug/Insect Repellent
Soothing Blend	●	●	●	×	×	×	×	×	×	Arthritis, Back Pain, Inflammation, Joint Pain, Muscle Aches, Tension
Topical Blend	●	●	●	×	×	×	×	×	×	Acne, Calluses, Dermatitis, Impetigo, Oily Skin
Women's Blend	●	●	●	●	●	●	×	×	×	Hormonal Balance, Perfume
Women's Monthly Blend	●	●	●	●	●	●	×	×	×	Hot Flashes, Hormones (Balancing), Menopause, Menstruation, PMS

● Safe to use without dilution as directed.

● Safe to use with moderate dilution.

● Safe to use with heavier dilution—consult with a physician before using if pregnant or ill.

× Not a generally recommended use.

✳ Avoid sunlight for several hours after topical use.

✳✳ Avoid sunlight for 12–24 hours after topical use.